CLINICIAN'S GUIDE TO PTSD

Clinician's Guide to **PTSD**

A COGNITIVE-BEHAVIORAL APPROACH

STEVEN TAYLOR

THE GUILFORD PRESS
New York   London

© 2006 The Guilford Press
A Division of Guilford Publications, Inc.
72 Spring Street, New York, NY 10012
www.guilford.com

Printed in the United States of America

This book is printed on acid-free paper.

Last digit is print number: 9 8 7 6 5 4 3 2

Library of Congress Cataloging-in-Publication Data
Taylor, Steven, 1960–
   Clinician's guide to PTSD : a cognitive-behavioral approach / Steven Taylor.
      p. ; cm.
   Includes bibliographical references and index.
   ISBN-13: 978-1-59385-326-6 (hardcover : alk. paper)
   ISBN 10: 1-59385-326-2 (hardcover : alk. paper)
   1. Post-traumatic stress disorder. 2. Cognitive therapy. I. Title. II. Title:
Clinician's guide to post-traumatic stress disorder.
   [DNLM: 1. Stress Disorders, Post-Traumatic—therapy. 2. Cognitive Therapy—
methods.   WM 170 T246c 2006]
   RC552.P67T39 2006
   616.85′21—dc22

                                                                      2006013543

*To my wife, Amy,
and our son, Alex*

About the Author

Steven Taylor, PhD, is a clinical psychologist and Professor in the Department of Psychiatry at the University of British Columbia. For 10 years he was Associate Editor of *Behaviour Research and Therapy* and now is Associate Editor of the *Journal of Cognitive Psychotherapy*, as well as being on the editorial boards of several journals. He has published over 180 journal articles and book chapters and 11 books on anxiety disorders and related topics. He served as a consultant on the text revision of the *Diagnostic and Statistical Manual of Mental Disorders* (DSM-IV-TR). Dr. Taylor has received career awards from the Canadian Psychological Association, the Association for Advancement of Behavior Therapy, the Anxiety Disorders Association of America, and the British Columbia Psychological Association. He is also a fellow of several scholarly organizations, including the Academy of Cognitive Therapy, the Canadian Psychological Association, and the American Psychological Society. Dr. Taylor is actively involved in clinical teaching and supervision. His clinical and research interests include cognitive-behavioral treatments and mechanisms of anxiety disorders and related conditions.

Preface

Much has been written on the treatment of posttraumatic stress disorder (PTSD). Why write another clinician's guide? There are several reasons why a fresh, empirically grounded guidebook is required. Most previous books have been narrow in focus, dealing only with a specific form of the disorder, such as rape-related PTSD. Clinicians rarely have the luxury of such a narrow specialization. Accordingly, a volume is needed that covers the many manifestations of PTSD, the common elements of treatment, and the special interventions needed for (1) particular types of trauma populations (e.g., interventions used particularly with formerly battered women), (2) various demographic groups (e.g., children and the elderly), and (3) particular clinical presentations (e.g., PTSD associated with other prominent clinical problems, such as severe guilt, anger, shame, chronic pain, dissociation, or substance abuse). The present volume aims to be comprehensive in this regard, covering both the science and art of cognitive-behavioral treatment of PTSD for various populations and clinical presentations. The nuts and bolts of interventions are described, along with useful variations on treatment methods.

The second reason for writing this book is that in recent years there have been many new and important developments in treating PTSD, including the development and refinement of cutting-edge treatment methods that, by virtue of their recent appearance in the PTSD treatment literature, have not found their way into most treatment guidebooks. Examples include cognitive methods for treating mental defeat and numbing, and interoceptive exposure techniques for treating maladaptive beliefs about PTSD symptoms. The present volume is a compendium of new and established treatment methods, including handouts for patients and troubleshooting sections for helping therapists deal with common problems that arise in implementing cognitive-behavioral interventions. Readers are provided with numerous clinical examples of how the interventions can be used, as well as detailed suggestions about how to select, organize, and implement behavioral interventions, such as the various forms of exposure exercises. It can be challenging to develop some types of exposure exercises, particularly live or situational exposure assignments. Creativity is needed— or at least a list of guiding examples developed by others. The chapter on situational exposure (Chapter 13) includes numerous examples, including a long list of movies that contain relevant material for use as exposure stimuli for various trauma populations. (I am greatly indebted to my cinephile colleagues for their assistance in compiling this list.)

A third reason for the present volume is that most cognitive-behavioral treatment guidebooks have neglected the biological side of PTSD. A comprehensive clinical guide should be one that provides the cognitive-behavioral clinician with information concerning the nature and treatment relevance of the various biological findings concerning PTSD. Findings regarding the question of whether stress damages the brain have great relevance for how we respond to patients who worry that they have stress-induced brain damage. Other important findings from the biological realm address the question of whether certain pharmacological agents, such as D-cycloserine, can augment the efficacy of cognitive-behavioral treatments. Such issues are covered in the present volume.

The fourth, and perhaps most important, need for a new treatment guidebook concerns the very nature of PTSD treatment in clinical practice. By virtue of the remarkable variety of clinical presentations of PTSD, including the many different ways this disorder can co-occur with other clinical problems, a simple treatment manual is inadequate. Clinicians cannot be expected to work, lockstep, through a fixed treatment protocol that dictates which intervention will be implemented in which treatment session. The reality of clinical practice requires a flexible, individually tailored, but empirically informed approach to developing treatment plans. The development of such an approach was a further goal in writing the present book, which advocates a case formulation approach, in which a formulation of the causes of a patient's problems is used to determine how empirically supported treatment protocols can be adapted to meet the needs of a particular patient. A case formulation is used to develop treatment plans for the many different constellations of comorbidity and other complicating factors for which there are no standardized, empirically supported manuals.

The present volume is intended for clinical trainees, such as clinical psychology graduate students, postdoctoral clinical psychology fellows, and psychiatry residents. It also is intended as a resource for mental health professionals wanting to learn more about cognitive-behavioral approaches to treatment. No one book, however, is sufficient to learn how to treat

PTSD; this volume is best used in the context of supervised training from a suitably qualified practitioner, such as a clinician with expertise in both PTSD and cognitive-behavioral therapy.

All clinical examples presented in the book were disguised to protect patient privacy and confidentiality. This was done according to the guidelines of the American Psychological Association and by using the procedures set out by Clifft (1986). The case illustrations either were disguised to eliminate identifying information or represent composite descriptions, combining material from several patients. Modification of the case material was done in such a way that it does not compromise the didactic value of these examples.

Several people deserve special thanks for their help in facilitating the completion of this volume. I am grateful to my wife and fellow clinical psychologist, Amy S. Janeck, PhD, for her encouragement and support, and for her many insights and suggestions concerning the various clinical problems and interventions tackled in this volume. Thanks also to Jim Nageotte, Senior Editor at The Guilford Press, for his sage advice and guidance. The four anonymous reviewers of the first draft of this book provided useful, constructive feedback. Their enthusiasm for the project made the revisions far less onerous than they otherwise might have been. Thanks also to my many clinical colleagues, research collaborators, and patients, who have all taught me a great deal over the years.

Contents

PART I

CONCEPTUAL AND EMPIRICAL FOUNDATIONS

CHAPTER I

Clinical Features
of Posttraumatic Stress Disorder

John was driving his three young children to the park when they were struck head-on by a driver attempting to overtake a truck on a sharp bend. John's car was wrecked and he developed posttraumatic stress disorder (PTSD), with the most severe symptoms being persistent nightmares of the accident, profound fear and avoidance of driving, and chronic tension, irritability, and guilt about not being able to swerve out of the path of the oncoming vehicle. His children received minor cuts and bruises, from which they quickly recovered. They had more difficulty overcoming the psychological impact of the crash. In the weeks afterward, the youngest, a 4-year-old girl, frequently complained of stomachaches and refused to be out of sight of her father for fear that something bad would happen. The two older boys, ages 7 and 8, had recurrent nightmares. During the day, the boys often engaged in stereotypical play, in which they pretended to be driving cars. They would crash into one other and both fall to the ground. The boys would then get up and run around pretending to shoot one another, shouting, "You're the bad man!" "No, you're the bad man!" Sometimes this escalated to the point that they physically fought with one another.

John and his children provide us with examples of the wide range of problems people often experience in the wake of traumatic experiences. We see these patients frequently in our practices, sometimes presenting with what might look like relatively simple anxiety or depressive problems, or anger management issues. But as we engage with these patients and families, a more complex pattern emerges, and we recognize the problems they present with as both intransigent and multilayered. How do we spot symptoms of PTSD and how do we differentiate it from other clinical problems? Furthermore, once we have a fair picture of the underlying causes of the patient's problems, just how should we treat them? This book delves into these very questions and provides as many answers as one can derive from the current scientific literature, and from the clinical experiences of the author and others. This book offers a perspective on how to think through the process of assessing and treating these patients, using cutting-edge, empirically informed cognitive-behavioral interventions.

DIAGNOSTIC CRITERIA

DSM-IV-TR tries to capture the diversity of posttraumatic stress reactions in the diagnostic criteria for PTSD (American Psychiatric Association [APA], 2000). The criteria are summarized in Table 1.1, which shows that the major symptom clusters are reexperiencing, avoidance/numbing, and hyperarousal. Recent research suggests that the criteria may need to be modified for DSM-V, to divide avoidance and numbing into separate clusters (Asmundson, Stapleton, & Taylor, 2004). This is because avoidance and numbing (1) are empirically distinct clusters or factors, (2) differ in their clinical correlates (numbing is more strongly correlated with depression), (3) differ in their prognostic significance (numbing, but not avoidance, predicts poor response to treatment in some studies), and (4) differ in their response to treatment (e.g., cognitive-behavioral treatments may have greater impact on avoidance than numbing) (Asmundson et al., 2004; Taylor, 2004; Taylor et al., 2003). Throughout this volume I distinguish between avoidance and numbing instead of grouping them together.

DIFFERENTIAL DIAGNOSIS

To diagnose PTSD, a sufficient number of symptoms must be present for a month or more. This can be contrasted with acute stress disorder, which is defined by the development of dissociative and PTSD symptoms within a month after exposure to a traumatic stressor (APA, 2000). Dissociative symptoms, which overlap to some degree with PTSD symptoms, may occur during or after exposure to the stressor. Dissociation refers to the breakdown in the normally integrated functions of consciousness, identity, memory, or perception of one's self or surroundings and is manifested by symptoms such as depersonalization, derealization, or psychogenic amnesia (APA, 2000). Dissociative symptoms consist of the following: a subjective sense of numbing, detachment, or absence of emotional responsiveness; reduction in awareness of surroundings; derealization; depersonalization; or dissociative amnesia. Acute stress disorder is diagnosed if the symptoms last a minimum of 2 days and a maximum of 4 weeks. If the symptoms persist beyond that time, then PTSD is diagnosed.

TABLE 1.1. DSM-IV-TR Diagnostic Criteria for PTSD

A. **Traumatic stressor:** The person has been exposed to a traumatic event in which both of the following were present:

    (1) the person experienced, witnessed, or was confronted with an event or events that involved actual or threatened death or serious injury, or a threat to the physical integrity of self or others

    (2) the person's response involved intense fear, helplessness, or horror. **Note:** In children, this may be expressed as disorganized or agitated behavior.

B. **Reexperiencing:** The traumatic event is persistently reexperienced in one (or more) of the following ways:

    (1) recurrent and intrusive distressing recollections of the event, including images, thoughts, or perceptions. **Note:** In young children, repetitive play may occur in which themes or aspects of the trauma are expressed.

    (2) recurrent distressing dreams of the event. **Note:** In children, there may be frightening dreams without recognizable content.

    (3) acting or feeling as if the traumatic event were recurring (includes a sense of reliving the experience, illusions, hallucinations, and dissociative flashback episodes, including those that occur on awakening or when intoxicated). **Note:** In young children, trauma-specific reenactment may occur.

    (4) intense psychological distress at exposure to internal or external cues that symbolize or resemble an aspect of the traumatic event

    (5) physiological reactivity on exposure to internal or external cues that symbolize or resemble an aspect of the traumatic event

C. **Avoidance and numbing:** Persistent avoidance of stimuli associated with the trauma and numbing of general responsiveness (not present before the trauma), as indicated by three (or more) of the following:

    (1) efforts to avoid thoughts, feelings, or conversations associated with the trauma

    (2) efforts to avoid activities, places, or people that arouse recollections of the trauma

    (3) inability to recall an important aspect of the trauma

    (4) markedly diminished interest or participation in significant activities

    (5) feeling of detachment or estrangement from others

    (6) restricted range of affect (e.g., unable to have loving feelings)

    (7) sense of a foreshortened future (e.g., does not expect to have a career, marriage, children, or a normal life span).

D. **Hyperarousal:** Persistent symptoms of increased arousal (not present before the trauma), as indicated by two (or more) of the following:

    (1) difficulty falling or staying asleep

    (2) irritability or outbursts of anger

    (3) difficulty concentrating

    (4) hypervigilance

    (5) exaggerated startle response

E. Duration of the disturbance (symptoms in Criteria B, C, and D) is more than 1 month.

F. The disturbance causes clinically significant distress or impairment in social, occupational, or other important areas of functioning.

Note. From American Psychiatric Association (2000). Copyright 2000 by the American Psychiatric Association. Reprinted by permission.

During the sexual assault, Hanna felt like she was caught in some terrible dream from which she could not awaken. Her body felt numb and unreal as the rapist pinned her down. At one point she felt as if she was floating above her body, watching the assault unfold as if she was a spectator. In the weeks after the assault, Hanna often had episodes in which she and her surroundings felt strange and unreal. For example, walking though a busy pedestrian shopping district one day, it was as if the world was draped with a gauze veil. Colors seemed pale and washed out, and the faces of the shoppers looked gray and indistinct. It was also as if her ears were plugged. Instead of hearing the noisy commotion of the marketplace, she felt as if the sounds were muted, as if they were coming from far away. Hanna was experiencing recurrent dissociative symptoms.

If symptoms of avoidance, numbing, or hyperarousal are present before exposure to the traumatic stressor, they are not counted toward a diagnosis PTSD and may be due to some other disorder. If the person develops PTSD-like symptoms but has not experienced a traumatic stressor, then a diagnosis of adjustment disorder can be made. A diagnosis of adjustment disorder may be changed to one of anxiety disorder "not otherwise specified" (NOS) if the symptoms persist for more than 6 months after the cessation of the stressor.

A person might experience a trauma but not develop enough symptoms to meet diagnostic criteria for full-blown PTSD. Clinical investigators often refer to this as "partial PTSD" (Kulka et al., 1990), although such a condition would be diagnosed in DSM-IV-TR as an adjustment disorder or anxiety disorder NOS.

CLINICAL COURSE

In the hours or days after a traumatic event, most people have at least some symptoms of PTSD (Blanchard & Hickling, 2004; Rothbaum, Foa, Riggs, Murdock, & Walsh, 1992). In at least half of all trauma survivors, complete recovery occurs within 3 months, even in the absence of treatment (APA, 2000). Symptoms lasting 1–3 months may be diagnosed as acute PTSD. If symptoms persist longer than 3 months, then PTSD is likely to be chronic. Symptoms may wax and wane over time, often in response to life stressors. PTSD may go into partial remission and reemerge later on, sometimes years later. Symptom reemergence may occur in response to reminders of the original trauma or be triggered by additional life stressors (APA, 2000).

Most cases of PTSD develop shortly after the traumatic event. However, in a minority (4–6%) of people the disorder does not develop until months or even years or decades afterwards (Bryant & Harvey, 2002; Gray,

Bolton, & Litz, 2004). Delayed-onset PTSD is defined by a delay interval of at least 6 months (APA, 2000). Research suggests that there may be two forms of delayed-onset PTSD, one in which the person has little or no psychopathology after the trauma (i.e., truly delayed onset; Gray et al., 2004), and another that would be more properly called "slowly developing" PTSD, consisting of posttrauma symptoms that gradually increase in severity (Bryant & Harvey, 2002). Stressors occurring after the trauma may contribute to the development of both forms of delayed onset PTSD (Ehlers, Mayou, & Bryant, 1998b; Green et al., 1990).

Miguel had witnessed many horrors during his tour of duty in Liberia as a Red Cross physician. Poverty, disease, and the sight of mutilated land mine victims were part of everyday life, and he was required to be in the company of military protection because of the risk of kidnapping. The impact of his experiences did not hit him until Miguel had returned home to the relative safety and luxury of California. He recovered from the physical exhaustion and sleep deprivation from the long hours working in Liberia and had also recovered from the various ailments, such as dysentery, that he had acquired over there. But as his body recovered, his mind turned more and more to dwell on the horrors and hardships he had encountered. Many things in his Californian town reminded him of Liberia, because they were the very opposite of what he had seen. The enormous, brightly lit display of fresh fruit and vegetables in his neighborhood supermarket, for example, reminded Miguel of the starvation and lack of clean drinking water in Liberia. During the months following his return to California, Miguel's PTSD gradually worsened in frequency and intensity, despite his efforts to force the tormenting memories from his mind.

PREVALENCE

The prevalence of PTSD depends, in part, on the prevalence of traumatic events where the person lives and works. In North America, the lifetime prevalence of PTSD is approximately 8% (APA, 2000), although it is higher among particular subgroups, such as people who have risky professions (e.g., people in the military, emergency services workers, police officers, sex-trade workers). For example, the lifetime prevalence of PTSD among combat veterans is 22–31% (Kulka et al., 1990; Prigerson, Maciejewski, & Rosenheck, 2002). The prevalence of PTSD is also higher in countries in which there is widespread persecution of ethnic groups or ongoing armed conflicts. According to one recent epidemiological survey, the lifetime prevalence of PTSD is 37% in Algeria, 28% in Cambodia, 16% in Ethiopia, and 18% in Gaza (de Jong et al., 2001).

Women have a higher lifetime prevalence of PTSD than men (10% vs. 5%; Kessler et al., 1995), even after controlling for frequency of exposure to traumatic events (Breslau, 2002). This may be due to differences in the types of trauma that men and women are most likely to experience. Men more often experience physical assault, and women more often experience sexual assault. Sexual assault, compared to physical assault, is more likely to cause PTSD in both genders (Kilpatrick & Acierno, 2003). This may be partly because rape has all kinds of stressful sequelae, such as sexually transmitted disease, unwanted pregnancy (in women), and aversive experiences that may arise when reporting the assault to police or testifying in court. Thus, the fact that sexual assault is more common among women than men may largely account for the gender differences in the lifetime prevalence of PTSD.

SOCIAL AND ECONOMIC COSTS

PTSD can have devastating social costs, including profound disruptions to families and relationships. Family members may find themselves "walking on eggshells" to avoid upsetting the person with PTSD. They may not be able to walk up unannounced behind the person without him or her becoming startled and distressed. Numbing and withdrawal can lead the family to feel estranged from the PTSD sufferer. PTSD-related anger and aggression may be associated with domestic violence. Such problems, along with hyperarousal-related concentration difficulties, can also impair occupational functioning.

Economic costs associated with PTSD include work absenteeism and health care costs. People with PTSD, compared to those without the disorder, are more likely to receive medical attention for emotional and general medical problems (Switzer et al., 1999; Tedstone & Tarrier, 2003; Walker et al., 2003). The latter includes medically unexplained symptoms (e.g., various forms of pain such as recurrent headache) and general medical conditions that may be associated with chronic hyperarousal (e.g., hypertension). When aggregated, the economic costs of PTSD are likely to be considerable (McCrone, Knapp, & Cawkill, 2003).

VARIETIES OF TRAUMA

What Qualifies as a Traumatic Stressor?

When PTSD was introduced in DSM-III (APA, 1980), it was said to arise only if the person had been exposed to a stressor that is generally outside the range of usual human experience. There were two problems with this definition. First, DSM-III presupposed that stressors could be objectively defined as traumatic. Although some stressors are likely to terrifying ordeals for virtually everyone (e.g., brutal rape or torture), the stressfulness of other events depends on how the person interprets them. Exposure to a natural disaster, such as a flood or hurricane, may be terrifying for one person, challenging but not traumatic for another, or an exciting adventure to yet another person. Accordingly, the person's appraisal of the event is integral in defining whether or not it is traumatic.

The second problem was that some events defined as traumatic under DSM-III are not "outside the range of usual human experience." Epidemiological surveys have shown that sexual and physical assaults are unfortunately common in many countries, including Western countries (Breslau, 2002).

In light of these problems, DSM-IV (American Psychiatric Association, 1994) (and DSM-IV-TR) revised the definition so that the event need not be outside the usual range of experience, and the person's reaction to the event was included in defining an experience as traumatic (see Table 1.1).

There is a long list of events that can be classified as traumatic stressors. *Direct experiences* can qualify as traumatic, such as military combat, violent personal assault (sexual assault, physical attack, robbery), being kidnapped, being taken hostage, a terrorist attack, torture, incarceration as a prisoner of war or in a concentration camp, natural or technological disasters, severe automobile accidents, being diagnosed with a life-threatening illness, or being a survivor of a botched medical or surgical procedure (e.g., awareness under anesthesia).

Torture provides a chilling illustration of the multifaceted nature of directly experienced traumatic experiences. There are several elements of torture that may act to accentuate its impact on PTSD symptoms (Silove, Steel, McGorry, Miles, & Drobny, 2002). The abuse is deliberate, and the perpetrators use methods that maximize fear, dread, and debility of the victim. The trauma is inescapable, uncontrollable, and often repetitive, and conditions between torture sessions (such as solitary confinement) undermine the recovery capacity of the victim. The torturer may attempt to induce feelings of guilt, shame, anger, betrayal, and humiliation, which can erode the victim's sense of security, integrity, and self-worth. Head injury or other lasting bodily damage may also be inflicted. For example, repeated beatings on the soles of one's feet can resulting in permanent damage (by damaging the spongy, cushioning tissue in the feet), making it painful to walk and thereby providing lasting reminders of the trauma.

Witnessed events can be traumatic, such as observing the serious injury or unnatural death of another person due to violent assault, accident, war or disaster, or unexpectedly witnessing a dead body or body parts after a flood or earthquake. For example, handling of bodies or bodily remains (e.g., as part of mortuary duty after airline accidents or as part of military graves registration duty) can be associated with PTSD (Deahl, Gillham,

Thomas, Searle, & Srinivasan, 1994; McCarroll, Ursano, Fullerton, Liu, & Lundy, 2001; Ursano & McCarroll, 1990). Participation in rescue work after disasters such as earthquakes can be similarly traumatizing, due to exposure to mutilated bodies, particularly bodies of children, or because of the inability to rescue loved ones (e.g., Şalcioğlu, Başoğlu, & Livanou, 2003).

Learning about events experienced by others can also be traumatizing, such as learning that a loved one has experienced a violent personal assault or serious injury. To illustrate, Bernice, a 45-year-old mother of two, learned of the violent gang-related death of her son. Although she obtained only sketchy details of the incident from the police and local newspapers, the information was enough for Bernice to imagine various scenarios about how her son was swarmed by assailants, beaten, and killed.

Given the current DSM-IV-TR definition of traumatic stressors, a range of other events could be defined as traumatic, even seemingly trivial ones. When the film *The Exorcist* was released in 1973, there were reports of people developing PTSD-like symptoms after seeing the film. After watching the movie, one person, for example, became frightened that the devil might possess him because of all the bad things he had done in life. He suffered from this fear for about four weeks, along with insomnia, irritability, decreased appetite, and inability to remove scenes of the film from his mind. Eventually, his problems resolved after he presented for treatment at a local hospital (Bozzuto, 1975).

Should such cases be defined as PTSD? Some have argued that distressing but relatively minor events genuinely qualify as traumatic stressors (Avina & O'Donohue, 2002; Weaver, 2001). McNally (2003b) referred to the increasingly liberal definition of the concept of traumatic stressor as *criterion bracket creep*. According to McNally, bracket creep is something that seriously imperils the credibility of the diagnosis of PTSD: "The more we identify noncatastrophic events as stressors deemed capable of producing PTSD, the less likely it is that we will ever discover any common mechanisms that mediate PTSD symptoms" (p. 280). Not all investigators share this view (e.g., Brewin, 2003). In fact, the liberal definition of a traumatic stressor (for diagnosing PTSD) is consistent with a diathesis-stress conceptualization of the disorder; the greater a person's diathesis (predisposition) for developing PTSD, the smaller the amount of stress required to precipitate the disorder. Thus, it seems unlikely that criterion bracket creep will threaten the credibility of the diagnosis of PTSD, nor will it impede our efforts to understand the basic mechanisms of the disorder. Consistent with this conclusion, research indicates that PTSD varies along a continuum of severity rather than being a categorical (present or absent) entity (Ruscio, Ruscio, & Keane, 2002), and studies show that even nontraumatic stressors can give rise to PTSD-like symptoms (Horowitz, 2001; Mol et al., 2005).

The Burden of Accumulated Adversity

Cumulative exposure to traumas increases the risk of PTSD (Fullerton, Ursano, & Wang, 2004). Exposure to lesser stressors before or after the traumatic event can also add to the burden of accumulative adversity (Alonzo, 1999). To illustrate, for both female and male soldiers, sexual harassment and racial discrimination have also been found to be incremental risk factors for PTSD (Fontana, Litz, & Rosenheck, 2000; Loo et al., 2001). The more stressful and less supportive the soldier's working environment, the greater the likelihood that a traumatic stressor will give rise to PTSD.

Stressors may be linked in a cascading fashion, where the traumatic event is followed by stressful sequelae. A rape survivor may believe that the sexual assault was the worst part of her experience but then encounter a nightmarish coda, where police, lawyers, parents, or friends accuse her of exaggerating or even fabricating the assault. In cases of childhood sexual abuse, the associated stressors can include the effects of disclosing the abuse, such as family disruptions (e.g., the removal of children from the family home by social workers) and blame from other siblings for "breaking up" the family. A survivor of genocide may be confronted with government officials who deny the atrocities ever happened. An adolescent with third-degree burns from a house fire may be mortified to find that she is frequently taunted with names like "Scarface" when she returns to school. A survivor of an aircraft accident may discover that the worst part of the ordeal is the way that he is treated in the hospital emergency room, where he lies cold and naked on a hospital gurney, awaiting some unknown surgical intervention while not knowing the nature or severity of his injuries. A factory worker may lose an arm in a chance industrial mishap and then have to endure insurance or worker's compensation hearings in which he is told it was his own fault. Such sequelae can be equally or even more disturbing than the actual traumatic event.

PTSD SYMPTOMS: A CLOSER LOOK

Many of the symptoms in Table 1.1 are self-explanatory, although some require further explanation and illustration in order to highlight their features and variants.

Reexperiencing

Recurrent, Intrusive Recollections

Recurrent, intrusive recollections and dreams are the most common reexperiencing symptoms (APA, 2000). Some patients report that every time they close their eyes they are met with unwanted images of the trauma. Intrusive recollections may also include other sensory experiences, such as smells, tastes, or sounds, as well as the emotions experienced at the time of the trauma, such as horror, dread, or helplessness (Foa & Rothbaum, 1998; van der Kolk, McFarlane, & Weisaeth, 1996; Vermetten & Bremner, 2003).

Some clinicians have made the controversial claim that intrusive recollections can come in the form of "body memories," that is, episodes in which the person has bodily sensations resembling those experienced at the time of the trauma, but occurring without conscious recollection of the trauma (Brown, Scheflin, & Hammond, 1998; Rothschild, 2000; van der Kolk, 1994). The problem with this idea is the difficulty determining what qualifies as a body memory. A person might have palpitations during a physical assault. Does that mean that all subsequent palpitations are body memories of the traumatic event? Clearly, no. Many bodily sensations that are purported to be body memories are simply manifestations of the person's psychophysiological reactions to a trauma cue, or to any other stressor for that matter (McNally, 2003b). Bodily sensations experienced during the trauma might be triggered by later exposure to trauma cues (e.g., chest pain; Salomons, Osterman, Gagliese, & Katz, 2004), but these are typically accompanied by conscious recollections of the trauma. Here, the person is simply recalling intense somatosensory aspects of the trauma along with other details of the trauma. This is not a body memory, as the term is used.

Nightmares

Some nightmares clearly qualify as reexperiencing symptoms. To give a historical example, in 1666 Samuel Pepys described what happened to him after surviving the Great Fire of London: "It is strange to think how to this very day I cannot sleep at night without great terrors of the fire; and this very night could not sleep to almost two in the morning through great terrors of the fire" (cited in Daly, 1983, p. 66). In other cases it can be more difficult to determine whether a patient's nightmares qualify as reexperiencing symptoms. As noted in DSM-IV-TR, reexperiencing symptoms in children may take the form of anxiety-evoking dreams that may not appear to be directly linked to the trauma. The same is observed in adults. Sexual assault survivors may report recurrent dreams about the actual assault, as well as other recurrent, threat-related dreams (e.g., nightmares of being chased or cornered by some malevolent character that they cannot clearly identify). A general rule of thumb is to classify thematically related dreams as reexperiencing symptoms.

Flashbacks

This is a widely used but often misunderstood term. The general public (and patients) typically equate flashbacks with intrusive recollections. Diagnostically, however, flashbacks are dissociative episodes in which the person believes, or behaves as if, the traumatic event were actually occurring; the person is reliving, not simply recalling, the event. Flashbacks are rare and typically last only a few moments (APA, 2000). They may involve hallucinatory phenomena, such as hearing cries of the dying or seeing images of the dead.

Reexperiencing and Trauma Cues

To understand the clinical nature of experiencing symptoms it is important to consider the manner in which the symptoms naturally occur. There is an endless range of stimuli that might trigger reexperiencing symptoms. Sometimes cues are subtle and highly idiosyncratic and can be easily overlooked by the clinician, especially for highly avoidant patients, who try to avoid thinking about and discussing aspects of their traumatic experiences. Patients might also be too embarrassed, ashamed, or disgusted to mention some trauma cues. Sexual arousal, for example, can trigger trauma memories in some survivors of sexual assault, especially if they found themselves becoming sexually aroused during the assault.

Visual stimuli are common trauma cues. One patient, a torture survivor who had broken glass ground into his torso and face, became extremely distressed whenever he saw broken glass. Gustatory, olfactory, and tactile stimuli can also serve as trauma cues. One patient, who was sexually abused by a neighbor, was given a candy bar as a "treat" after each episode of abuse. Thereafter, whenever she tasted candy she recalled the abuse, along with a vivid recollection of the taste of semen. The smell of cooked or rotting meat can trigger memories of burned or decaying corpses in veterans of combat or survivors of natural disasters.

Avoidance

Common Forms of Avoidance

These include the avoidance of trauma cues, as well as avoidance of things that resemble or symbolize the trauma. For example, avoiding watching television news coverage of wars (for combat veterans), avoiding banks (for people who have been in hold-ups), avoiding having contact with one's parents or siblings (for survivors of childhood physical or sexual abuse).

Subtle Avoidance

Some forms of avoidance can be quite subtle. A survivor of domestic violence, for example, might talk in a whisper and refrain from making eye contact in order to avoid "provoking" men by seeming too assertive. Avoidance can extend to attempts to avert the experience of trauma-related bodily sensations (Taylor, 2004). Bodily sensations associated with extreme hyperarousal, such as palpitations, shortness of breath, and dizziness, commonly occur during or shortly after traumatic experiences. These sensations may combine to take the form of peritraumatic panic attacks. Such bodily sensations can subsequently become cues or reminders of the traumatic event (Wald & Taylor, 2005b). Such patients may try to refrain from physical exertion as a means of avoiding the feared bodily sensations.

Adaptive versus Maladaptive Avoidance

Not all forms of avoidance are maladaptive. Some forms of trauma-related avoidance can be highly adaptive, for example, avoiding dangerous parts of town. These patterns of behavior should not be classified as PTSD symptoms. The distinction between adaptive and maladaptive avoidance is neglected in DSM-IV-TR, although it is important when it comes to treatment planning. We don't want to encourage patients to engage in objectively dangerous exposure exercises.

Numbing

Restricted Range of Affect and Diminished Interest in Activities

People suffering from emotional numbing may be unable to experience loving feelings toward significant people in their lives. They may have lost their sense of humor and enjoyment of things they formerly found entertaining. Their emotional palette may consist of a blend of aversive emotions (e.g., anxiety, anger, sadness) interspersed with periods in which they feel nothing at all.

Some people with severe emotional numbing describe feeling dead inside, while others report that it is as if "someone has turned down the volume" on their emotional resonance with the world. Phenomenologically, numbing and dissociation overlap with one another. The numbing of one's emotional resonance with others, particularly with significant others, can be associated with a sense that the world around oneself is unreal, as if the person were viewing the world as a spectator rather than a participant.

Detachment and Estrangement from Others

Finding that other people cannot understand what one has been through can lead to a feeling of estrangement from others. One patient had recently returned from peacekeeping duty in a strife-torn Eastern European country. Prior to deployment he enjoyed a full and active social life. Upon returning home he felt suspicious and disconnected from people. If he met someone new in a local bar, he tended to see them as a potential adversary—someone who could produce a weapon and might need to be "subdued." He tried to explain to his longtime friends how his military experiences had led him to see a side of humanity that most civilians would never see, and how this had changed his worldview. His friends didn't seem to understand. This compounded his sense of alienation.

Sense of a Foreshortened Future

As a result of trauma exposure, people may come to see themselves as vulnerable to harm and may come to regard the world as malevolent. This can lead them to conclude that they are unlikely to live long enough to have a normal life span.

Hyperarousal

Insomnia

There are various forms of insomnia associated with PTSD, including initial insomnia (difficulty falling asleep) and middle insomnia (difficulty staying asleep; Krakow et al., 2001a). Middle insomnia may be a product of heightened arousal, or it may be due to recurrent nightmares that awaken the person. Similarly, initial insomnia may reflect an arousal problem, or it may be specifically associated with worry about sleep (e.g., worry about having terrifying nightmares).

Hypervigilance

Here, the person is clearly watchful and may appear to be highly alert or vigilant. One might choose to sit in particular locations in public places—for example, in the corner of a restaurant, with one's back to the wall and facing the door—in order to scan for threat, or express an exaggerated concern for the safety of oneself, or one's home or significant others. The person might also engage in checking rituals, such as checking that the doors and windows are safely secured at night.

Concentration Difficulties

The person might find that special effort is required to concentrate on television programs or to read newspapers, or might lose track of conversations. The person might fail to complete activities because he or she loses focus and becomes distracted. Concentration difficulties can arise because the person is preoccupied with intrusive thoughts of the trauma, or because he or she is scanning the environment for threat instead of focusing on the task at hand. Concentration difficulties may be compounded by excessive daytime sleepiness due to insomnia.

Exaggerated Startle Response

People with an exaggerated startle response may report that they often feel "jumpy" and that it takes them some time to calm down after being startled. Exaggerated startle response is important because of its potential interpersonal or other consequences. For example, combat veterans with exaggerated startle responses may "reflexively" become physically aggressive when startled. Exaggerated startle is also an important problem for people with PTSD arising from road traffic collisions (Fairbank, DeGood, & Jenkins, 1981). One patient, for example, became startled when a truck suddenly roared past her while she was driving on a freeway. As she startled she jammed her foot on the brake and her car went into a spin. Other vehicles were able to avoid her car and nobody was injured. Fortunately, such incidents are rare.

Irritability and Anger

People with trauma-related irritability or anger may find that they become enraged at the slightest provocation. They may become unusually irritated or angry about being exposed to unwanted noise, such as the sound of a television in a neighboring apartment, or the sound of car alarms going off at night. Survivors of crime, torture, or genocide may angrily ruminate over fantasies of revenge or reparation (Wilson, 2001), especially if they were humiliated as a result of the event (Lee, Scragg, & Turner, 2001).

ASSOCIATED FEATURES

Trauma-Related Guilt

Guilt can be defined as an unpleasant feeling such as remorse or regret, accompanied by the belief that one should have thought, felt, or acted differently, based on an internalized set of standards (Kubany & Manke,

1995). People who have lived through traumatic events may experience painful feelings of guilt about the things they did or didn't do. Trauma-related guilt is common among various trauma populations, including combat veterans, survivors of spouse abuse, and rape or incest survivors (Glover, 1984; Kubany et al., 1996). A combat veteran, for example, may feel guilty about the things he or she did in order to survive, such as leaving wounded comrades behind as the enemy advanced. A rape survivor may experience guilt about not fighting back against the assailant, even though it might have been dangerous to do so. A survivor of domestic violence may feel guilty for not having left the relationship sooner.

Trauma-Related Shame

Shame and guilt are related but distinct emotions. Guilt involves a focus on the wrongness or badness of one's actions, whereas shame involves a global labeling that one is a bad person (e.g., "I feel so dirty and ugly"; Tangey, 1990). Thus, shame can be a painfully devastating emotion in which the whole self is damned, leaving the person feeling worthless and powerless, along with a desire to hide or escape from others (Gramzow & Tangey, 1992; Tangey, 1991). Trauma-related shame is an important but often overlooked associated feature of PTSD.

Other Comorbid Conditions

PTSD is commonly comorbid with many psychiatric disorders, including other anxiety disorders, mood disorders, and substance use disorders (Breslau, Davis, Andreski, & Peterson, 1991; Kessler et al., 1985; Kilpatrick et al., 2003). To illustrate, Breslau et al. (1991) found that 83% of people with PTSD also had at least one other disorder, most commonly substance abuse or dependence (43%), major depression (37%), or agoraphobia (22%).

It could be argued that the high rates of depression in people with PTSD are a function of symptom overlap; some numbing and hyperarousal symptoms overlap with depressive symptoms. However, PTSD and depression are commonly comorbid even after symptom overlap has been taken into consideration (Blanchard, Buckley, Hickling, & Taylor, 1998).

The high co-occurrence of PTSD with substance use disorders, such as alcohol abuse or dependence, may reflect inappropriate, albeit intermittently effective, stress reduction strategies (Kilpatrick & Acierno, 2003). Consistent with this, most studies have found that PTSD precedes substance abuse or dependence, although in some cases substance use disorders precede PTSD (Jacobsen, Southwick, & Kosten, 2001). In the latter situation, substance intoxication, and consequent foolhardiness or impaired judgment, may increase the risk of getting into a dangerous (traumatic) situation.

Some trauma populations are at risk for other forms of comorbidity. Survivors of industrial accidents or road traffic collisions are at increased risk for accident-related injuries (e.g., tissue and nerve damage) accompanied by chronic pain (Asmundson, Coons, Taylor, & Katz, 2002). Burn patients are also at increased risk for chronic pain as a result of tissue damage. Survivors of sexual assault may experience tissue damage and chronic pain as a result of forced penetration. Pain itself may be traumatizing and may serve as a reminder of the trauma. PTSD hyperarousal symptoms can be associated with heightened muscle tension or muscle spasms, and resulting pain. Thus, pain and PTSD can mutually exacerbate one another (Asmundson et al., 2002; Sharp & Harvey, 2001).

PTSD also may be associated with features of personality disorders (APA, 2000), particularly the features called "complex PTSD" or "disorders of extreme stress, not otherwise specified." These features resemble borderline personality traits (e.g., impaired affect modulation, self-destructive and impulsive behavior, identity disturbance, dissociative tendencies, impaired relationships) (APA, 2000; Herman, 1997). Such personality pathology has been identified in PTSD patients who have endured various forms of chronic or repetitive traumas (Jongedijk, Carlier, Schreuder, & Gersons, 1996; McLean & Gallop, 2003; Roth, Newman, Pelcovitz, van der Kolk, & Mandel, 1997) and in some cases in which the person has experienced a discrete, single-episode trauma (Taylor, Carleton, & Asmundson, 2006). Personality pathology may predate trauma exposure and PTSD, or, in other cases, personality disturbance and PTSD may both be consequences of traumatic events.

An advantage of the concept of complex PTSD is that it captures some of the comorbidity commonly seen in patients with a history of repeated interpersonal trauma. Disadvantages are the vagueness and the heterogeneity of traits and symptoms subsumed by the concept. Cluster analytic research involving measures of personality pathology suggests that there could be multiple forms of complex PTSD (Allen, Huntoon, & Evans, 1999).

PTSD ACROSS THE LIFESPAN

Children

The experience of, and reactions to, traumatic events depends on the person's level of cognitive development. If children are too young to understand what is happening to them (e.g., a developmentally inappropriate sexual experience without actual injury or perceived violence), then they may not experience the event as traumatic and therefore may not develop PTSD. However, PTSD may later emerge if they come to recognize what has happened to them (Foa, Steketee, & Rothbaum, 1989; Kilpatrick et al., 1989).

Children old enough to interpret events as traumatic (e.g., 4–7 years or older) generally have emotional responses similar to those of adults (Caffo & Belaise, 2003). To illustrate, Fletcher (1996) conducted a meta-analysis of 34 samples totaling 2,697 of such children who had experienced trauma. Children were comparable to adults in terms of the prevalence of PTSD and in the frequency of PTSD symptoms. The rates of diagnosed PTSD did not differ markedly across developmental levels. However, there are some differences in the way that PTSD symptoms are manifested (APA, 2000; Salmon & Bryant, 2002). Young children typically do not have the sense that they are reliving the traumatic event. Instead, reliving may be expressed through repetitive drawings or play (e.g., the reenacting of the car crash described in the opening vignette). Nightmares of the event may evolve over time into distressing dreams of monsters or other threats to oneself, or of rescuing others. There also may be "omen formation," consisting of the belief that one can foretell future ominous events. Hyperarousal symptoms may be expressed as headaches or stomachaches. Adolescents and adults may show these various features, but they are more common in children.

Trauma-related avoidance in children can have important interpersonal repercussions. Many children (and adolescents) who survive traumatic events find it difficult to discuss their feelings with family members or peers and may interpret reticence on the part of peers to ask about the event as a form of rejection (Yule, 2001). Parents may mistakenly believe that the child has forgotten about the traumatic event because he or she doesn't talk about it; it is common for young children to tell outsiders (e.g., a therapist) about the details of traumatic events while keeping them from their parents for fear of upsetting them (Yule, 2001).

Disorders that are commonly comorbid in childhood PTSD include phobias (e.g., fear of the dark or fear of using the toilet alone; Scheeringa et al., 1995), separation anxiety, oppositional disorder, and mood disorders. These may impair the growth of academic skills and friendships (McCloskey & Walker, 2000).

It has been claimed that very young children (e.g., 1–3 years of age) can develop PTSD-like syndromes (Keren & Tyano, 2000; Scheeringa, Zeanah, Myers, & Putnam, 2003). This is controversial, partly because of the difficulty in determining whether a given problem behavior is trauma related or whether it is due to other factors (e.g., the emergence of the fear of strangers is a normal milestone in childhood development; Cox & Taylor, 1999). Abused infants or toddlers may exhibit developmental delays, such as learning disorders, language disorders, motor disorders, poor emotional regulation, and poor socialization skills (Streeck-Fischer & van der Kolk, 2000). The cause of these deficits is unclear. It is possible that they could be a result of psychological abuse, or they could be due to more basic deprivations (e.g., poor nutrition, or being raised in an unstimulating environment in which learning opportunities are limited, or head injury associated with physical abuse).

The Elderly

There are few consistent variations in the clinical features or prevalence of PTSD across the adult life span (Norris et al., 2002). The greatest distinguishing feature of PTSD in the elderly is its apparent emergence or worsening in late life, after decades of having few or no symptoms (Hyer, Summers, Braswell, & Boyd, 1995; Peters & Kaye, 2003; van Achterberg, Rohrbaugh, & Southwick, 2001). Various explanations have been offered, including job retirement with loss of daily structure and social contact (and increased time to dwell on past experiences) and increased exposure to death or other losses reminiscent of past trauma (van Achterberg et al., 2001). The organizational practices of long-term care facilities may confront the person with a variety of trauma cues that he or she had managed to avoid throughout much of adulthood. For survivors of childhood sexual abuse, for example, old-age institutions can have many features reminiscent of childhood abusive settings. Residents may have little or no privacy, they may be exposed to naked bodies of other residents, and they have little control over who touches them or how (e.g., being handled, toileted, bathed, or checked) (Peters & Kaye, 2003).

Several case studies have described the worsening or apparent emergence of PTSD among trauma survivors with dementia (Johnston, 2000; Mittal, Torres, Abashidze, & Jimerson, 2001; van Achterberg et al., 2001). To illustrate, one case involved a 95-year-old woman who had probable Alzheimer's disease (van Achterberg et al., 2001). She had apraxia, agnosia, and was no longer able to recognize family members. When she was 22 years old she survived the sinking of the *Titanic*. Throughout her life she refused to talk about her involvement in this famous event. Aside from long-standing avoidance, her family could not recall any evidence of other PTSD symptoms, such as nightmares or hyperarousal (although she may have had some symptoms but avoided mentioning them). In the nursing home, she began to have periods of extreme agitation, accompanied by vivid reexperiencing: "For example, when placed in the day room with other residents, she would become markedly distressed, calling out 'The water is coming up! Go to the lifeboats! Save the children! We'll all be dead!' " (van Achterberg et al., 2001, p. 206).

The mechanism of dementia-related PTSD emergence or exacerbation remains to be elucidated, although there are several plausible possibilities. In some cases the person's PTSD has been in full or partial remission until the onset of dementia. Neurodegeneration of memory pathways may disinhibit recollections of trauma memories (Mittal et al., 2001) or disinhibit previously "extinguished" fears of trauma-related stimuli (see Chapter 4 on the role of the orbital frontal cortex in inhibiting limbic system activity). Another possibility is that with dementia-associated impairment in memory for recent events, longer-term memories such as long-standing traumatic memories may become more salient. With a dementia-related decline in reality testing, recollections of the trauma may increasingly take the form of dissociative reliving of the event (flashbacks).

CULTURAL CONSIDERATIONS

Is PTSD a culturally universal syndrome or it is culturally bound to contemporary Western society? Historical sources have identified PTSD symptoms in trauma survivors in various wars, including the Civil War and World Wars I and II (Dean, 1997; Kardiner, 1941; Lerner, 2003). There is also evidence of PTSD symptoms in antiquity, such as in the Epic of Gilgamesh, written between 2027 and 2003 B.C. (Ben-Ezra, 2002; Birmes, Hatton, Bruner, & Schmitt, 2003). These findings are not surprising because the fundamental features of PTSD symptoms—such as the acquisition of trauma-related fear and avoidance, and increased vigilance for threat—likely arise from basic survival mechanisms.

PTSD has been identified in a range of contemporary cultures, including the cultures in Afghanistan, Cambodia, China, Colombia, Ecuador, Fiji, Japan, Mexico, Nepal, South Africa, Sudan, Somalia, Sri Lanka, and Vietnam (Elbert & Schauer, 2002; Marsella, Friedman, Gerrity, & Scurfield, 1996; Shrestna et al., 1988). McCall and Resick (2003) demonstrated that PTSD could be identified in a radically non-Western culture, the Kalahari Bushmen, who are African hunter-gatherers. PTSD symptoms (related to domestic violence) were assessed by administering the diagnostic interviews in the difficult, click-laden Kalahari language. Despite this obstacle, PTSD symptoms could be readily identified.

After reviewing studies from a wide range of Western and non-Western societies, Marsella et al. (1996) concluded that they could not find any ethnocultural group in which PTSD could not be identified, although the prevalence rates varied from one culture to another. Thus, PTSD is not simply a syndrome bound to Western culture. Other studies have compared U.S. cultural subgroups of people seeking treatment for PTSD (e.g., African Americans vs. Caucasians) and found few differences on measures of psychopathology (Monnier, Elhai, Frueh, Sauvageot, & Magruder, 2002; Trent, Rushlau, Munley, Bloem, & Driesenga, 2000; Zoellner, Feeny, Fitzgibbons, & Foa, 1999).

There are, however, some ways in which the disorder or its associated features may differ over time and culture. Posttraumatic conversion reactions, such as mutism, aphonia, or paralysis, were more common in previous wars (e.g., World Wars I and II) than they are today (Kardiner, 1941; Lerner, 2003). Such disorders are only occasionally seen today (Rothbaum & Foa, 1991; Wald, Taylor, & Scamvougeras, 2004b). So there is some connection between historical epoch, culture, and PTSD, but this connection is mild at most, with cultural influences limited to the less common conversion symptoms (Ben-Ezra, 2003). This does not mean, however, that the treating clinician should ignore the patient's cultural background. The latter is important, for example, in establishing a therapeutic relationship, as discussed in later chapters

RISK FACTORS FOR PTSD

Estimates indicate that 40–60% of community adults have been exposed to trauma (Kessler et al., 1995; Yehuda & Wong, 2001), yet only a fraction develop PTSD (8%: APA, 2000). This suggests that trauma alone is insufficient to cause PTSD and that other factors must be taken into consideration. One of the first steps in identifying vulnerability factors is to identify risk factors. These are variables that predict the development of PTSD. A risk factor need not play a causal role—it could simply be a correlate of a causal factor. One should not confuse risk factors with causal factors, although the former can provide clues about the latter.

There have been many studies of PTSD risk factors. The results have been synthesized in two major meta-analyses (Brewin, Andrews, & Valentine, 2000; Ozer, Best, Lipsey, & Weiss, 2003). Four categories of predictors were found to be significant predictors of PTSD: (1) historical features such as family psychiatric history, low intelligence, family instability, and personal past history of PTSD or trauma exposure (i.e., traumas arising prior to the index trauma associated with the current episode of PTSD); (2) severity of the index trauma; (3) threat-relevant psychological processes during and immediately after the trauma (e.g., perception of threat, dissociative symptoms); and (4) life stressors and low social support after the trauma.

Factors closer in time to the traumatic event (e.g., perception of threat) tend to be stronger predictors of PTSD than historical factors (e.g., personality traits) (Ozer et al., 2003). The strongest predictor, investigated only in the Ozer et al. (2003) meta-analysis, was peritraumatic dissociation, that is, the experience of dissociative symptoms during or immediately after the trauma (e.g., the sense that time has slowed down, perceiving one's environment to be unreal, or feeling that one's body is unfamiliar or unreal). Although the various predictors were statistically significant, the effect sizes were not generally large; none of the risk factors was necessary or sufficient for developing PTSD (Ozer & Weiss, 2004). For example, although peritraumatic dissociation is a risk factor for PTSD, many people who dissociate do not develop PTSD, and many cases of PTSD arise in people who do not experience peritraumatic dissociation (Harvey & Bryant, 2002).

Many of the risk factors for PTSD in children are similar to those for adults, including the level of exposure, extent of disruption of social support systems, and pretrauma levels of psychopathology (Caffo & Belaise, 2003). Parental distress and psychopathology are also predictors of childhood PTSD (Davis et al., 2000). Parental modeling might play a role, especially for a traumatic event that has afflicted the entire family. Children who observe their parents becoming highly distressed by the trauma may be more likely to become distressed themselves. Consistent with this, persistent maternal preoccupation with the trauma and other trauma-related family disruptions have been found to predict PTSD in children (Pynoos & Nader, 1993). Persistent separation from parents immediately after a natural disaster (such as a hurricane or flood), along with the loss of the child's home, pets, toys, and friends also predicts PTSD in children (Pynoos & Nader, 1993; Vernberg, La Greca, Silverman, & Prinstein, 1996). For children living in families marred by severe marital conflict, PTSD symptoms can develop as a result of witnessing violence of one parent inflicted on the other (Rossman & Ho, 2000).

SUMMARY

PTSD is a complex and often chronic disorder that commonly co-occurs with many other disorders, including other anxiety disorders, mood disorders, and substance use disorders. PTSD takes similar forms across the life span, although PTSD in children differs in some ways from that of adults. PTSD takes a similar form across diverse cultures. Many people are exposed to traumatic events and yet only a few develop PTSD. Various risk factors have been identified, such as peritraumatic dissociation and low social support.

CHAPTER 2

Cognitive and Behavioral Features of PTSD

What the Research Tells Us

Cognitive-behavioral theories and research are tightly intertwined; empirical findings give rise to models of PTSD, and the models influence the directions pursued by empirical investigations. Even so, it is expedient to review theories and research separately, rather than wade through a dense forest of conjecture, evidence, counterconjecture, and further evidence. We will begin by reviewing the current state of knowledge on the cognitive and behavioral features of PTSD, including cutting-edge discoveries as well as established findings. Armed with this information, we will then consider, in the following chapter, which models are most promising.

We will begin by reviewing two empirical approaches used to study cognitive processing abnormalities in PTSD. The first has examined whether PTSD is associated with general information processing abnormalities, independent of the content of the information being processed. The second approach has focused on content-related abnormalities, such as selective attention to, or biased recall of, information that is specifically trauma related. Later sections of the chapter will review the role of beliefs in PTSD and the role of behavioral (e.g., interpersonal) factors.

GENERAL INFORMATION PROCESSING

Global Intelligence

The strongest evidence for the relationship between global intelligence and PTSD comes from longitudinal research, which has shown that lower premorbid IQ predicts subsequent PTSD, even after controlling for trauma severity (Macklin et al., 1998). The reasons for the IQ–PTSD relationship may have to do with working memory capacity (discussed below) and problem-solving ability. A facet of intelligence is the ability to solve problems, and recovering from the effects of trauma is most certainly a problem to be solved (McNally, 2003a). People with higher IQ may have better cognitive ability to cope with the emotional impact of traumatic experiences (Schnurr, Rosenberg, & Friedman, 1993). In fact, problem-focused coping is correlated with positive outcome following trauma (Sutker, Davis, Uddo, & Ditta, 1995; Wolfe, Keane, Kaloupek, Mora, & Wine, 1993). People with higher IQ and superior language skills also may be those most likely to impose meaning on their traumatic experiences, thereby facilitating their recovery (Macklin et al., 1998).

Attention and Memory

Numerous studies have found that people with PTSD, compared to various types of controls (including trauma-exposed, non-PTSD controls), have deficits in sustained attention (e.g., Beckham, Crawford, & Feldman, 1998; Sutker et al., 1995; Vasterling, Brailey, Constans, & Sutker, 1998). Several studies have documented impairments in various aspects of memory, including acquisition and recall (e.g., Bremner, Vermetten, Afzal, & Vythilingam, 2004; Bustamante, Mellman, David, & Fins, 2001; Koenen et al., 2001). The deficits were not attributable to age or education, or to comorbid mood, anxiety disorders, or substance use disorders.

PTSD is also associated with deficits in working memory, that is, the ability to hold and manipulate information in short-term storage (Brewin & Holmes, 2003; Koenen et al., 2001). Individual differences in working memory capacity appear to be related to the ability to prevent unwanted thoughts or memories from intruding into consciousness. People with greater working memory capacity are better at suppressing unwanted thoughts when instructed to do so under experimental conditions (Brewin & Beaton, 2002; Brewin & Smart, 2005). This may partly explain why lower intelligence, which is strongly related to working memory capacity, is a risk factor for PTSD (Brewin & Holmes, 2003). The patterns of memory impairment suggest dysfunction of the frontal lobe or hippocampus (Golier & Yehuda, 2002; Koenen et al., 2001), which is implicated in the memory encoding and retrieval (see Chapter 4).

Autobiographical Memory

Autobiographical memory consists of recollections of episodes from one's past (e.g., "Memory of the birth of my son, Alex, at St. Paul's Hospital on August 7, 2004") and factual knowledge about oneself (e.g., "Knowledge that I am a father") (Conway, Singer, & Tagini, 2004). People with PTSD, compared to people exposed to traumatic events without developing PTSD, have "overgeneral" autobiographical memories in that their recollections are vague and lacking in detail (Harvey, Bryant, & Dang, 1998; McNally, Litz, Prassas, Shin, & Weathers, 1994; McNally, Lasko, Macklin, & Pitman, 1995). To illustrate, when asked to retrieve specific memories in response to cue words (e.g., *happy*), they recall general categories of memories ("When I was kayaking") rather than specific episodes ("The kayaking trip I took to the Queen Charlotte Islands last summer"). Overgeneral memory retrieval is not mood-state dependent and may be a stable cognitive style or trait (Brittlebank, Scott, Williams, & Ferrier, 1993; Henderson, Hargreaves, Gregory, & Williams, 2002). Difficulty accessing one's "autobiographical database" of nontraumatic memories may hamper attempts to solve problems in everyday life and may underlie difficulties envisioning one's future, which is a feature of PTSD (McNally, 1998a). Overgeneral autobiographical memory may be due to hippocampal abnormalities associated with PTSD (McNally, 1998a; see Chapter 4).

THREAT-SPECIFIC PROCESSING

Fear Conditioning

PTSD is characterized, in part, by the acquisition of fears of harmless, but trauma-related stimuli, that is, a process of learning to associate harmless stimuli with danger. To illustrate, Sam was held hostage by an escaped convict wearing an orange jumpsuit. Thereafter, whenever he encountered people wearing orange clothing (e.g., road construction workers wearing orange reflective clothing or people in orange-colored Halloween costumes) he became panicky and had a powerful urge to flee from the situation. Such cases raise the question of whether people with PTSD differ from control groups in terms of fear conditioning. Some, but not all, experiments show that people with PTSD, compared to controls, more readily acquire conditioned fears and have slower habituation of electrodermal response to neutral auditory stimuli (Orr et al., 2000; Rothbaum, Kozak, Foa, & Whitaker, 2001; but cf. the null findings of Grillon & Morgan, 1999; Peri, Ben-Shakhar, Orr, & Shalev, 2000). The null results may be due to methodological problems with those studies (Orr, Metzger, Miller, & Kaloupek, 2004).

Why is PTSD apparently associated with heightened fear conditioning and slower extinction? Heightened conditionability may be due to failure of cortical inhibitory control over conditioned responses (Gurvits et al., 2000). This could result from abnormalities predating trauma exposure, or it could be a consequence of dysregulations arising from the development of PTSD.

Attentional Bias

Several studies have investigated whether people with PTSD, compared to controls, differ in their attentional biases for trauma-related information. Here, the modified Stroop test is the most widely used method. The participant is presented with a series of words, each written in a different colored ink. The goal is to name the color of the ink as quickly and accurately as possible, while ignoring the meaning of the word. Stroop interference is demonstrated when the meaning of the word interferes with the speed with which the person can name the color of the ink. Using this procedure one can assess the degree of interference produced by different types of words, for example, trauma-related words, (e.g., *rapist*) compared to emotionally neutral words (e.g., *apple*). The degree of interference is an index of the degree to which the meaning of the word draws the person's attention and thereby disrupts processing, even when the purpose of the task is not to focus on the meaning of the word. Thus, Stroop interference is a marker of attentional bias toward information pertaining to the person's current concerns (Williams, Watts, MacLeod, & Mathews, 1997).

Studies using the modified Stroop procedure have demonstrated trauma-related interference in various PTSD populations, including PTSD survivors of combat, sexual assault, or motor vehicle accidents (e.g., McNally, Amir, & Lipke, 1996; Moradi, Neshat-Doost, Taghavi, Yule, & Dalgleish, 1999; Vrana, Roodman, & Beckham, 1995). Another experimental paradigm, the dot probe method, has also demonstrated attentional bias in PTSD (Bryant & Harvey, 1997). This bias could be partly due to involuntary retrieval of traumatic memories (McNally, 1998a). Trauma-related information (e.g., trauma words) may serve as retrieval cues, causing traumatic memories to be involuntarily accessed, thereby interfering with other ongoing tasks. Consistent with this, the degree of Stroop interference increases with the severity of reexperiencing symptoms but not with the severity of numbing or avoidance symptoms (Cassiday, McNally, & Zeitlin, 1992). Thus, "hyperaccessibility" of traumatic memories appears linked to the attentional bias. Cognitive-behavioral therapy reduces this bias (Foa, Rothbaum, Riggs, & Murdock, 1991).

Memory Retrieval

Reexperiencing of traumatic events is a cardinal feature of PTSD, suggesting that people with PTSD too easily and involuntarily recall traumatic events. Reexperiencing symptoms mainly consists of sensory impressions rather than thoughts. They may consist of all sensory modalities, although they are most often visual (Ehlers & Steil, 1995; Ehlers et al., 2002). Intrusive memories commonly consist of stimuli that were present immediately before the traumatic event happened or shortly before the moments that had the largest emotional impact (i.e., when the meaning of the traumatic event became apparent; Ehlers et al., 2002). Ehlers and colleagues suggested that intrusive memories are about stimuli that through temporal association with the trauma acquired the status of warning signals, that is, stimuli that if encountered again would indicate impending danger. This may explain why intrusive memories are often accompanied by a sense of serious current threat.

Experimental studies provide evidence of memory bias for trauma information. People with PTSD, compared to controls, have enhanced memory for trauma-related material, compared to neutral material (e.g., better recall of trauma-related words, such as *combat*, compared to neutral words, such as *carrot*) (Paunovic, Lundh, & Öst, 2002; Vrana et al., 1995). Persistent rumination about the trauma may undermine the retrieval of nontraumatic material and facilitate recall of traumatic material (McNally, Metzger, Lasko, Clancy, & Pitman, 1998).

Are Trauma Memories Indelible?

Animal research suggests that emotional memories are remarkably long-lasting and may even be indelible (LeDoux, 2000). This suggests that fear extinction may not involve the erasure or modification of memories but rather involves the inhibition of old (fear) memories with new memories (e.g., memories that the previously feared conditioned stimulus (CS) no longer predicts danger). This hypothesis is consistent with the well-established finding that the return or relapse of previously extinguished fears can readily occur, even by a single pairing of the conditioned and unconditioned stimulus (UCS) (Vermetten & Bremner, 2002b). Similarly, people who have recovered from PTSD are at heightened risk, compared to people who have never had the disorder, to develop PTSD in the future if confronted with new stressors (APA, 2000).

Research on humans suggests that memories for traumatic experiences are reasonably accurate and well-retained for very long periods (Koss, Tromp, & Tharan, 1995). However, the human research also raises the possibility that trauma memories may not be entirely indelible; they are subject to some degree of modification over time. This is consistent with the research on memory in general, which shows that recollections are constructive and malleable and are influenced by a variety of factors, including the purpose and context of retrieval (Schacter, 2002).

The malleability of trauma memories has been demonstrated in longitudinal studies of military personnel, in which soldiers recalled the nature and frequency of their trauma exposure at Time 1 (shortly after the trauma) and at Time 2 (e.g., a year or more later). The most commonly reported finding is an increase in the reported frequency of stressors on the second assessment, compared with the first (King et al., 2000a; Roemer, Litz, Orsillo, Ehlich, & Friedman, 1998; Southwick, Morgan, Nicolaou, & Charney, 1997b). Human conditioning research also suggests that the reevaluation of an aversive (unconditioned) stimulus can alter the memory representation of that stimulus (Davey, 1992); the memory representation of the traumatic event can be altered in light of subsequent information. Thus, it appears that trauma memories can be altered to some extent.

Are Trauma Memories Fragmented?

Although people with PTSD tend to show better recall of trauma-related than emotionally neutral material, their recollections of traumatic events are typically far from perfect. Clinically, their recollections sometimes appear to be fragmentary, with details missing and jumbled recollection of the exact order of events. If trauma memories are fragmented, then this may make it difficult for the person to impose meaning on the traumatic experience and to psychologically "place it in the past," alongside other autobiographical memories (Horowitz, 1975).

Some studies have reported findings that purportedly provide evidence that trauma memories tend to be fragmented (e.g., Amir, Stafford, Freshman, & Foa, 1998; Foa, Molnar, & Cashman, 1995b; Tromp, Koss, Figueredo, & Tharan, 1995). Other studies have failed to replicate the results (e.g., Berntsen, Willert, & Rubin, 2003; Reviere & Bakeman, 2001). The findings said to be evidence of fragmented memories have been questioned on methodological grounds (Berntsen et al., 2003; McNally, 2003a, 2003b). To illustrate some of these problems, Tromp et al. (1995) claimed that rape memories were less vivid and detailed than memories for other sorts of unpleasant experiences. But Tromp et al. did not report the age of the different kinds of memories; differences in vividness and detail could be an artifact of the rape memories being older than the other memories. Foa et al. (1995b) compared rape memories before and after exposure therapy and found that a reduction in the fragmentation in the organization of the narrative was positively related to a reduction in the level of trauma-related anxiety. However, it was not clear whether fragmentation of the articulated narrative (assessed by repetitions, unfinished thoughts, and speech fillers) reflects fragmentation in the memory as opposed to practice in recounting the memory (Berntsen et al., 2003). Amir et al. (1998) measured the reading level of rape narratives and found that reading level correlated negatively with PTSD symptoms 12 weeks but not 2 weeks posttrauma. Reading level is a questionable (and unvalidated) measure of memory fragmentation, and other researchers have failed to replicate Amir et al.'s findings (Zoellner, Alvarez-Conrad, & Foa, 2002).

Traumatic Amnesia

Amnesia for important parts of the traumatic event is included in DSM-IV-TR as one of the diagnostic features of PTSD. Yet, the very existence of traumatic amnesia is controversial, and the preponderance of clinical and experimental evidence indicates that people generally encode and retrieve traumatic events all too well (McNally, 2003a). It has been suggested that traumatic amnesia could arise from deliberate attempts to suppress upsetting memories (Golier & Yehuda, 2002). However, research suggests that attempts at suppressing upsetting thoughts lead to a paradoxical increase in their frequency (see below). Another speculation is that failure to recall elements of traumatic events is due to unconscious repression (van der Kolk et al., 1996). But this fails to explain why traumatic amnesia, as a PTSD symptom, is characterized by the failure to recall only some aspects of the trauma. The person may fail to recall important details of the trauma, but he or she can recall the fact that the trauma happened (APA, 2000).

A more plausible explanation for traumatic amnesia (as a DSM-IV-TR symptom of PTSD) concerns attentional narrowing. When a person is highly aroused, his or her attentional field is narrowed to focus on the central features of the threat, and the person thereby fails to encode peripheral features (Easterbrook, 1959). This is illustrated by the "weapon focus" phenomenon (McNally, 2003b). When a bank teller is involved in an armed holdup, he or she may recall the weapon that was used but be unable to describe the assailant's features. This is because the teller was focusing on (and thereby encoding into memory) the weapon but not focusing on other features, such as the characteristics of the assailant. This suggests that psychogenic amnesia as a PTSD symptom may not really be amnesia at all; it may simply be a failure to encode (attend to) particular aspects of the traumatic event.

Is traumatic amnesia more likely for survivors of recurrent trauma? Contrary to some clinical impressions (e.g., Terr, 1991), there is no scientific evidence that exposure to repeated trauma leads to impairments in recalling the events. People may have difficulty remembering specific episodes of abuse, particularly if they have gone through a great many episodes, but they typically have no difficulty recalling that they were abused and can readily recall particular, unusually aversive episodes (McNally, 2003b).

Avoidance and Thought Suppression

Avoidance of trauma-related stimuli, which is a diagnostic feature of PTSD, prevents the person from being exposed to corrective information. For example, by striving to avoid social activities (despite a desire for an intimate relationship), a survivor of sexual assault fails to learn how to distinguish safe from potentially risky relationships, thereby perpetuating her fear of dating. Thus, the use of avoidance behaviors has been shown to predict the persistence of other PTSD symptoms (Dunmore, Clark, & Ehlers, 2001).

One form of avoidance is the deliberate attempt to suppress unwanted trauma-related thoughts. Research indicates that this sort of avoidance can produce a paradoxical increase in the frequency of trauma-related thoughts and thereby perpetuate reexperiencing symptoms (e.g., Davies & Clark, 1998; Dunmore et al., 2001; Shipherd & Beck, 1999). This may occur because distraction is used as a means of thought suppression (e.g., focusing one's attention on reading a book in an effort to drive unwanted memories out of consciousness). As a result, the distractors (e.g., books) become reminders or retrieval cues for the unwanted thoughts (Wegner, 1994).

Ruminative Thinking

Rumination consists of persistently thinking about the trauma and its aftermath, along with repeatedly asking oneself questions like "Why did this happen to me?", "How could I have prevented it from happening?", and "Was it my fault?" People who believe that they have been wronged by others during the trauma may also ruminate about ways of seeking justice or achieving retribution (e.g., revenge fantasies). The extent to which a person ruminates about the traumatic event is positively correlated with the severity of his or her PTSD symptoms (e.g., Murray, Ehlers, & Mayou, 2002). After rumination develops, as a consequence of trauma exposure and PTSD, it may play a role in maintaining hyperarousal symptoms such as irritability or anger (Rusting & Nolen-Hoeksema, 1998).

How do rumination and thought suppression fit together? They seem to be mutually exclusive cognitive processes. It may be that some people tend to ruminate over the trauma, whereas other people tend to engage in thought suppression. Alternatively, a trauma survivor might engage in periods of rumination interspersed with periods of thought suppression and other forms of avoidance. This alternating pattern is consistent with evidence that reexperiencing and avoidance symptoms alternate with one another (Creamer, Burgess, & Pattison, 1992; Herman, 1997; Horowitz, 2001). These alternating patterns may arise from mechanisms for processing or making sense of the traumatic experience in a controlled, dosed fashion.

BELIEFS ASSOCIATED WITH PTSD

Various types of beliefs have been associated with PTSD. These include basic assumptions about the self and the world, and assumptions about the meaning or consequences of one's PTSD symptoms. Although the beliefs can be highly idiosyncratic, several themes have emerged in the research literature.

Beliefs about the Self and World

Shattered Assumptions

Drawing on social psychology research, Janoff-Bulman (1992) argued that people ordinarily operate on the basis of unchallenged, unquestioned assumptions about themselves and the world (e.g., "My world is predictable, meaningful, and fundamentally just" and "Bad things don't happen to good people like me"). When trauma strikes, the person's assumptions about the self and world may be shattered, thereby leading to confusion, distress, and attempts to make sense of what happened. The person may try to fit the traumatic experience into their belief system (assimilation) or alter their beliefs, sometimes dramatically, in light of the experience (accommodation).

Although some research supports Janoff-Bulman's view that poor posttrauma adjustment and PTSD symptoms arise from events that shatter the person's assumptions, the relationship between pretrauma beliefs and posttrauma adjustment is much more complex. For people who have always held negative beliefs about themselves (e.g., "I'm not worthy of good things"), traumatic events may "confirm" their beliefs, rather than shatter them. In such cases, traumatic events can lead to psychopathology because they strengthen dysfunctional beliefs (Brewin & Holmes, 2003). Consistent with this, longitudinal research indicates that the tendency to hold dysfunctional beliefs prior to trauma exposure predicts the tendency to develop PTSD after trauma exposure (Bryant & Guthrie, 2005). Conversely, strongly optimistic pretrauma beliefs can serve as a buffer against the effects of trauma (Ali, Dunmore, Clark, & Ehlers, 2002). The factors that lead to shattering versus buffering of optimistic beliefs are currently unknown.

Beliefs about the World

PTSD is correlated with various beliefs about the dangerousness of people and the world (Foa, Ehlers, Clark, Tolin, & Orsillo, 1999c). Examples include "The world is a dangerous place" and "People can't be trusted." Severity of PTSD is also correlated with beliefs that one is alienated from other people (Ehlers, Maercker, & Boos, 2000). A sense of alienation can arise from experiences of being blamed, mistreated, or not being believed or emotionally supported after the trauma, (Ehlers et al., 1998a). Ehlers and colleagues proposed that this sense of alienation is different from PTSD numbing symptoms, although the two appear to overlap considerably.

Self-Related Beliefs

People with PTSD, compared to people who have been subjected to stressors without developing PTSD, are characterized by negative beliefs about themselves (e.g., "I am incompetent," "I can't trust myself"). The strength of these beliefs is correlated with the severity of PTSD symptoms (Ehlers et al., 2000; Foa et al., 1999c).

PTSD, especially when it arises from interpersonal traumas such as rape or torture, is correlated with a sense of *mental defeat* (Dunmore, Clark, & Ehlers, 1999; Dunmore et al., 2001; Ehlers et al., 2000). Mental defeat is a complex concept that has cognitive and motivational elements. It refers to "the perceived loss of all autonomy, a state of giving up in one's own mind all efforts to retain one's identity as a human being with a will of one's own" (Ehlers et al., 2000, p. 45). Trauma survivors who experience mental defeat may describe themselves as being an object, as having been destroyed, or as ceasing to care whether they live or die.

Beliefs Associated with Trauma-Related Anger, Guilt, or Shame

Anger

Two types of beliefs have been associated with anger. The first are beliefs that the trauma survivor has been wronged by others (e.g., "They had no right to do this to me," "Others should be punished for what they've done"). Such beliefs are correlated with, or predict, the severity of PTSD symptoms (e.g., Ehlers et al., 1998b). The second type of beliefs are *meta-cognitions*, that is, beliefs about the value of dwelling on anger thoughts (Simpson & Papageorgiou, 2003). Positive meta-cognitive beliefs include beliefs that dwelling on anger thoughts helps persons understand, prepare for, and cope with threatening situations and also helps justify their aggressive behavior (e.g., "Others are not likely to take advantage of me if I have been dwelling on my angry thoughts," "Dwelling on what happened prevents me from blaming myself"). Negative meta-cognitive beliefs concern the adverse emotional impact of dwelling on anger thoughts, as well as the detrimental effect on social and occupational functioning (e.g., "My anger builds up, last longer, and gets me into trouble when I dwell on my angry thoughts," "Dwelling on my memory of the event gets me worked up and stops me going about my usual daily tasks") (Simpson & Papageorgiou, 2003). As the examples suggest, patients with anger problems are more likely to try to regulate their anger if they hold stronger negative than positive meta-cognitive beliefs. That is, if they believe their anger is more of a liability than an asset.

Guilt

Many trauma survivors exaggerate or distort the importance of their roles in traumatic events and experience excessive guilt as a consequence (e.g., "I should have realized that the situation would be dangerous," "I should fought back against the rapist"). According to Kubany and Manke (1995), trauma survivors tend to draw four kinds of faulty conclusions about their role in trauma: (1) many survivors believe they "knew" what was going to happen before it was possible to know, or that they dismissed or overlooked clues that "signaled" what was going to happen (*hindsight bias*, i.e., outcome knowledge tends to bias the person's recollections of what they actually know before events occurred); (2) many survivors believe that their trauma-related actions were less justified than would be concluded on the basis of an objective analysis of the facts (*justification distortion*); (3) many survivors accept an inordinate share of responsibility for causing the trauma or related negative outcomes (*responsibility distortion*); (4) many survivors believe they violated personal or moral convictions even though their intentions and actions were consistent with their convictions (*wrongdoing distortion*).

These faulty conclusions appear to arise from various types of reasoning errors (Kubany & Manke, 1995), such as the following.

- Failure to recognize that different decision-making "rules" apply when time is precious than in situations that allow extended contemplation of options.
- Weighing the merits of actions taken against options that only came to mind later on.
- Weighing the merits of actions taken against ideal or fantasy options that did not exist.
- Focusing only on the "good" things that might have happened if an alternative action had been taken.
- Tendency to overlook "benefits" associated with actions taken.
- Failure to compare available options in terms of their perceived probabilities of success before outcomes were known.
- Ignoring to the totality of forces that cause traumatic events.

- Equating a belief that one could have done something to prevent a traumatic event with a belief that one caused the event.
- Confusion between responsibility as accountability (e.g., "doing one's job") and responsibility as power to cause or control outcomes. (i.e., having been given a job or "put in charge" does not mean that one has complete control).
- Tendency to conclude wrongdoing on the basis of the outcome rather than on the basis of one's intentions (before the outcome was known).
- Failure to realize that strong emotional reactions are not under voluntary control (i.e., not a matter of choice or willpower).
- Failure to recognize that when all available options have negative outcomes, the least bad choice is a highly moral choice.

Shame

A person can experience shame about one's social presentation (*external shame*; e.g., "I'm a hideous freak because I lost my arm in the accident") or about one's sense of self (*internal shame*; e.g., "I'm weak and disgusting because I was raped") (Lee et al., 2001). A person with PTSD may experience both sorts of shame, for example, "I'm weak and inadequate for not resisting the mugger, and other people despise me for my cowardice." Such shame-related beliefs can give rise to various behavioral patterns including submissiveness and efforts to escape, hide, or conceal oneself (e.g., avoiding eye contact, hiding one's face, or lowering one's head; Kaufman, 1989).

The various cognitive factors linked to guilt, as described above, could also contribute to trauma-related shame. However, this has yet to be empirically investigated. Nor is it known whether meta-cognitive beliefs play an important role in shame or guilt.

Beliefs about Symptoms

The persistence of PTSD in longitudinal studies is associated with, at initial assessment, the tendency to regard PTSD symptoms as harmful, shameful, or indications that one could go crazy (e.g., "Palpitations lead to heart attacks," "Flashbacks mean I'm going crazy"; Dunmore et al., 2001; Halligan, Michael, Clark, & Ehlers, 2003; Steil & Ehlers, 2000). People with PTSD also tend to interpret symptoms (e.g., anxiety or intrusive thoughts) as indications or predictors of danger in one's environment (Engelhard, Macklin, McNally, van den Hout, & Arntz, 2001; Engelhard, van den Hout, Arntz, & McNally, 2002).

People with PTSD are not just frightened of the symptoms of this disorder. Compared to controls, they tend to be more frightened of arousal-related sensations in general (i.e., sensations that may be associated with anxiety, anger, or other emotions), because they believe the sensations are associated with harmful somatic, psychological, or social consequences (Taylor, 1999). This is known as *anxiety sensitivity*, which is a vulnerability factor associated with anxiety disorders in general, and particularly PTSD and panic disorder (Taylor, 2004). The severity of anxiety sensitivity is correlated with the severity of PTSD symptoms, and longitudinal research shows that reductions in anxiety sensitivity predict reductions in PTSD symptoms (Fedoroff, Taylor, Asmundson, & Koch, 2000). Accordingly, interventions that reduce anxiety sensitivity, such as interoceptive exposure (Chapter 12), can reduce PTSD symptoms (Wald & Taylor, 2005a, 2005b).

COGNITIVE FACTORS IN AVOIDANCE AND NUMBING

Avoidance and emotional numbing can be empirically distinguished from one another and may have different underlying mechanisms (Chapter 1). Some theorists suggest that avoidance is driven largely by controlled processing (i.e., processes under conscious control, such as expectations of danger), whereby beliefs about safety and danger determine what the person strives to avoid. In comparison, emotional numbing may arise from some automatic (nonconscious) psychobiological mechanism, such as catecholamine depletion (van der Kolk, Greenberg, Boyd, & Krystal, 1985) or conditioned opioid-mediated analgesia (Foa, Zinbarg, & Rothbaum, 1992). Emotional numbing may be a variation of conditioned analgesia, triggered by trauma cues (Foa et al., 1992). In fact, there is evidence of conditioned analgesia after exposure to trauma-related stimuli in PTSD (Pitman, van der Kolk, Orr, & Greenberg, 1990).

It is possible that controlled processes also play a role in numbing. Numbing might occur as a result of deliberate attempts to suppress hyperarousal symptoms. The person might attempt to deliberately suppress emotional experience and expression, regardless of the valence of the emotion. Positive emotional experiences may be suppressed because some of these emotions (e.g., excitement or happiness) can be physiologically arousing. As noted earlier, people with PTSD tend to be frightened of arousal-related bodily sensations.

Consistent with the possibility that controlled processes are involved in numbing, the severity of numbing symptoms is correlated with deliberate attempts to suppress emotions (Litz et al., 1997; Tull & Roemer, 2003). Despite these findings, the causes of numbing—cognitive or otherwise—remain poorly understood.

DO COGNITIVE FACTORS PLAY A ROLE IN DISSOCIATIVE SYMPTOMS?

As with numbing, there are very few empirical data on the causes of dissociative symptoms such as derealization and depersonalization. It has been speculated that dissociative symptoms are indicative of a problem with the organization or structure of mental contents (Spiegel, 1996), or that dissociation is a coping response to intrusive images and fears (Foa & Rothbaum, 1998). Persistent dissociation after a trauma predicts the persistence of PTSD (Halligan, Clark, & Ehlers, 2002; Murray et al., 2002). Such findings are consistent with the view that persistent dissociation interferes with the cognitive and emotional processing of traumatic events (Ehlers et al., 2003; Foa & Hearst-Ikeda, 1996). Dissociation during attempts to recall the trauma, for example, could interfere with the access of these memories. The causes of persistent dissociation and the nature of its possible effects in perpetuating PTSD remain to be further investigated. Clinically, it appears that dissociation may sometimes be automatic and in other cases may be a controlled (intentional) process intended to avoid awareness of distressing stimuli.

INTERPERSONAL FACTORS

The way that people with PTSD interact with their social environment can influence the nature, severity, and persistence of their symptoms. The person's social milieu is shaped by the way significant people in the person's life react to the following:

- The fact that a person has been involved in a traumatic event. The person may be shunned, stigmatized, blamed, or disbelieved (e.g., "You were asking for trouble by wearing that outfit to the nightclub").
- The development of PTSD symptoms (e.g., implying that the person is morally weak, emotionally frail, or otherwise inferior for developing symptoms).
- The fact that the trauma survivor "looks OK" but is socially or occupationally impaired by PTSD (e.g., "Why don't you stop complaining and just get over it?").

Reactions such as these can be stressful in themselves, thereby adding to the burden of stress experienced by the trauma survivor. Also, some trauma survivors are persuaded to believe these unfair criticisms, which adds to their distress (Foa & Rothbaum, 1998).

Other interpersonal factors also can exacerbate PTSD, including too little social interaction and too much of particular sorts of interactions. Low social support is a risk factor for PTSD (Chapter 1), perhaps because it is more difficult to cognitively process (i.e., come to terms with or extract meaning from) a traumatic event if one does not have a supportive person with whom to discuss the traumatic event (Hyman, Gold, & Cott, 2003; Tremblay, Hebert, & Piche, 1999). Thus, social support can help correct dysfunctional beliefs, such as those to do with danger, safety, and the self.

Sometimes, significant others avoid discussing the trauma because it distresses them or because they believe it would greatly distress the trauma survivor. The trauma survivor, in turn, may misinterpret this as a sign that other people don't care or actually blame him or her for the trauma, leading to beliefs like "I'm all alone," "They don't want to know what happened to me," or "Everyone thinks it was my fault" (Foa & Rothbaum, 1998). This can prevent the trauma survivor from disclosing his or her traumatic experiences to other people.

Living in an environment in which one is exposed to high *expressed emotion* also can exacerbate PTSD and can hamper the treatment of this disorder (Tarrier & Humphreys, 2004). High expressed emotion is characterized by an environment in which family members are hostile, critical, and overinvolved with the patient's day-to-day life.

PTSD is often associated with depression, mistrust of others, and heightened irritability or aggression (Chapter 1). These can lead to interpersonal problems, just as interpersonal problems can exacerbate PTSD. To illustrate, a survivor of a bank robbery may feel hypervigilant, tense, irritable, and preoccupied with proper banking protocols and procedures. As a result, conflicts with coworkers are more likely to occur, thereby worsening hyperarousal symptoms. Conversely, some survivors of assault feel fragile and helpless and have difficulty asserting themselves or saying no to sexual advances, thereby increasing their risk of being involved in future abusive relationships (Najavits, 2002).

SUMMARY

A number of cognitive and behavioral features distinguish people with PTSD from controls. These are summarized in Table 2.1. PTSD is associated with a complex array of cognitive abnormalities and behavioral problems. People with PTSD have trouble focusing on daily activities, and their attention is readily directed to trauma-related stimuli. People with PTSD tend to have significant deficits in recalling everyday events and yet have vivid, intrusive recollections of traumatic experiences. PTSD is associated with negative beliefs about oneself and the world, and many people with

TABLE 2.1. Cognitive-Behavioral Characteristics of PTSD

Domain	Major findings
General information processing	
Global intelligence	Low IQ predicts risk of developing PTSD, even after controlling for trauma exposure.
Attention and memory	PTSD is associated with impairments in everyday attention and memory.
Autobiographical memory	In PTSD, memories of past events, including neutral events, tend to be overgeneral (vague and lacking in details).
Trauma-related processing	
Attentional bias	In PTSD, attention is biased toward the detection of trauma-related stimuli.
Fear conditioning	There is some evidence that PTSD is associated with enhanced acquisition of conditioned fears and slower extinction.
Retrieval of trauma-related memories	Retrieval of trauma-related memories is enhanced in PTSD, particularly the sensory aspects of these memories.
Persistence of trauma memories	Trauma memories are fairly well retained over time, although some alteration in memories can occur.
Memory fragmentation	There is no clear evidence that trauma memories are fragmented in PTSD, although this issue is controversial.
Traumatic amnesia	The occurrence of traumatic amnesia in PTSD is controversial. Further research is required.
Avoidance	Deliberate attempts to suppress trauma-related recollections and other forms of avoidance are associated with the persistence or worsening of various PTSD symptoms.
Ruminative thinking	Persistently thinking about the trauma and its meaning (e.g., "Why me?") is correlated with PTSD.
Beliefs	
Shattered assumptions	PTSD is associated with traumatic events that strongly refute positive, previously held assumptions (e.g., "My world is safe, predictable, and just").
Beliefs about world	PTSD is associated with strong beliefs that the world is dangerous. Such beliefs may be induced or strengthened by traumatic events.
Beliefs about self	Beliefs that one is incompetent or inferior are associated with PTSD. Beliefs that one no longer has autonomy or a will of one's own (mental defeat) is also associated with PTSD.
Trauma-related anger, guilt, shame	Beliefs about the trauma-related wrongdoing of oneself or others are associated with PTSD.
Beliefs about symptoms	PTSD is associated with beliefs that one's symptoms are dangerous or harbingers of catastrophe.
Avoidance and numbing	Avoidance appears to be a controlled (intentional) process, determined by beliefs about safety and danger. Emotional numbing may arise from either automatic or deliberate attempts to dampen emotional arousal.
Dissociative symptoms	Little is known about causes. Symptoms may be automatic responses to threat, or they may be deliberate coping responses.
Behavioral (interpersonal) factors	Posttrauma reactions by other people (e.g., low social support, blame, or shunning) are associated with PTSD.

PTSD believe that their symptoms will have harmful consequences. PTSD sufferers may try to avoid trauma cues, such as by trying to suppress unwanted recollections of the trauma. Such avoidance can perpetuate or worsen PTSD. Behavioral factors and PTSD can mutually influence one another; PTSD symptoms (e.g., anger or withdrawal) can impair interpersonal functioning, and aversive posttrauma social environments (e.g., low social support or criticism and shunning by others) can exacerbate PTSD. A challenge for any theory of PTSD is to explain how the various cognitive-behavioral features fit together, and which might be causes and which might be consequences of PTSD.

CHAPTER 3

Cognitive-Behavioral Models

Only a fraction of people exposed to traumatic events go on to develop PTSD, and, of those, only some develop chronic PTSD. To understand why these patterns occur, we need to consider the possible predisposing, precipitating, perpetuation, and protective factors in PTSD. Predisposing factors are diatheses or vulnerability factors. For people with a few or no predisposing factors, extremely severe stress is needed to cause PTSD; for people with a very strong vulnerability, milder stressors can be sufficient to give rise to the disorder. Precipitating factors are those stimuli or circumstances involved in triggering PTSD. These include trauma exposure. Perpetuating factors are those that maintain the disorder. Protective factors prevent problems from developing, persisting, or getting worse. They may not be present in every case.

There are many different theories of PTSD but comparatively few that provide clear, detailed descriptions of the mechanisms thought to cause the disorder. Few theories have been subject to extensive empirical evaluation. Among the most prominent psychological approaches are four cognitive-behavioral approaches, including novel and established theories, which are the focus of this chapter. We will review the conditioning model (e.g., Keane, Fairbank, Caddell, Zimmering, & Bender, 1985), emotional processing model (Foa & Rothbaum, 1998), dual representation model (Brewin et al., 1996), and Ehlers and Clark's (2000) cognitive model. In evaluating each model, we will consider issues such as the following: Does the model offer a clear description of its conceptual elements, such as the processes thought to maintain PTSD? Is the model able to account for the various findings reviewed in Chapter 2, or does it neglect important areas of research? Is the model parsimonious? Is the model consistent with what is currently known about the treatment of PTSD?

CONDITIONING MODEL

A number of theorists have proposed a conditioning model of PTSD, with their origins in Mowrer's (1960) two-factor theory. Mowrer proposed that fears are acquired by classical conditioning and maintained by operant conditioning. To illustrate, a life-threatening jungle attack by enemy insurgents is a traumatic unconditioned stimulus (UCS), which evokes an unconditioned response (UCR: fear or pain). An association is learned (classically conditioned) between the UCS and innocuous stimuli (CSs: e.g., humid weather, areas of dense undergrowth, or people from the enemy's ethnic background). Once the associations are learned, each CS evokes a conditioned response (CR: fear). The person learns that fear can be minimized by performing *safety behaviors*, that is, by avoiding or escaping from CSs, which prevents the classically conditioned fear from being extinguished. Safety behaviors can also involve checking and reassurance-seeking, as means of avoiding feared stimuli. Conditioning also involves learned associations between the presence of particular stimuli and the absence of the fear-evoking UCS. Stimuli that predict the absence of the UCS are known as *safety signals*.

Mowrer's theory is elegant and parsimonious, but it has difficulty accounting for several aspects of fear acquisition and maintenance, particularly the evidence that fear and avoidance are influenced by cognitive factors, such as expectations. Accordingly, Mowrer's theory was reformulated to propose that the CS and UCS are cognitively represented in long-term memory (Rescorla, 1988). According to this revision, UCS–CS links are acquired when CSs, present before or during the occurrence of the UCS, are perceived as *predictors* of the UCS. To illustrate, for a tsunami survivor who has PTSD, the beach and sound of lapping waves (CSs) are cognitively represented as predictors of a destructive tidal wave (UCS). The strength of the conditioned fear response is determined by the strength of the UCS–CS link and by the aversiveness of the UCS. The strength of the link is influenced by the subjective probability that the CS will lead to a given UCS. Fear of CSs can be acquired by higher-order conditioning (stimulus generalization), whereby the person fears stimuli that are associated with a CS (Keane et al., 1985). Thus, recollections of the trauma can become higher-order CSs with fear-evoking properties. The revised conditioning approach also entails a revised view of operant conditioning of avoidance behavior (Seligman & Johnston, 1973). According to this view, avoidance is not directly determined by the experience of fear, but by the individual's *expectation* of whether a given behavior will protect him or her from harm.

As applied to PTSD, the conditioning model proposes that reexperiencing and hyperarousal symptoms occur because trauma exposure has resulted in a plethora of fear-evoking CSs—both external (e.g., reminders of the trauma) and internal (recollections)—which activate the cognitive representation (memory) of the UCS. There are so many CSs that complete avoidance is rarely possible. The person tries to escape the CSs, which means that exposure to each CS is too brief for the CR to be extinguished (Keane et al., 1985).

How does the conditioning model account for delayed-onset PTSD, in which the person may have few or no symptoms after the trauma and then, months or years later, develop full-blown PTSD? The concept of UCS reevaluation can be invoked (Davey, 1992). That is, the person acquires information that causes him or her to reevaluate the threat value of the trauma (UCS). A rear-end road traffic collision, for example, that was initially appraised as minor might be reappraised as life-threatening if the person learns that his or her make of car has been known to burst into flames from such accidents, as a result of rupturing the gas tank. Another example is the case of woman who was raped but did not develop PTSD symptoms until some months later, when she learned that her attacker had killed another rape victim. This led her to reinterpret the life-threatening nature of her own rape (Kilpatrick et al., 1989).

Comment

The conditioning model provides a plausible explanation of conditioned fear and avoidance of trauma-related stimuli and is associated with an effective treatment (imaginal and situation exposure; see Chapter 5). However, the model fails to account for individual differences in conditionability. Why, for example, are people with PTSD more readily conditioned to fear stimuli than normal controls, as we saw in Chapter 2? The conditioning model also has difficulty accounting for emotional numbing. Numbing symptoms are said to somehow arise from chronic avoidance of trauma reminders and reactions (Keane et al., 1985). Keane et al. attempted to explain the diminished interest in social and leisure activities as resulting from a contrast effect; for example, combat veterans returning from war are less interested in civilian pursuits because these activities are not as stimulating as wartime events. This explanation isn't plausible for PTSD arising from other traumas (e.g., rape, torture, or accident-related PTSD). The conditioning model also doesn't account for the role of dysfunctional beliefs in PTSD (Chapter 2). Despite these limitations, the concepts entailed in conditioning are important and have found their way into some of the other models of PTSD reviewed in this chapter.

EMOTIONAL PROCESSING MODEL

The emotional processing model (Foa & Kozak, 1986; Foa et al., 1989; Foa & Rothbaum, 1998) proposes that PTSD arises from a fear structure in long-term memory, containing representations of feared stimuli (e.g., being alone at night), response information (e.g., palpitations, trembling, fear, safety-seeking behaviors), and meaning information (e.g., the concept of danger). In the network the three types of information—stimuli, responses, and meaning elements—are interlinked. For example, conditioned links among stimuli (e.g., links between "adult men" and "weapons") and links between stimuli and meaning elements (e.g., "sleeping with the lights off" and "danger"), as well as other types of links (e.g., stimulus–response or response–meaning links). Links can be innate (i.e., UCS–UCR links) or acquired by processes such as conditioning (CS–UCS links and CS–CR links). In PTSD, many of these links represent erroneous associations (e.g., "smell of aftershave" linked with "danger"). Fear structures are activated by incoming information that matches information stored in the network (i.e., matches a stimulus, response, or meaning element). Activation of the network evokes fear and motivates avoidance or escape behavior.

As with the conditioning model, the emotional processing model holds that traumatic events are so intense that they cause fear conditioning to a wide range of stimuli (e.g., sights, sounds, odors, and bodily sensations associated with the trauma). Thus, a multitude of stimuli and responses are represented in the fear structure. Trauma-related stimuli serve as reminders of the trauma, activating the fear structure and thereby producing hyperarousal and intrusive recollections of the trauma.

Avoidance and emotional numbing are said to arise from mechanisms for deactivating the fear structure in the short term (e.g., via conditioned analgesia; Foa et al., 1992). They prevent the structure from being modified and thereby contribute to the persistence of PTSD in the longer term. Avoidance also prevents dysfunctional beliefs (meaning elements) from being corrected.

Compared to phobias, PTSD is characterized by fear structures that (1) contain more stimulus–danger associations, leading to the belief that the world is very dangerous; (2) contain stronger (more intense) physiological and behavioral response elements; (3) contain more associations that represent erroneous generalizations about the self or world (e.g., association between tattoos and knives); and (4) have a lower threshold for activation; that is, the fear structure is readily activated because of the wide range of triggering stimuli, thereby leading to "frequent bursts of arousal (e.g., startle) and reexperiencing of the events (e.g., nightmares, flashbacks), alternating with attempts to avoid or escape fear (e.g., numbness, behavioral avoidance, depersonalization)" (Foa et al., 1989, p. 167).

Foa and Rothbaum (1998) elaborated the emotional processing model by including the schema concept, which is the person's store of abstracted knowledge and beliefs about a given topic, such as the self. The model, in its current form, consists of "memory records" (fear structures) that interact with (e.g., influence) schemas. Chronic PTSD is said to be associated with strong negative schemas involving beliefs that one is totally incompetent and that the world is highly dangerous. Such beliefs are said to produce chronic hyperarousal, extreme fear, and widespread avoidance.

People with rigid pretrauma beliefs are said to be more vulnerable to PTSD. Such beliefs include rigid positive beliefs about the self as being highly competent and the world as being very safe, which become shattered by the trauma. In such cases the person may radically shift his or her beliefs, from a self-view of competent to incompetent, and from a world-view of safe to dangerous. Rigidly negative pretrauma beliefs (e.g., self as incompetent and world as dangerous) are also said to be relevant to PTSD because such beliefs are strengthened by the trauma. Appraisals of one's reactions or behaviors during or after the trauma are also emphasized as important contributors to PTSD (e.g., "I'm to blame for being raped because I didn't fight back"), as well as interpretations of PTSD symptoms (e.g., acquired fears, exaggerated startle) as indications that one is weak, bad, or going crazy. Beliefs about the reactions of others are also implicated in the development of PTSD (e.g., "People think I'm overreacting"). In contrast to people who have rigid positive or negative pretrauma beliefs, people who make finer discriminations about degrees of competence and safety are said to be more resilient to trauma because they are better able to interpret the trauma as an unusual experience, without broad implications about competence or safety. As with the conditioning model, the emotional processing model invokes the concept of stimulus reevaluation to account for delayed-onset PTSD.

According to Foa and colleagues, effective treatment of PTSD requires exposure to corrective information. This includes interventions such as (1) imaginal exposure to the trauma until emotional extinction occurs, thereby breaking, weakening, or inhibiting the link between trauma-related stimuli and conditioned emotional arousal; (2) situational exposure to distressing but harmless stimuli, which teaches the person that the stimuli are not dangerous (i.e., incorporates safety information into the fear structure); and (3) cognitive restructuring to help the person make sense out of the traumatic event and to modify maladaptive beliefs.

Comment

Several investigators have proposed network models of PTSD (e.g., Chemtob, Roitblat, Hamada, Carlson, & Twentyman, 1988), although

Foa's emotional processing model is the most widely used and best-articulated approach. The model provides a cogent account of most PTSD symptoms and is consistent with the goals and procedures of empirically supported cognitive-behavioral treatments for PTSD (Chapter 5). Despite these strengths, the model also faces some challenges. The model emphasizes the modification of memories by the incorporation of corrective information. Research suggests that the mechanism may be more one of memory inhibition than memory modification. Fear memories can be modified to some degree, as in the case of UCS reevaluation (Davey, 1992). However, the research suggests that, more generally, fears are extinguished not by altering fear memories but by overriding or inhibiting them with new memories (Chapter 4), that is, the inhibition of one memory network by another.

DUAL REPRESENTATION MODEL

The emotional processing model emphasizes a verbal-propositional memory system, as illustrated by the networks of propositional links between stimulus, meaning, and response elements. Imagery in this model is not completely neglected; it could be stored in memory records. However, imagery is not accorded special status. In comparison, the dual representation model places a great emphasis on imagery (Brewin, 2001; Brewin et al., 1996; Brewin, McNally, & Taylor, 2004). The model proposes that there are two memory systems—*verbally accessible memory* (VAM) and *situationally accessible memory* (SAM)—which operate in parallel. The VAM system represents verbal information that was consciously perceived, as expressed in oral or written descriptions of the trauma. The amount of information contained in VAM is restricted because input is through limited-capacity serial processes such as attention. Attention is narrowed by high levels of arousal (Chapter 2), which further restricts the amount of information contained in VAM. Thus, VAM representations encode only the conscious contents of what the person attends to, such as conscious evaluations of the trauma and reevaluations afterward, when the person considers the consequences and implications of the event. VAM representations can be deliberately retrieved and "edited," and interact with the rest of the autobiographical knowledge base, so that the trauma is represented with a complete personal context comprising past, present, and future (Brewin, 2001).

SAM representations contain information that is not recorded in the VAM system. The SAM system contains information obtained from extensive, lower-level perceptual processing of information (e.g., sights and sounds of the traumatic event) "that was apprehended too briefly to be consciously recalled" (Brewin et al., 2004, p. 105), along with peri-traumatic emotions and bodily sensations. The SAM system does not use a verbal code, so SAM representations are difficult to communicate to others and are not necessarily integrated with autobiographical knowledge. Recollections of SAM representations are triggered by matching stimuli in the environment, and so it can be difficult for the person to control the triggering of these memories, because the people are not able to always avoid reminders. Because SAM representations are so detailed and emotion-laden, involuntarily triggered, and not necessarily integrated with autobiographical knowledge, retrieval of these memories can give the person a sense of suddenly reliving an event. Thus, trauma-related flashbacks and dreams are said to be products of the SAM system. Other forms of reexperiencing symptoms—in which the person involuntarily recalls the trauma but retains the sense that he or she is recalling something that happened in the past—presumably could arise from SAM representations that are integrated to some extent with autobiographical knowledge.

The dual representation model proposes that SAM and VAM memories coexist, and that these memory systems interact with one another. SAM and VAM representations compete with one another; the memory system that is more strongly activated will win in its effects on either activating or inhibiting fear (Brewin, 2001). Activation of SAM representations also provides raw material for the progressive development or modification of VAM representations of the trauma. Conversely, intentional "editing" of VAM representations (e.g., by deliberately pondering the meaning of the trauma) can somehow enable the person to block the automatic, unwanted retrieval of SAM representations (Brewin, 2001).

Comment

The rationale for proposing that PTSD arises from two distinct memory systems, rather than a single trauma memory, is based on the claim that trauma images are experienced as vivid and compelling, and yet the person supposedly provides impoverished or confused verbal descriptions of the trauma (Brewin et al., 2004). The claim for this distinction is controversial; there is no compelling evidence for fragmented verbal memories in PTSD (Chapter 2). People with PTSD do report periods in which they have trauma-related imagery and periods in which their recollections are in more of a verbal or narrative form (Hellawell & Brewin, 2004), but that is not evidence for two separate memory systems. The results could reflect differences in the degree and scope of activation of memory elements from a single memory system. The nature of recollections (sensory vs. verbal) may be due to differences in retrieval strategies rather than reflecting differences in memory systems. For example, people might experience more "verbal" recollections when they retrieve the meaning information stored in memory, and they might report more "sensory" recollections when retrieving stimulus information from the same memory network. Differences in encoding conditions (e.g., encoding favoring either sensory or verbal information) also influence the nature of material stored in memory without requiring distinct memory systems.

A further concern is that the dual representation model focuses largely on flashbacks, which are the rarest PTSD symptoms (APA, 2000). The model provides no explanation for more common PTSD symptoms such as emotional numbing. Also, it is unclear how the model accounts for recurrent, trauma-related dreams. Such nightmares are supposedly a product of SAM activation. But SAM is purportedly triggered by environmental cues, so it is unclear why nightmares should persistently occur while the person is asleep, shielded from external reminders of the trauma.

Another problem is the claim that SAM encodes memories that are not consciously attended to. If memories are not encoded (attended to), then it is unclear how they can be represented in memory. There is also no persuasive evidence that people with PTSD have memories (putative SAM representations) that they are unable to verbally articulate. In other words, there is no persuasive evidence that the SAM system contains information that is not stored in the VAM system. Because the dual representation model does not explicitly include representations of abstracted knowledge such as schemas, "it is less convincing in its account of the transformation of meaning following trauma and the operation of some pretrauma risk factors such as previous psychiatric history" (Dalgleish, 2004, p. 240). The model has little to say about how VAM and SAM interact with one another (Dalgleish, 2004), and the model also fails to provide a cogent explanation for delayed-onset PTSD. In summary, the dual representation model is an interesting approach, but it encounters numerous difficulties, which make it less compelling as an explanation of PTSD than the emotional processing model.

EHLERS AND CLARK'S COGNITIVE MODEL

One of the most complex models, which contains elements of the other models reviewed in this chapter, is Ehlers and Clark's (2000) cognitive model. It includes conditioning, schemas, dysfunctional beliefs, and verbal and situational memories as explanatory constructs. The emphasis of the model is on factors contributing to the maintenance of PTSD. Ehlers and Clark proposed that PTSD becomes persistent when the person processes the traumatic event in a way that leads to a sense of serious, current threat. This produces fear and avoidance of trauma-related stimuli, as well as hyperarousal. The sense of current threat is said to arise from various factors including, among other things, the following:

- During traumatic events, people who go on to develop chronic PTSD tend to be those who engage in data-driven (sensory) processing of the event rather than conceptually driven processing (i.e., processing the meaning and implications of the event).
- This is associated with a disturbance of autobiographical memory, characterized by poor elaboration and contextualization, strong associative memory, and strong perceptual priming. This prevents the person from putting the traumatic event in the past.
- Also implicated are excessively negative appraisals, in which the probability or cost of further aversive events is overestimated, and the competency of the self is underestimated. Such negative appraisals include particular interpretations of the trauma, its consequences, and the world, and appraisals of PTSD symptoms (e.g., "I'm not safe anywhere," "I attract danger," "These symptoms mean I'm losing my mind"). Such appraisals generate strong emotions such as anxiety, anger, shame, or guilt. They also motivate the person to engage in maladaptive coping strategies.
- Maladaptive coping strategies, used to avoid sources of threat, serve to reduce distress in the short term, but in the longer term they perpetuate the sense of pervasive threat. This is because these coping strategies prevent the negative appraisals from being corrected. Maladaptive coping strategies include avoidance of trauma stimuli, attempts to suppress unwanted, trauma-related thoughts, abuse of arousal-dampening drugs or alcohol, and other efforts to avoid distress and harm.

Trauma memories are said to be readily triggered (resulting in re-experiencing symptoms) because these memories are not adequately integrated into the autobiographical memory knowledge base. The latter is purportedly organized by themes and personal epochs, in which memories for events are integrated (elaborated and contextualized) by being interconnected with one another (e.g., spatial and temporal connection: event X was followed by event Y, and both occurred at location Z). A memory is highly integrated into autobiographical memory if it has a lot of interconnections (associations) with other memories. This facilitates intentional retrieval of a memory (such as searching for memories on the basis of theme or epoch) and inhibits retrieval that is triggered purely by sensory cues. Integration also gives memories, when recalled, the sense that they happened in the past, in a given epoch (i.e., the time and place of the recalled event is also retrieved). Trauma memories are said to lack this contextual information (e.g., lacking interconnections with other memories, such as memories of the aftermath of the event, such as "I did not die"), thereby giving the person the sense that he or she is reliving the trauma (flashbacks). The "here and now" quality of the memory also contributes to the person's sense of current threat.

The model further implicates the role of conditioned associations among stimuli (S) and responses (R): "We propose that a further problem in persistent PTSD is that S-S and S-R associations are particularly strong for traumatic material. This makes triggering of memories of the event and/ or emotional responses by associated stimuli even more likely" (Ehlers & Clark, 2000, p. 325).

The trauma memory and threat appraisals are said to mutually influence one another; retrieval of the memory can lead to, or strengthen, appraisals that one is in danger, and threat-relevant appraisal can bias recall, such that it is easier to recall congruent (threat-relevant) memories. The poor elaboration of the memories is also said to make it difficult to integrate information that might disconfirm negative appraisals. Deliberate rumination to try to understand the trauma (e.g., "Why did this happen?" "Why me?") is also said to perpetuate PTSD.

Comment

Ehlers and Clark's model is consistent with many of the findings reviewed in the previous chapter. The fact that the model contains many of the constructs included in other models means that the explanatory power of the Ehlers and Clark model is as good as or better than some of the other models. However, the Ehlers and Clark model has several important drawbacks. First, it is substantially less parsimonious that the other models reviewed in this chapter. Second, some of the explanatory mechanisms are highly speculative or implausible. Ehlers and Clark (2000) speculated that low premorbid intelligence predicts PTSD because low intellectual ability may be related to a less conceptual and more data-driven processing of the trauma. This does not seem plausible because the task of interpreting the meaning of a trauma is relatively straightforward. One does not need a high IQ to know that being shot at by the enemy is potentially bad for your health, or that being robbed at gunpoint is a dangerous situation. Indeed, as we saw in Chapter 1, children of 3 years of age (and perhaps younger) can interpret an event as threatening and develop PTSD.

Third, the claim that PTSD arises from a preponderance of data-driven processing is questionable. Although it is possible that there is a preponderance of data-driven processing during quickly unfolding events, it seems implausible that there would be little meaning-based processing during traumatic events that gradually unfold over time, such as being tortured or held hostage. Even for rapidly occurring events, people who develop PTSD commonly report that during the event they knew that something terrible was going to happen, even though they felt confused about what to do. Thus, meaning-based processing commonly occurs during traumatic events associated with PTSD, even though the full implications of the event might not be apparent until later on. This is so common that the threat-related *interpretation* of the traumatic event is a cardinal feature required for the diagnosis of PTSD (APA, 2000).

Fourth, the model does not offer a persuasive explanation of many PTSD symptoms, including emotional numbing and dissociative symptoms. Finally, the model fails to explain why some of the putative causal factors are present for some people but not others. For example, why do only some people interpret stressful events as life threatening, and why do only some people ruminate about the meaning of such events? Related to this point, Dalgleish (2004) observed that the model generally lacks the ability to make unique, testable empirical predictions.

> Although the model emphasizes the key role of negative appraisals in the maintenance of PTSD, it generally does not elucidate, a priori, that certain appraisals would be toxic and others benign, nor how this might vary across individuals. Indeed, such specificity would be difficult without a much fuller explication of the more generic-meaning representations that contextualize any appraisal that an individual would make. (p. 244)

ETIOLOGICAL SPECIFICITY

A challenge for any model of PTSD is to explain why, after a traumatic event, a person develops PTSD instead of some other disorder (e.g., major depression), and to explain why PTSD is commonly comorbid with other disorders, such as other anxiety disorders and mood disorders. Such patterns of comorbidity suggest that disorder specific and nonspecific etiological factors are necessary to fully account for PTSD and its relationship with order disorders.

As we saw in Chapter 2, research suggests that people with PTSD, compared to controls, tend to have lower IQs and deficits on neurological and neuropsychological tests. Such deficits are not specific to PTSD. Neuropsychological impairments, for example, have been identified in other disorders such as obsessive–compulsive disorder, panic disorder, and bulimia nervosa (e.g., Alarcón, Libb, & Boll, 1994; Jones, Duncan, Brouwers, & Mirsky, 1991; Lucas, Telch, & Bigler, 1991). Neither is overgeneralized autobiographical memory limited to traumatic events or to PTSD; it has also been observed in people with major depression (Brittlebank et al., 1993; Williams & Scott, 1988). Deficits such as these might be predisposing factors for various disorders.

PTSD is associated with trauma-specific processing deficits such as biased attention toward threat cues and superior memory for trauma-related information. Again, these deficits are not specific to PTSD. Such "concern-specific" biases have been associated with a number of disorders, including mood disorders, panic disorder, generalized anxiety disorder, and eating disorders (McNally, 1998b; Williams et al., 1997). People with eating disorders, for example, display attentional bias toward food-related information. These results raise the question of whether the concern-related cognitive biases in PTSD and other disorders are consequences rather than causes of the disorder. Once the disorder develops, the person may become preoccupied with the symptoms (e.g., preoccupation with intrusive traumatic memories) and therefore develop attention and memory biases for information relating to these symptoms.

Self-denigrating beliefs, including beliefs about incompetence, low self-worth, and self-blame, are not specific to PTSD; they are associated with various forms of psychopathology, such as other anxiety disorders and mood disorders (Beck & Emery, 1985; Beck, Rush, Shaw, & Emery, 1979). Beliefs that arousal-related symptoms are dangerous (i.e., elevated anxiety sensitivity) is similarly not specific to PTSD (Taylor, 1999). The fact that all sorts of cognitive factors appear to play a role in various disorders may partially explain why PTSD is commonly comorbid with many other disorders. Possibly more specific to PTSD are the various types of trauma-related beliefs about the dangerousness of the world, along with the presence of readily triggered trauma memories. The cognitive-behavioral models of PTSD generally fail to consider that PTSD likely arises from a mix of disorder-specific and disorder-nonspecific factors.

RELATIVE STRENGTHS AND LIMITATIONS OF THE MODELS

Table 3.1 summarizes the strengths and weaknesses of the models reviewed in this chapter. The models generally focus on precipitating and perpetuating factors, with less attention to predisposing and protective factors. Each model is consistent with at least some of the empirical findings reviewed in the previous chapter. All the models can account for the effects of interpersonal factors (e.g., blame, shunning, and low social support) on PTSD. The models predict that the effects of interpersonal factors are mediated by factors such as dysfunctional beliefs and appraisals or exposure to danger or safety cues that may influence the activation of memories and fears. All the models suggest that exposure therapy would be a useful treatment, and all but the conditioning model suggest that cognitive restructuring would be beneficial.

TABLE 3.1. Strengths and Limitations of Four Leading Psychological Models of PTSD

	Conditioning model	Emotional processing model	Dual representation model	Ehlers and Clark's cognitive model
Ability of model to account for . . .				
Reexperiencing	+	+	+	+
Avoidance	+	+	+	+
Numbing	?	+	−	−
Hyperarousal	+	+	?	+
Trauma-related anger and guilt	?	+		+
Dissociative symptoms	−	+/?	−	?
Persistence of PTSD symptoms	+	+	+	+
Delayed-onset PTSD	+	+	−	−
Comorbidity with other disorders	−	+/?	−	+/?
Consistency with empirical findings regarding . . . [a]				
Global intelligence and PTSD	−	−	−	?
General attention and memory disturbance	−	−	−	−
Overgeneral autobiographical memories	−	−	−	+/?
Threat-focused attentional bias	+	+	?	+
Heightened fear conditioning in PTSD	−	−	−	−
Recall bias for trauma-related memories	−	+	+	+
Traumatic amnesia	−	−	−	−
Ruminative thinking as a perpetuating factor	−	+	−	+
Dysfunctional beliefs	−	+	?	+
Known predisposing or risk factors	−	+/?	−	?
Known protective factors (e.g., social support)	−	?	−	?
Interpersonal exacerbating factors (e.g., criticism)	−	+	?	+
Explanatory power. Ability to explain . . .				
Delayed-onset PTSD	+	+	−	+
Hot versus cold cognition	−	+	−	−
Fluctuating insight in PTSD	−	?	+	?
Anger and guilt in PTSD	−	+	−	+
Data on the efficacy of cognitive-behavioral treatments [b]	−	+	+	+
Model parsimony	+	+	+	−
Number of + ratings	8	20	7	15

Note. +, good; ?, uncertain or equivocal; −, poor; +/?, support in some areas but not others.
[a] See Chapters 1 and 2 for a review of these findings.
[b] Reviewed in Chapter 5.

The models differ in some important respects, including their underlying assumptions. The emotional processing model emphasizes the importance of memory modification, despite evidence that fear reduction appears to be largely due to the process of inhibition of fear memories, with memory modification playing a more minor role. The dual representation model is based on the controversial assumption that there are two distinct memory systems. Ehlers and Clark's model is based, in part, on the questionable assumption that trauma memories are fragmented. The emotional processing model does include the possibility of disorganized autobiographical memory (Foa & Riggs, 1993), although this is not an important feature of the model.

The dual representation model, compared to the other models, has the greatest difficulty accounting for delayed-onset PTSD. The other models account for this in terms of changes in beliefs or reevaluation of the trauma, based on the accrual of new information. Only the emotional processing model offers a cogent explanation of numbing symptoms.

It is unclear how some of the models would distinguish between "hot" and "cold" cognition (Dalgleish, 2004). That is, on some occasions a person may become extremely distressed when recalling the trauma, but on other occasions he or she may be able to recall the event while experiencing little or no emotion. The hot–cold distinction is less of a problem for the emotional processing model than the other models. The emotional processing model suggests that hot cognition corresponds to full activation of the fear network, whereas cold cognition represents partial activation (e.g., activation of some of the stimulus elements), without activation of meaning or response elements. Clinically, this is seen in patients who try to narrate "just the facts" of their trauma, as if they were reading a police report, while deliberately trying not to think about the meaning of the event or how they felt at the time.

The models also differ in whether they provide an explanation of the fact that insight fluctuates in PTSD. People with the disorder are able to acknowledge, at least in their calmer moments, that their fears are excessive. Yet, when exposed to trauma cues they may believe that they are in real danger and may even have a flashback, in which they actually believe that they are back in the traumatic situation. Only the dual representation model offers an explicit explanation of these fluctuations in insight. However, the other models could be readily amended to include an explanation. For example, people may have dual belief systems (Beck & Emery, 1985) or dual representation of a given CS (i.e., paired with danger vs. paired with safety; Bouton, 2002). The relative dominance of danger- versus safety-related representations may depend, in part, on the nature of triggering cues in the environment (danger vs. safety cues).

The emotional processing model and Ehlers and Clark's model, compared to the other models, provide the most persuasive explanations of intense trauma-related anger or guilt, which is commonly comorbid with PTSD. In terms of the emotional processing model, for example, PTSD plus strong guilt could arise from particular constellations of beliefs, such as beliefs that the self is incompetent and blameworthy (e.g., "I shouldn't be so inadequate; it's my fault that I'm so weak"). Similarly, PTSD plus strong anger could arise from beliefs about the dangerousness and injustice in the world (e.g., "It's not fair that there are so many dangerous people in the world; it shouldn't be that way!").

A major problem of the Ehlers and Clark model, compared to the other models, is its lack of parsimony. A limitation of all the models is that they were developed for adults, and they fail to consider how developmental factors such as the person's level of cognitive development could influence the risk and manifestation of PTSD in children.

SUMMARY

Four leading cognitive-behavioral models of PTSD are the conditioning model, the emotional processing model, the dual representation model, and Ehlers and Clark's cognitive model. The models overlap in various ways and each has some degree of supporting evidence. The models are broadly consistent with the efficacy of cognitive-behavioral treatments, as reviewed in Chapter 5, although the conditioning model would not lead us to expect that cognitive restructuring would be a potent intervention. Each model has its own set of empirical and conceptual difficulties, and none provides a comprehensive account of PTSD. How should we choose among the models reviewed in this chapter? Choosing a guiding model is important for developing a case formulation and treatment plan. The most promising approaches are the emotional processing model and the Ehlers and Clark model. On balance, the former model seems to have the advantage, because it is more parsimonious and associated with fewer empirical and conceptual problems. Accordingly, the treatment approaches described in the remainder of this volume are based largely on the emotional processing model, modified to emphasize a wider range of dysfunctional beliefs in PTSD, such as beliefs about symptoms (including anxiety sensitivity) and beliefs associated with mental defeat. It should be noted that the treatment methods described in this book are also broadly consistent with the Ehlers and Clark model.

CHAPTER 4

Neurobiology for the Cognitive-Behavioral Therapist

In recent years there has been a flood of important studies on the neurobiology of PTSD, which have unfortunately been neglected by many cognitive-behavioral writers. There are several reasons why the cognitive-behavioral therapist should have a basic knowledge of the neurobiology of PTSD. First, it gives one a more complete understanding of the underpinnings of PTSD. Second, such knowledge can help the therapist understand how treatments—both pharmacological and psychosocial—might exert their effects at a biological level. Third, such knowledge can be used for the purposes of patient psychoeducation.

If the cognitive-behavioral therapist can answer the patient's questions about the biological basis of PTSD, then the therapist is likely to have greater credibility in the eyes of the patient. A question like the following is commonly voiced by patients: "My doctor says that PTSD is caused by a biochemical imbalance. If that is true then how can cognitive-behavioral therapy help me?" The therapist can also use knowledge of the psychobiology of PTSD to address catastrophic thoughts about the effects of the trauma. For example, a patient might ask, "I saw on TV that stress can damage the brain; does this mean my brain has been irrevocably damaged?"

The findings discussed in this chapter have emerged from a range of research paradigms, including animal studies, studies of humans with brain damage, pharmacological challenge studies (e.g., studies of the effects of drugs that stimulate particular neurotransmitter or neurohormonal systems), and functional neuroimaging studies (e.g., PET scans) of normal and clinical human samples. This chapter will begin by reviewing the neurobiology of the normal stress and fear responses because this provides the basis for understanding how these processes can go awry in PTSD. This will be followed by a review of what is currently known about the brain structures, circuits, neurotransmission, and brain–behavior links that are most relevant for understanding PTSD and its treatment.

NEUROBIOLOGY OF FEAR AND STRESS

Overview

Although fear and stress can be conceptually distinguished, the two have many features in common. Phenomenologically, both are associated with apprehension and hyperarousal, although stress (when defined as a response) is a broader concept, entailing irritability and a tendency to be easily upset and agitated (Lovibond, 1998). Fear and stress both involve the detection of threatening stimuli and the transduction of this information into neurobiological responses. Fear is an emotion experienced in anticipation of exposure to some specific pain or danger, whereas stress reflects an individual's physiological and affective responses during the process of coping with (e.g., adapting to or warding off) aversive stimuli. Given the similarities between fear and stress, it is not surprising that they have similar neurobiological correlates. Figure 4.1 shows the anatomical location of the major brain structures implicated in fear and stress, while Figure 4.2 provides a schematic illustration of how the structures are interrelated.

In humans and many other animals there are four distinct, biologically based fear responses, which often proceed in the following sequential pattern: (1) freezing, (2) fleeing, (3) fighting, and (4) tonic immobility (Bracha, Ralston, Matsukawa, Williams, & Bracha, 2004; Gray, 1988). Freezing is a "stop, watch, and listen" pattern of vigilance, where the individual voluntarily ceases activity and scans for danger, in preparation for action. As

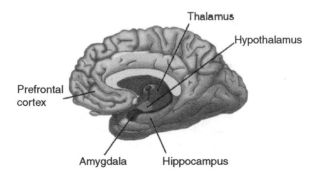

FIGURE 4.1. Major brain structures involved in fear and stress.

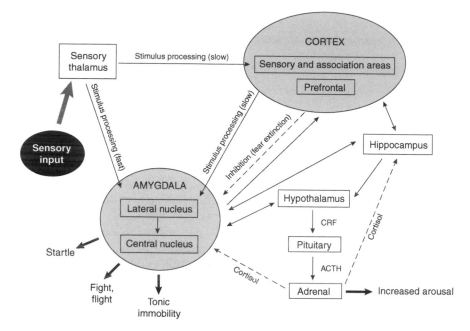

FIGURE 4.2. Schematic diagram of circuits involved in fear and stress. CRF, corticotropin-releasing factor; ACTH, adrenocorticotropic hormone.

danger looms, there is an attempt to flee. When this is not possible there is an attempt to fight. If fleeing or fighting are not viable options, then tonic immobility occurs. The latter is a "play dead" response, which often occurs when entrapment is perceived or when there is direct physical contact with a predator (Moskowitz, 2004). Unlike the freeze response, tonic immobility is an involuntary state of profound, reversible motor inhibition.

Fast and Slow Circuits

Fear and stress both involve the activation of primitive, threat-related autonomic and somatic reflexes, as well as the involvement of more complex cortical processes (Lang, Bradley, & Cuthbert, 1998; LeDoux, 2000). There are two major brain circuits—a fast pathway (also known as the "low road") and slower pathway ("high road")—which operate in parallel to detect and process threat-related stimuli (Fellous, Armony, & LeDoux, 2002; see Figure 4.2). The rapid pathway is from the thalamus to the amygdala. It entails the rudimentary processing of stimuli (processing of raw sensory features) and provides a quick assessment of potential danger. The slower pathway is from the thalamus to the primary somatosensory cortices, the insula, the anterior cingulate, and the prefrontal cortex (Charney, 2004). The slower pathway involves a more elaborated processing (e.g., processing of whole objects), thereby enabling assignment of significance based on prior experience with complex stimuli (Charney, 2004).

The Amygdala

The amygdala plays an important role in processing the emotional significance of stimuli, including the acquisition of fears of particular stimuli and the contexts in which the stimuli occur (Davis & Whalen, 2001; Pare, Quirk, & LeDoux, 2004). Such learning appears to be a result of synaptic plasticity in the amygdala, in which learning is reflected in structural changes in neurons, such as the growth of dendritic spines, which results in changes in the way neurons stimulate or inhibit one another (Lamprecht & LeDoux, 2004).

Animal research suggests that N-methyl-D-aspartate (NMDA) receptors in the amygdala are important for the expression of conditioned fear responses (Lee et al., 2001; Walker & Davis, 2002). Because NMDA receptors in the amygdala are critical for fear conditioning, and because extinction, like fear conditioning, is a form of learning, researchers have investigated the possibility that NMDA receptors in the amygdala might also be involved in fear extinction. In fact, research indicates that NMDA receptors in the amygdala play an important role in conditioned fear extinction. The findings also raise the possibility that NMDA agonists, like D-cycloserine, might facilitate fear extinction (Davis, Myers, Ressler, & Rothbaum, 2005; see Chapter 5). (Agonists are substances that bind to, and activate, a receptor.)

The amygdala also activates the autonomic nervous system and the hypothalamic–pituitary–adrenal axis. The latter plays an important role in the stress response. The amygdala plays an important role in the expression of defensive behaviors, such as startle responses, fight or flight reactions, avoidance, and tonic immobility (Davis & Whalen, 2001; Fellous et al., 2002; Yehuda, 2002a).

Amygdala–Hippocampal Interactions

The amygdala provides output to the hippocampus. There is some evidence that the latter plays a role in contextual learning (e.g., learning about the contexts in which threatening stimuli are likely to occur; Sotres-Bayon, Bush, & LeDoux, 2004), although the importance of the hippocampus for contextual learning remains a matter of debate (Gewirtz, McNish, & Davis, 2000). What is not contentious is the fact that the hippocampus plays an important role in declarative memory, that is, memory for facts or events, such as conscious recollection of traumatic events. The amygdala appears to be involved in giving declarative memories their emotional flavor (Fellous et al., 2002). Declarative memories are not stored "in" any particular brain region; rather, the storage of these memories involves interconnections among a number of brain structures, including regions of the amygdala and hippocampus and cortical regions such as the frontal lobes (Cahill & McGaugh, 1998).

Amygdala–Frontal Lobe Interactions

The amygdala receives input from the frontal cortex. Research indicates that fear extinction is mediated by medial prefrontal cortical inhibition of amygdala activity (Vermetten & Bremner, 2002b). Cortical involvement in fear conditioning is clinically relevant because it provides a mechanism by which cognitive factors influence the magnitude of the stress (Charney, 2004). Input from the hippocampus, such as inputs relaying context-related information, to the medial prefrontal cortex may facilitate the control of the medial prefrontal cortex over the amygdala (Sotres-Bayon et al., 2004).

The amygdala sends inputs, directly and indirectly, to the prefrontal cortex. Once the amygdala is activated by sensory input from the thalamus or cortex, it can begin to regulate the cortex and could thereby facilitate the processing of danger stimuli (LeDoux, 2000), such as by promoting hypervigilance for threat (Davis & Whalen, 2001). Under normal circumstances, the prefrontal cortex and amygdala orchestrate the control of emotional states by regulating one another; these interactions may be compromised in emotional disorders such as PTSD (Sotres-Bayon et al., 2004).

Autonomic Nervous System

One of the most immediate fear or stress responses is the activation of the sympathetic branch of the autonomic nervous system, which causes increases in heart rate and blood pressure, as well as increases in blood flow and glucose availability to skeletal muscles (Yehuda, 2002b). The parasympathetic branch of the autonomic nervous system operates independently to constrain the effects of sympathetic activation.

The major hormones of the sympathetic nervous system are adrenaline and noradrenaline (also called epinephrine and norepinephrine, respectively). The locus ceruleus, located in the brain stem, is a major site of noradrenergic neurons, which provide output to many regions of the brain, including the prefrontal cortex, hippocampus, amygdala, thalamus, and hypothalamus (Vermetten & Bremner, 2002a). Noradrenergic outputs influence a range of functions, including attention and scanning for danger (McFarlane, Yehuda, & Clark, 2002). Noradrenergic outputs also influence memory formation (Vermetten & Bremner, 2002a), perhaps by their effect on attention, which influences the encoding of stimuli into memory. Noradrenergic output generally facilitates memory formation in a dose-dependent way; the higher the level of noradrenergic output, the greater the facilitating effects on memory. However, at high levels of noradrenergic output, memory formation is impaired (Cahill & McGaugh, 1998).

Hypothalamic–Pituitary–Adrenal Axis

The sympathetic nervous system and the hypothalamic–pituitary–adrenal (HPA) axis are functionally interrelated. Sympathetic activation has stimulatory effects on the HPA axis, and the HPA axis can have stimulatory or inhibitory effects on the autonomic nervous system (Vermetten & Bremner, 2002a). The sympathetic nervous system and the HPA axis are both involved in enhancing declarative memory for stressful events (Cahill & McGaugh, 1998), thereby helping the individual prepare to deal with (e.g., master or avoid) similar situations in the future.

Stress, particularly acute stress, usually causes an increase in catecholamines (adrenaline and noradrenaline) and cortisol. The greater the severity of the stressor, the higher the resulting levels of catecholamines and cortisol (Yehuda, 2002b). Compared to the speed of response of the amygdala and the autonomic nervous system, the cortisol response is slower, occurring some minutes later (Vermetten & Bremner, 2002a). The cortisol response ultimately dampens the initial stress response (Yehuda, 2002b). That is, catecholamines facilitate sympathetic nervous system activation, whereas cortisol dampens or shuts down sympathetic activation and other neuronal defensive reactions that have been initiated by stress (Yehuda, 2002b).

It is important for the organism that cortisol secretion is not excessive and sustained, because this can have deleterious effects, including immunosuppression, insulin resistance, and cardiovascular disease (Karlamangla, Singer, McEwen, Rowe, & Seeman, 2002). The hippocampus regulates the shut-down process by negative feedback (Vermetten & Bremner, 2002b). Thus, as stress-activated biological reactions shut down as a result of cortisol inhibition, cortisol levels also suppress the further release of cortisol itself. Once the acute stressor has passed, and no external threat is detected, this process of negative feedback leads to the restoration of basal hormone levels (Yehuda, 2002b).

Other Neuromodulatory Systems

Several neurotransmitter or neurohormonal systems have been implicated in fear and stress. Important neurotransmitters include glutamate and gamma-aminobutyric acid (GABA). Glutamate has an excitatory effect on neurons, while GABA is the major inhibitory neurotransmitter in the nervous system. Glutamate plays a role in synaptic plasticity and memory formation. Stress increases glutamate outflow to the prefrontal cortex and hippocampus. The release of GABA is also influenced by stress and might serve as a mechanism of stress coping by reducing arousal (Vermetten & Bremner, 2002a).

The serotonergic system also plays an important role in fear and stress. The raphe nucleus, located in the midbrain, contains serotonin neurons that send outputs to all areas of the cerebral cortex, amygdala, hippocampus, hypothalamus, midbrain, cerebellum, and regions of the brain stem. Serotonin is involved in the regulation of a range of things, including fear, mood, arousal, vigilance, aggression, impulsivity, sleep, analgesia, and food intake (Vermetten & Bremner, 2002a, 2002b). Serotonin also regulates stress-induced HPA activity (Stowe & Taylor, 2002). Stress-induced serotonin release may have either anxiogenic or anxiolytic effects, depending on the region of the brain involved and the receptor subtype activated (Charney, 2004). Serotonergic output to the amygdala and hippocampus by the dorsal section of the raphe is believed to mediate anxiogenic effects via 5-HT_2 receptors. In contrast, the median raphe output to hippocampal 5-HT_{1A} receptors may facilitate the disconnection of previously learned associations with aversive events or suppress formation of new associations, thus providing resilience to aversive events (Vermetten & Bremner, 2002b).

The dopaminergic system has also been implicated in fear and stress. The major locations of dopamine neurons are the ventral tegmental areas and the substantia nigra, both located in the midbrain. They provide output to various brain regions, including the amygdala, hippocampus, hypothalamus, basal ganglia, and prefrontal cortex. The effects of dopamine are broad. Dopamine is involved in the regulation of motor activity, cognition (e.g., attention and memory), emotion (e.g., the hedonic impact of rewards, which can influence learning), and neuroendocrine secretion (Vermetten & Bremner, 2002a). Dopamine output to the amygdala and prefrontal cortex may contribute to the acquisition, expression, and extinction of conditioned fear (Charney, 2004). Dopamine, through its output to the prefrontal cortex, appears to play a role in the optimal functioning of working memory, that is, short-term memory that stores information currently being used or attended to. Stress exposure increases dopamine release and metabolism in the prefrontal cortex and thereby influences working memory. There appears to be an optimal range for stress-induced increases in dopamine release in the prefrontal cortex to facilitate adaptive behavior. Too much dopamine release in the prefrontal cortex produces cognitive impairment, such as impairment in working memory, while too little prefrontal cortical dopamine impairs the extinction of conditioned fear (Charney, 2004).

Other neuromodulators of fear and stress include neuropeptides. These are a class of protein-like molecules consisting of short chains of amino acids produced in the brain. Some neuropeptides function as neurotransmitters while others function as hormones. The neuropeptides that are thought to modulate the stress response include endogenous opioids (e.g., beta-endorphin), cholecystokinin, neuropeptide Y, and oxytocin. For example, stress is associated with an increased release of beta-endorphin, which can lead to feelings of analgesia (Vermetten & Bremner, 2002a).

Tonic Immobility

Tonic immobility has been identified in a third to two-thirds of sexual assault cases (Burgess & Holmstrom, 1976; Galliano, Noble, Travis, & Puechl, 1993; Heidt, Marx, & Forsyth, 2005). It has also been described in survivors of airline disasters (Gallup & Rager, 1996) and may occur in response other traumatic events. Tonic immobility is an unlearned, defensive reflex (Klemm, 1977). It is characterized by extreme fear and inability to move. Common features include reduced vocalization, intermittent eye closure, rigidity and paralysis, muscle tremors in the extremities, chills, and unresponsiveness to pain. There is no apparent loss of consciousness, and occasional movements of the head and legs, vocalization, and eye closure preclude it from being described as complete immobility (Moskowitz, 2004). Tonic immobility may be associated with peritraumatic dissociation (Heidt et al., 2005). The duration of tonic immobility is variable, ranging from a few seconds to hours, depending on the species and environmental conditions (Olsen, Hogg, & Lapiz, 2002).

Tonic immobility may enhance survival because some predators do not attack immobile prey. Or if they attack, the occurrence of tonic immobility causes predators loosen their grip on captured prey, thereby increasing the chances of escape. Some predators lose interest in seemingly dead prey (Moskowitz, 2004). The adaptive value of tonic immobility is not limited to situations of physical assault. Some rapists may become extremely violent if the victim fights back (Marshall, Laws, & Barbaree, 1990), and therefore tonic immobility may save the life of the assault victim. In some cases tonic immobility may even abort the sexual assault because some rapists lose interest in victims who are immobile and unresponsive (Burgess & Holmstrom, 1976).

Various brain structures and neurotransmitter systems are involved in modulating tonic immobility, including the amygdala, hypothalamus, frontal lobes, brain stem, and serotonergic, noradrenergic, GABAergic, and endogenous opioid systems (Moskowitz, 2004; Olsen et al., 2002; Silva, Gargaro, & Brandao, 2004).

NEUROBIOLOGY OF PTSD

Overview

A comprehensive knowledge of the neurobiology of PTSD involves understanding how PTSD may arise from a combination of normal and dysregulated neurobiological mechanisms. Not all posttraumatic stress reactions may be due to neurobiological abnormalities.

Some PTSD symptoms may represent normal reactions to extreme stressors. Although the majority of people exposed to traumatic stressors do not develop PTSD, they may experience a period of PTSD-like symptoms over the weeks after the traumatic event, but these symptoms quickly subside (Flynn & Norwood, 2004; see also Chapter 1). The symptoms of PTSD are also similar to the symptoms of "ordinary" stress (e.g., sleeplessness, irritability, avoidance, intrusive thoughts regarding the stressor; Horowitz, 2001; Mol et al., 2005). Thus, most people exposed to traumatic stressors show similar symptoms and patterns of remission to people exposed to lesser stressors. This suggests that for most people, the neurobiology underlying the response to traumatic stressors is similar to the neurobiology of the normal fear and stress responses.

But why do some people develop PTSD in response to traumatic stressors, while most other people recover from trauma? To fully understand the neurobiology of PTSD it is necessary to understand the neurobiological dysregulations and biological vulnerability factors associated with this disorder.

PTSD is not a categorically discrete entity; the severity of the symptoms of this disorder varies along a continuum (Ruscio et al., 2002). This suggests that there may be numerous neurobiological dysregulations or abnormalities involved in the disorder, which each additively contribute to the risk for PTSD. The following sections focus largely on how the neurobiology of PTSD might deviate from the processes involved in normal fear and stress.

Amygdala and Medial Prefrontal Cortex

Neuroimaging research has implicated dysregulations in at least three important brain regions in PTSD: the amygdala, medial prefrontal cortex, and hippocampus (Nutt & Malizia, 2004). In PTSD, the amygdala appears to be hyperreactive to trauma-related stimuli. Although the amygdala functions differently in PTSD, compared to controls, it is unclear whether the source of the problem is with the amygdala or whether it lies elsewhere. Nevertheless, increased activity of the amygdala seems to play a role in PTSD symptoms such as hyperarousal (e.g., exaggerated startle response) and trauma-related fear and avoidance (see Figure 4.2).

In normal individuals, the suppression of declarative memories is associated with heightened activity of the dorsolateral prefrontal cortex and decreased activity of the hippocampus (Anderson et al., 2004). This raises the possibility that dysregulations in the frontal or hippocampal systems may be associated with intrusive recollections (reexperiencing symptoms) in PTSD. Consistent with this, neuroimaging studies show that PTSD is associated with lower than normal activation of the medial prefrontal cortex upon exposure to threatening stimuli, which occurs while the amygdala is hyperactivated (Nutt & Malizia, 2004).

Given that amygdala inhibition by the prefrontal cortex plays a role in fear extinction (as discussed earlier), it has been suggested that the neuroimaging findings indicate that PTSD is associated with insufficient amygdala inhibition by the medial prefrontal cortex (Pare et al., 2004). This could account for the persistence of trauma-related fear and avoidance that characterizes PTSD. Insufficient inhibition may also play a role in reexperiencing symptoms such as flashbacks (Nutt & Malizia, 2004). This could occur if heightened activity of the amygdala leads to the repeated stimulation of fear memories. It is unclear, however, whether this "inhibition insufficiency" is something that predisposes a person to develop PTSD or whether it is an acquired consequence of trauma exposure.

The Hippocampal Controversy: Does Stress Damage the Brain?

Animal research and experimental studies of humans have demonstrated that moderate levels of stress can impair learning and memory (Sapolsky, 2000), and that this appears to arise from the effects of glucocorticoids (e.g., cortisol in humans). Glucocorticoids are important for successfully coping with stress because they mobilize stored energy, increase cardiovascular tone, and suppress energy costly anabolism, such as growth, tissue repair, reproduction, digestion, and immunity. Prolonged release of glucocorticoids can damage the hippocampus, because this structure is rich in receptors that are heavily occupied by glucocorticoids during times of stress (Sapolsky, 2000).

Such findings suggested the hypothesis that exposure to traumatic stress and subsequent PTSD are associated with damage to the hippocampus. Such findings, if borne out by research, could explain why PTSD is associated with various types of memory deficits (Chapter 2). Neuroimaging findings initially provided some support for these conjectures. Several neuroimaging studies found that people with PTSD, compared to controls, had smaller hippocampi, and that smaller hippocampal volume was correlated with poorer performance on memory tests (Bremner, 2001). Other studies, however, failed to find that PTSD was associated with smaller hippocampal volume (Grossman, Buchsbaum, & Yehuda, 2002).

The strongest evidence against the hippocampal damage hypothesis came from a twin study, which found evidence that smaller hippocampal volume may be a *predisposing* factor for PTSD rather than a consequence of any trauma- or PTSD-related hippocampal damage (Gilbertson et al., 2002). That study compared two groups of monozygotic twins. In Group 1, one twin had been exposed to combat and developed PTSD, while the co-twin had no trauma exposure and no PTSD. In Group 2, one twin had combat exposure but did not develop PTSD, and the co-twin had no combat exposure or PTSD. Consistent with some of the previous research, people with combat exposure and PTSD had smaller hippocampal volume than people with combat exposure and no PTSD. However, the hippocampal volume of people with combat exposure and PTSD was not different from the volume of their nonexposed, non-PTSD co-twins. In other words, the hippocampal volumes of twins in Group 1 all tended to be smaller than those of Group 2. Although the findings challenged the idea that traumatic stress or PTSD produces hippocampal damage, the results are consistent with the idea that smaller hippocampal volume is a risk factor for PTSD for people exposed to traumatic stress.

How can these findings be reconciled with animal research that clearly shows that stress increases the secretion of glucocorticoids, and that glucocorticoids damage the hippocampus? The answer is suggested by research on cortisol levels in people with PTSD versus controls. Most studies suggest that cortisol levels are not elevated in PTSD, and that in many cases cortisol levels are abnormally low (Yehuda, 2004). Thus, without hypersecretion of cortisol, there is no cortisol-induced damage to the hippocampus. This is further evidence of how the neurobiology of PTSD differs from that of the normal stress response. The implications of low cortisol levels in PTSD are discussed later in this chapter.

In summary, the available research suggests that traumatic stress or chronic PTSD does not damage the hippocampus. Although many people with PTSD, compared to controls, have smaller hippocampal volume (and associated memory difficulties and lower intelligence), these are probably pretrauma differences that could be vulnerability factors for PTSD (see Chapter 2 for a discussion of how memory and intelligence might be vulnerability factors for PTSD). Smaller hippocampal volume may also be associated with other possible risk factors for PTSD, such as impairments in contextual learning and extinction (Grossman et al., 2002), which involve difficulty learning to identify contextual cues that predict whether or not a fear-evoking stimulus is likely to occur in a given situation.

Autonomic Nervous System

A meta-analysis of psychophysiologic studies of PTSD indicates that this disorder, compared to various control groups, is associated with elevated resting heart rate and heightened diastolic blood pressure (Buckley & Kaloupek, 2001). People with PTSD, compared to controls, also show enhanced startle response to neutral stimuli (e.g., to sudden loud tones) and to trauma-related cues (Yehuda, 2002a; Metzger et al., 1999). Taken together, these findings suggest that PTSD is associated with chronically heightened activity of the sympathetic branch of the autonomic nervous system. This is consistent with reports of many PTSD patients, who report that they are particularly sensitive to stressors, including mild stressors (Yehuda, 2002b).

Cortisol and the HPA Axis

Normal stress responses are associated with an increase in the secretion of cortisol, and yet many (but not all) studies have found that PTSD, particularly chronic PTSD, is associated with low or nonelevated levels of cortisol (Yehuda, 2004; Young & Breslau, 2004). Abnormally low cortisol responses to trauma are evident immediately after trauma exposure in people who go on to develop PTSD (Delahanty, Raimonde, & Spoonster, 2000; McFarlane, Atchison, & Yehuda, 1997; Yehuda, McFarlane, & Shalev, 1998). This suggests that in people at risk for PTSD, there is a failure of cortisol to shut down the stress response (e.g., a failure to shut down the activation of the autonomic nervous system) (Yehuda, 2002b).

According to Yehuda (2004), the absence of elevated cortisol indicates that PTSD in general— or perhaps a particular subtype of PTSD—is characterized by heightened sensitivity of the HPA axis, where there is a strong negative feedback to the release of cortisol (recall that cortisol is regulated via negative feedback; release of cortisol leads to the subsequent inhibition of cortisol release). The stronger negative feedback may be due to heightened receptor sensitivity, perhaps due to an increased number of pituitary glucocorticoid receptors (Yehuda, 2002b).

Noradrenergic Dysregulation

Heightened activity of the sympathetic nervous system may be partly due to dysregulation (heightened response) of the noradrenergic neurotransmitter system. This system plays a role in fear and arousal, so dysregulation could lead to the excessive fears and hyperarousal seen in PTSD. Given the role of the noradrenergic system in memory consolidation (McFarlane et al. 2002), it is also possible that heightened activation of this system, in response to a traumatic stressor, could lead to "overconsolidated" or readily recalled trauma memories (Pitman, 1989). In this way, noradrenergic dysregulation could lead to reexperiencing symptoms.

There are several lines of evidence suggesting that the noradrenergic system is dysregulated in PTSD. People with this disorder have increased levels of catecholamines such as noradrenaline under resting and stimulated conditions (Geracoti et al., 2001; Yehuda, 2002a; Young & Breslau, 2004). Pharmacological challenge research provides further evidence of noradrenergic dysregulation. Here, investigators administer a drug that stimulates a given neuromodulatory system and see whether patients differ from controls in their responses. If the groups differ, then this is taken to suggest that the functioning of the neurotransmitter system in patients differs from that of controls. Such research suggests noradrenergic dysregulation in PTSD (Southwick et al., 1997a).

Serotonergic Dysregulation

There is evidence that the serotonergic system may also be dysregulated in PTSD (Southwick et al., 1997a). This system modulates a variety of brain structures and neurotransmitter systems. For example, it influences activity of the locus ceruleus, which is the major source of noradrenergic neurons in the brain. Therefore, dysregulated control of the noradrenergic system by the serotonergic system could lead to PTSD symptoms such as hyperarousal and reexperiencing symptoms. This could occur even in circumstances where there is nothing inherently wrong with the noradrenergic system. Serotonergic hypofunction could also be associated with symptoms commonly associated with PTSD, such as irritability, aggression, and depression (Stowe & Taylor, 2002).

Other Neuromodulators

Dysregulations in other neuromodulatory systems have also been suggested to play a role in PTSD, including dysregulations in the dopaminergic, GABAergic, and endogenous opioid systems (Stowe & Taylor, 2002). It has been speculated that reduced activity in the dopamine system, in the prefrontal cortex, could lead to excessive, persistent fear of trauma-related cues (Charney, 2004; Morrow, Elsworth, Rasmusson, & Roth, 1999).

Dysregulation in the endogenous opioid system, such as a heightened release of endogenous opioids in response to stress, could play a role in emotional numbing. In support of this conjecture, Vietnam veterans with PTSD exposed to trauma videos experienced a 30% decrease in pain sensitivity on subsequent exposure to heat stimuli (van der Kolk, Greenberg, Orr, & Pitman, 1989). This effect was reversible with naloxone administration, suggesting an opioid-mediated response (Pitman et al., 1990). This is consistent with the finding of elevated cerebrospinal fluid beta-endorphin in PTSD (Baker et al., 1997).

GENETIC FACTORS IN PTSD

Studies of monozygotic and dizygotic twins have been conducted to investigate the heritability of trauma exposure and the heritability of PTSD symptoms among those twins who have been exposed to traumatic stressors (Jang, Stein, Taylor, Livesley, & Asmundson, 2003; Lyons et al., 1993; Stein, Jang, Taylor, Vernon, & Livesley, 2002; True et al., 1993). These studies suggest that genetic factors are moderately important in exposure to assaultive trauma and in combat exposure. Assaultive trauma refers to exposure to various forms of interpersonal violence, such as physical or sexual assault. Exposure to nonassaultive trauma (e.g., natural disasters, motor vehicle accidents) was not heritable. Genetic factors also are moderately important in influencing exposure and in PTSD symptoms.

Why would exposure to combat or assaultive trauma be heritable? Trauma exposure per se is unlikely to be inherited. More likely, trauma exposure is influenced by the genes underlying certain personality characteristics, which influence the likelihood that a person will get into a potentially traumatizing situation. A history of conduct disorder is a risk factor for PTSD (Breslau & Davis, 1992; Ozer et al., 2003); people who engage in impulsive or antisocial behaviors (e.g., stealing cars, frequenting dangerous parts of town, associating with felons) are at increased risk of being traumatized. Consistent with this, Jang et al. (2003) found that the genes associated with antisocial personality traits predicted the risk of exposure to assaultive trauma. The strength of association, however, was modest, with genetic factors accounting for 5–11% of the observed relationship between personality and trauma exposure.

Two broad genetic factors may play a role in PTSD. One factor likely represents the genes underlying antisocial or impulsive behavior, which shape the person's risk of trauma exposure. Such genes are insufficient in themselves in causing PTSD, because they fail to explain why PTSD develops in only a fraction of people exposed to trauma. The second genetic factor that likely plays a role in PTSD is probably defined by the genes that contribute to negative emotionality or neuroticism, that is, genes that play a role in a person's tendency to experience fear or anxiety.

Despite the evidence suggesting the role of genetic factors in PTSD, one should not lose sight of the fact that the heritabilities are modest (accounting for about a third of the variance), and environmental factors play a substantial role in determining the risk for this disorder. Such factors may include early (pretrauma) learning experiences that influence the formation of dysfunctional beliefs or poor coping skills (see Chapter 2), or early exposure to unpredictable, uncontrollable stressors, which could sensitize the HPA axis and autonomic nervous system (Nemeroff, 2004).

Kendler and colleagues (e.g., 1995) have shown that some psychiatric disorders (e.g., anxiety and mood disorders) have genetic and environmental factors in common with one another. The same may be true for PTSD, which has not yet been investigated in this manner. Based on previous research (e.g., Kendler et al., 1995), it is likely that PTSD arises from a combination of disorder-specific factors (i.e., genetic and environmental factors specific to PTSD) and nonspecific factors (genetic and environmental factors that play a role in PTSD and other disorders).

IMPLICATIONS FOR CBT

The research on the neurobiology of PTSD can be shared, in a summarized form, with patients to help them realize that their symptoms are not due to some weakness or failing on their part; the symptoms arise from the interaction between genetic predispositions and environmental events. Similarly, it can be useful to provide patients (and their significant others) with information about the causes of particular types of posttraumatic stress response. Exaggerated startle response, for example, is not a sign of timidity or cowardice; it is an involuntary defensive reflex, which is readily activated in PTSD. A useful therapeutic goal is to ensure that patients and their significant others do not become alarmed about the patient's startle response.

Unless the person is becoming startled in situations where this could be risky (e.g., becoming startled while driving in a manner that makes driving hazardous), an exaggerated startle reflex is no more dangerous than a bout of hiccups. Even in those circumstances where it might be dangerous (e.g., if it impairs driving), CBT can reduce or dampen the startle response (Fairbank et al., 1981).

Corrective information can be similarly provided for people who experienced tonic immobility at the time of the trauma. Some assault survivors feel guilty, ashamed, or confused because they did not fight back against the assailant. To illustrate, women who felt paralyzed during a sexual assault are likely to blame themselves and feel intense guilt and self-derogation (Meyer & Taylor, 1986). Guilt, self-blame, and shame can be reduced by educating patients about the fact that tonic immobility is a defensive reflex, and therefore they need not blame themselves about how they behaved during the assault. Assault survivors can also be assured that the failure to fight back against the assailant (due to tonic immobility) in no way implies "consent" for the assault. In some cases it may be necessary to convey this information to the survivor's significant others, who may otherwise blame the person for not fighting back (Heidt et al., 2005).

People with PTSD sometimes report that they are not as resilient to stress as they were before the traumatic event. They may find themselves to be more reactive to even minor stressors. Such patients could be educated about the nature of the stress response systems (HPA axis and autonomic nervous system), and how the sensitivity of these systems can change. Exposure to unpredictable, uncontrollable stress can sensitize these systems, whereas graded exposure to predictable, controllable stress (as in CBT exposure exercises) can reduce stress sensitivity (Dienstbier, 1989; Nemeroff, 2004). It is important that PTSD patients understand that their stress hyper-responsiveness is not a fixed trait; CBT can help them improve their stress resilience. Physical exercise is also another useful means of improving stress resilience (Dienstbier, 1989).

Some patients (and some clinicians) may ask how CBT could possibly be helpful with PTSD, because this disorder has been shown to be "genetic," and is a "brain disease" according to neuroimaging studies. Patients (and sometimes their doctors) who firmly believe that PTSD is simply a "biological" disorder may be reluctant to try CBT, thereby unnecessarily narrowing their treatment options. There are several responses that the cognitive-behavioral therapist could make to these claims. First, there are several neuroimaging studies of anxiety and mood disorders showing that CBT normalizes patterns of brain activation (e.g., Baxter et al., 1992; Furmark et al., 2002; Goldapple et al., 2004). In a sense, CBT and pharmacotherapies are both somatic interventions.

Some patients (and clinical practitioners) believe that if a disorder is "genetic" then it is not amenable to psychosocial interventions. If this belief presents a barrier to the implementation of CBT, then the patient could be educated that genes do not necessarily define one's destiny. For some disorders that are strongly genetic, the most effective available treatment is an environmental intervention. To illustrate, phenylketonuria is a genetic disorder that results in a deficiency of the enzyme phenylalanine hydroxylase (Thompson, 1995). This disorder is effectively managed by an environmental intervention—a phenylalanine-restricted diet (Brown & Guest, 1999). Another example is obesity, which is a substantially heritable condition (Bulik, Sullivan, & Kendler, 2003). Among the most effective treatments for obesity are environment interventions, such as physical exercise and behavior therapy (Avenell et al., 2004). Similarly, CBT is effective for PTSD, even though the disorder is moderately heritable.

The finding that PTSD is associated with smaller hippocampal volume has been widely reported in the popular press, which has led some PTSD patients to despair that they have stress-induced brain damage. The finding that hippocampal volume is not a result of stress may be reassuring to patients. Further good news is the evidence that the hippocampus can regenerate lost neurons (Bendel et al., 2005). In this regard the hippocampus is unusual compared to other brain structures. Preliminary evidence suggests that treatment with popular and effective pharmacotherapies for PTSD—the selective serotonin reuptake inhibitors—can increase hippocampal volume in people with PTSD (Vermetten, Vythilingam, Southwick, Charney, & Bremner, 2003). It is not yet known whether other effective PTSD treatments have a similar salubrious effect on hippocampal volume. However, given that CBT and medications produce many of the same changes in brain function, as revealed by neuroimaging research, it is quite possible that CBT also may increase hippocampal volume.

SUMMARY

PTSD probably arises from a mix of normal and dysregulated neurobiological processes. The risk for developing PTSD and the subsequent severity and chronicity of the disorder may depend on the nature and number of processes that are involved in a given individual, for example, the number of risk-imparting genes a person possesses, or the number of neurotransmitter systems that become dysregulated after trauma exposure.

Knowledge of the neurobiology of PTSD can aid the cognitive-behavioral therapist in several ways. It can help the therapist understand how the cognitive abnormalities and models of PTSD, discussed in Chapters 2 and 3, may be related to brain structures and processes. Knowledge of the neurobiology of PTSD can also help the therapist provide psychoeducation to the patient, for instance, information that the patient is not to blame for defensive, reflexive reactions like tonic immobility and reassurance that trauma exposure is unlikely to damage the patient's brain. The neurobiologically informed clinician can help patients treated with a combination of CBT and pharmacotherapy understand how these treatments may be complementary, and how they may exert their therapeutic effects on similar or interconnected brain structures and processes.

CHAPTER 5

Treatments

A Review of the Research

The therapist needs to choose from a wide range of options to determine which interventions to use with which patient. An evidence-based approach can help guide the process. In this chapter we will focus primarily on research on the efficacy of different forms of CBT. This chapter reviews what is currently known about the merits of CBT in relation to other treatments, with particular attention to clinically important questions such as the following:

- Are CBT methods useful for PTSD prevention or early intervention?
- What are the most effective CBT interventions for acute or chronic PTSD? To optimize outcome, these could be emphasized in treatment packages, while the less effective interventions could be de-emphasized or dropped altogether.
- What are useful guidelines for selecting, sequencing, and integrating cognitive-behavioral and other interventions?
- How common are CBT side effects and other adverse outcomes?
- Is CBT effective for special populations such as children and the elderly, and how should treatment be adapted to such groups?
- What are the most promising directions for further improving the efficacy of CBT?

CBT COMPARED TO OTHER TREATMENTS

Controlled Trials and Meta-Analyses

There are several CBT protocols, typically involving some combination of imaginal exposure, situational exposure, cognitive restructuring, and anxiety management techniques such as relaxation training and breathing retraining. Most CBT protocols contain some form of exposure therapy, typically a combination of imaginal and situational exposure.

Numerous studies, including carefully designed, randomized controlled trials, have shown that various forms of CBT are effective in treating PTSD, with gains generally maintained at follow-ups of a year or more (Chard, 2005; Foa et al., 2005; Taylor, 2004). There have been comparatively fewer direct comparisons of CBT with other sorts of interventions. Meta-analytic research, which pools outcome studies to compare treatment effects, has therefore been conducted to estimate the comparative efficacy of treatments. Such research indicates that CBT protocols, as a group, tend to have lower dropout rates than pharmacotherapies, and that CBT is equally effective in the short term as the most potent PTSD pharmacotherapies, the selective serotonin reuptake inhibitors (SSRIs) (van Etten & Taylor, 1998).

Meta-analytic research suggests that CBT tends to be more effective than supportive counseling and short-term psychodynamic therapy. Meta-analysis also suggests that CBT and eye movement desensitization and reprocessing (EMDR) have comparative efficacy, and that EMDR and the various forms of CBT do not differ in treatment dropout (Hembree et al., 2003; van Etten & Taylor, 1998). More recent research, which circumvented many of the methodological problems in previous EMDR studies, suggests that CBT is more effective and works faster than EMDR in reducing symptoms, and that EMDR is no more effective than relaxation training (Taylor et al., 2003).

Expert Consensus Guidelines

The above-mentioned results are consistent with the conclusions drawn from a group of internationally recognized PTSD experts (Ballenger et al., 2000; Foa, Davidson, & Frances, 1999b). The expert consensus, based on a combination of research evidence and clinical experience, was that either SSRIs or psychosocial interventions using exposure therapy are the first-line interventions. The expert consensus also was that exposure therapy is the most effective and fastest acting psychotherapeutic technique, and that the methods with the fewest negative side effects are anxiety management techniques, psychoeducation, and cognitive restructuring. The expert consensus also offered the following guidelines (Foa et al., 1999b):

- Regardless of patient age and PTSD severity or duration, treatment should begin with either psychotherapy alone (e.g., CBT) or a combination of psychotherapy and medications.
- When PTSD is comorbid with major depression, bipolar disorder, or anxiety disorders, use combination treatment from the start.
- When PTSD is comorbid with substance abuse or dependence, either

treat PTSD and substance problems simultaneously or treat the substance problems first.

- Exposure therapy is recommended for reexperiencing and avoidance symptoms.
- Cognitive restructuring is recommended for numbing, irritability, anger, guilt, and shame.
- Cognitive restructuring, with or without exposure therapy, is recommended for hyperarousal symptoms.
- For children and younger adolescents, treatment might involve play therapy, along with psychoeducation, anxiety coping skills, and cognitive restructuring.
- Older adolescents can benefit from the same cognitive-behavioral interventions as younger adults.
- If a trial of psychosocial treatment is insufficient, try adding medication or switching to another psychotherapy technique.

The guidelines did not discuss the treatment of mental defeat (defined in Chapter 2). Research suggests that cognitive restructuring may be effective for reducing this problem (Ehlers et al., 1998a).

Prevention and Early Intervention

Prevention and early intervention for PTSD are important because we, as treating clinicians, often find ourselves in a position where we have to decide how best to help someone presenting with symptoms associated with a very recent trauma (e.g., a survivor of a holdup occurring a few days earlier). People who have just experienced a traumatic event could develop PTSD. Accordingly, programs have been developed to prevent PTSD (and other psychopathology) in trauma-exposed populations.

One approach is to intervene shortly after the person has been exposed to a trauma. Among the most widely used of these early interventions are the various forms of psychological debriefing, such as critical incident stress debriefing (Mitchell & Everly, 2000). Debriefing is implemented in a single session, 24–48 hours posttrauma, to *all* available trauma survivors, regardless of whether they are distressed, either individually or in groups. The trauma survivor is presented with information about common reactions to trauma (e.g., PTSD symptoms) and asked to provide the debriefer with a detailed description of the trauma. The debriefer encourages emotional expression and advises the person to discuss the trauma with others. Avoidance of trauma-related stimuli is discouraged, and the person is encouraged to seek further help if symptoms persist.

Despite the widespread use of psychological debriefing, little information about its effects has been available until recently. Research indicates that debriefing, compared to no intervention, is either ineffective or possibly harmful in that it seems to perpetuate PTSD symptoms (Bisson, 2003; National Institute of Mental Health [NIMH], 2002; van Emmerik et al., 2002). There is also no evidence that EMDR has any particular benefits in treating people shortly after trauma exposure (NIMH, 2002). A more promising approach is to determine whether the patient has PTSD symptoms and desires treatment and, if so, to then implement a 4–5 session CBT program 2–4 weeks posttrauma. Research indicates that the latter is effective in reducing symptoms and reducing the risk of developing full-blown PTSD (e.g., Bisson, Shepherd, Joy, Probert, & Newcombe, 2004; Bryant, Sackville, Dang, Moulds, & Guthrie, 1999; Foa, Hearst-Ikeda, & Perry, 1995a).

ADVERSE EFFECTS OF CBT

Most treatments, whether they are psychosocial or pharmacological, have side effects, such as transient increases in PTSD symptoms. Initial symptom exacerbation during CBT can be a result of increased exposure to trauma-related stimuli; that is, patients are encouraged to become less avoidant (e.g., through the use of exposure exercises), so they increasingly come in contact with stimuli that evoke distress and trigger memories of the traumatic event (reexperiencing symptoms).

How frequent and severe are CBT side effects? In a small series of cases selected to illustrate problems with exposure therapy, Pitman et al. (1991) reported that exposure sometimes exacerbated various forms of psychopathology, including trauma-related anger and guilt, anxiety symptoms, and comorbid substance use disorders. In a randomized, controlled trial of people seeking treatment for PTSD, Tarrier et al. (1999a) reported that 31% of patients treated with imaginal exposure experienced a worsening of PTSD symptoms from pre- to posttreatment. The validity of Tarrier's findings has been debated (Devilly & Foa, 2001; Tarrier, 2001). In a study comparing exposure, EMDR, and relaxation training, Taylor et al. (2003) found that symptom worsening occurred in fewer than 7% of patients and did not vary with the type of treatment. Foa, Zoellner, Feeny, Hembree, and Alvarez-Conrad (2002) found that symptom worsening was similarly rare during imaginal exposure and situational exposure. Symptom worsening tended to be mild and transient and was unrelated to treatment dropout. By the end of treatment, patients who had symptom worsening during treatment made comparable treatment gains to patients who did not experience symptom worsening (Foa et al., 2002).

In summary, side effects consisting of symptom worsening sometimes occur during psychosocial treatments for PTSD. Sometimes these side effects are significant (Pitman et al., 1991), but for the majority of patients side effects are mild and transient (Foa et al., 2002; Taylor et al., 2003).

When serious side effects or other forms of symptom worsening occur, then cognitive restructuring may be particularly helpful (Pitman et al., 1991).

Who is most likely to experience adverse effects? Patients who have substance use disorders (either currently or in recent remission) may be at risk for an exacerbation of these disorders during PTSD treatment. Other pretreatment characteristics have generally failed to identify patients who are at risk for symptom worsening. Therapist skill may be an important factor in limiting CBT side effects (Taylor et al., 2003). Skilled therapists may be better able to guide the pacing and difficulty of exposure exercises. Some lesser skilled therapists might push patients to attempt exposure exercises that are too distressing to endure, resulting in aborted (and brief) exposures to intensely distressing stimuli. Such experiences of failed exposure may intensify the patient's avoidance of trauma cues.

PROGNOSTIC FACTORS

Studies of prognostic factors have produced many inconsistent findings. In part, the inconsistencies may be due to differences in sample size, and hence differences in statistical power. Studies with small samples (and low power) will only be able to identify the most robust predictors, while studies with larger samples will be able to identify more subtle predictors. The research on prognostic factors is still in its infancy, and so the following review can only offer tentative conclusions.

Concerning treatment dropout, pretreatment variables, such as PTSD severity, severity of associated symptoms, trauma characteristics, receipt of disability benefits, trauma-related litigation, and demographic features, are unreliable predictors, significant in some studies but not in others (e.g., Tarrier et al., 1999a; Taylor, 2004; Taylor et al., 2001). Treatment credibility, assessed early in treatment, is also an inconsistent predictor of attrition, being a significant predictor in some trials but not others (Tarrier et al., 1999a; Taylor, 2004; van Minnen, Arntz, & Keijsers, 2002).

With regard to predicting treatment outcome, the following are unreliable predictors: demographic features, trauma-related disability benefits and litigation, trauma characteristics, concurrent use of psychotropic medication, pretreatment clinical features (e.g., PTSD symptoms, duration of trauma, duration since trauma, depression, dissociation, guilt, shame, substance abuse history, comorbid Axis I disorder), and personality variables (e.g., Başoğlu et al., 2003; Forbes, Creamer, Hawthorne, Allen, & McHugh, 2003; Taylor, 2004). Pretreatment dysfunctional beliefs are similarly unreliable or nonsignificant predictors of outcome (Livanou et al., 2002). Although PTSD-related compensation seeking and litigation generally do not predict outcome (e.g., Brooks & McKinlay, 1992; Grace, Green, Lindy, & Leonard, 1993; Taylor et al., 2001), there are occasional exceptions of patients who simulate PTSD symptoms and fail to adhere to treatment in the hope of receiving a large financial settlement (Simon, 2003).

Clinical lore suggests that the patient's pretreatment level of anger (either severity of trauma-related anger or anger proneness in general) predicts the outcome of PTSD treatment. Anger has been implicated in poor outcome for CBT in some studies (e.g., Foa, Riggs, Massie, & Yarczower, 1995c; Forbes et al., 2003; Taylor et al., 2001) but not in others (e.g., Cahill, Rauch, Hembree, & Foa, 2003; Taylor, 2004; van Minnen et al., 2002). Pretreatment trauma-related guilt is similarly an unreliable predictor of PTSD treatment outcome (Taylor, 2004). It is possible that only very severe trauma-related anger or guilt predicts poor response to PTSD treatments, but this remains to be empirically established.

PTSD is often comorbid with chronic pain in survivors of road traffic collisions, industrial accidents, and other cases of traumatic injury. Studies examining the predictive importance of chronic pain suggest that severe pain (arising from, for example, soft tissue injury) predicts poor outcome for PTSD treatments, even when treatments include techniques for managing pain such as relaxation training (Taylor et al., 2001; Wald, Taylor, & Fedoroff, 2004a). Such patients may be best treated in programs that integrate PTSD treatment with multidisciplinary pain management. When PTSD is comorbid with milder forms of recurrent pain (e.g., occasional tension-related headaches or muscle spasms), then pain and PTSD can both be managed by incorporating simple pain management strategies (e.g., relaxation exercises) into conventional CBT for PTSD (Wald et al., 2004a).

The patient's interpersonal environment may have important implications for PTSD treatment. Tarrier et al. (1999b) found that poor outcome for imaginal exposure or cognitive restructuring for PTSD tended to occur when patients lived with angry or critical significant others (i.e., lived in environments with high expressed emotion). Under these circumstances it may be necessary to target the expressed emotion directly, such as by including couple or family interventions that target this problem.

In summary, to date there are few variables that reliably predict the outcome of CBT for cases in which PTSD is the primary presenting problem. Patients who are most likely to benefit from CBT tend to show treatment-related gains within the first few sessions (van Minnen & Hagenaars, 2002).

CBT ACTIVE INGREDIENTS

Although CBT is generally useful, it is far from universally efficacious. For patients treated with cognitive-behavioral protocols, 15–45% still meet criteria for PTSD by the end of a typical (e.g., 8–12 week) course of treatment

(Taylor et al., 2003; van Minnen et al., 2002). Treatment efficacy may be improved by better understanding the efficacy of particular cognitive-behavioral interventions.

A number of component studies have been conducted in order to gauge the efficacy of various cognitive-behavioral interventions. Component studies address two questions: (1) Is a given intervention effective, compared to no treatment or compared to placebo? (2) Is the efficacy of a treatment package improved, for the average patient, if a given intervention is added to the package? Implicit in Question 2 is the assumption that treatment duration is fixed; to add a treatment component means that there will be less therapy time available for other components. For a program of exposure, consisting of eight hourly treatment sessions, for example, adding cognitive restructuring will mean that there is less time available for exposure. The goal behind Question 2 is to identify the most efficient, powerful combination of interventions for a given treatment duration. An intervention may be effective (compared to no treatment), even though the intervention need not find a place in the most efficient, powerful package of interventions.

Research addressing Question 1 has compared cognitive restructuring plus imaginal exposure to supportive counseling plus imaginal exposure (Bryant, Moulds, Guthrie, Dang, & Nixon, 2003). Previous studies have shown that supportive counseling is largely a placebo (e.g., Foa, Rothbaum, Riggs, & Murdock, 1991), so this intervention can be used as a "filler task." Bryant et al.'s study found that the treatment package that included cognitive restructuring was more effective than the package that included counseling. This suggests that cognitive restructuring is better than placebo in reducing PTSD, although it does not show that restructuring should be included in the most efficient and effective treatment package.

Studies have also shown that imaginal exposure, situational exposure, cognitive restructuring, and their combination are more effective than no treatment at all and are more effective than interventions that are largely placebos, such as supportive counseling or some forms of relaxation training (e.g., Foa et al., 1991; Marks et al., 1998; Taylor et al., 2003).

Research addressing Question 2 has shown that treatments combining imaginal and situational exposure tend to be more effective than treatments consisting of imaginal exposure alone (Devilly & Foa, 2001). Other studies addressing Question 2 have generally failed to show, for a fixed treatment duration, that a treatment package consisting of exposure (imaginal and/or situational exposure) can be improved by adding cognitive restructuring or anxiety management techniques (e.g., relaxation training), at least when outcome is assessed in terms of reductions in PTSD or depressive symptoms (e.g., Foa, 2000; Foa et al., 1999a, 2005; Paunovic & Öst, 2001). It is possible that combination treatments are most effective for some patients whereas simpler protocols (e.g., exposure alone) are most effective for other patients. There is some indication that trauma-related guilt is more effectively reduced by combined exposure plus cognitive restructuring, compared to exposure alone (Resick, Nishith, Weaver, Astin, & Feurer, 2002). Cognitive restructuring may also be particularly useful for severe trauma-related shame and mental defeat (e.g., Ehlers et al., 1998a).

Case studies and a handful of uncontrolled and controlled trials suggest that other interventions can be usefully added to exposure protocols for PTSD, depending on the nature of the presenting problems. The addition of anger management training (Novaco, 1975) is promising for people with PTSD and severe anger (Chemtob, Novaco, Hamada, & Gross, 1997). Cognitive-behavioral interventions for panic disorder, such as interoceptive exposure (i.e., exposure to arousal-related bodily sensations; Taylor, 2000), are useful additions for people with PTSD, even for patients who don't have comorbid panic attacks (Wald & Taylor, 2005a, 2005b).

INTERVENTION SELECTION AND SEQUENCING

A range of useful methods are currently available. How should the cognitive-behavioral practitioner select among these for use in a specific case? In what order should the interventions be used? Should some methods be used sequentially, or should they be integrated so that they are administered at the same time? Some interventions logically seem to precede others. Breathing retraining or some other method for reducing arousal, for example, is typically implemented prior to exposure exercises. This is so that patients will be able to regulate the degree of arousal they experience, to prevent them from feeling emotionally overwhelmed. Similarly, training in relapse prevention logically occurs at the end of therapy, once the patient has learned skills in managing or reducing PTSD symptoms.

The ordering of other interventions is less clear. Cognitive restructuring could be implemented before exposure exercises in order to facilitate exposure. That is, the distress associated with trauma memories can be lessened by restructuring maladaptive, trauma-related beliefs (e.g., "I'm in danger if I go to a bar"). In these circumstances exposure becomes easier to accomplish. Cognitive restructuring could also be performed during exposure. This could be done, for example, by asking the patient to articulate negative thoughts during imaginal or situational exposure (the "think aloud" method), which the therapist could then challenge during exposure. Cognitive restructuring could also be performed after exposure.

That is, exposure exercises could be used as a means of eliciting dysfunctional beliefs, which then would be targeted with cognitive restructuring.

At the present time, little is known about the best way to combine cognitive restructuring with exposure. The development of a case formulation of the patient's problems can also guide the selection of interventions (see Chapter 8).

SPECIAL POPULATIONS

Studies indicate that cognitive-behavioral interventions are efficacious for diverse trauma populations, such as survivors of physical and sexual assault (including child and adult survivors of childhood assault), survivors of terrorism and torture, survivors of motor vehicle accidents and natural disasters, refugees, torture survivors, and combat veterans (e.g., Başoğlu, Ekblad, Baarnhielm, & Livanou, 2004; Ehlers et al., 2003; Taylor, 2004). Special issues arise in the treatment of particular populations, as discussed in the following sections.

Children and Adolescents

Research indicates that cognitive-behavioral interventions can reduce PTSD in children and adolescents (e.g., Cohen, 2003; Farrell, Hains, & Davies, 1998; King et al., 2000b). It is unclear whether the efficacy of CBT varies with the age of the child or adolescent. In a small study of abuse-related PTSD in 19 girls age 3–16 years, Deblinger, McLeer, and Henry (1990) found no relationship between age and treatment response. This may have been because the flexibility of their treatment permitted the children to choose from various forms of exposure that may differ in their developmental appropriateness (e.g., exposure therapy conducted by doll playing, drawing, or reading). These findings are consistent with the PTSD practice guidelines from the American Academy of Child and Adolescent Psychiatry (1998), derived from a combination of empirical research and expert consensus:

• Interventions should include some discussion of the trauma, stress management techniques, exploration and correction of inaccurate attributions regarding the trauma, and inclusion of parents in treatment.
• As in the treatment of traumatized adults, the therapist should not coerce the child to participate in exposure exercises. Persistent talking about traumatic memories with children who are very embarrassed or highly resistant may not be indicated and may in fact worsen symptoms.

Indirect methods of addressing traumatic issues, such as art and play techniques, may be helpful in these situations.

• Stress management skills are useful because they may give the child a sense of control over unwanted thoughts and feelings. Such skills also allow the child to approach the direct discussion of the traumatic event with confidence that this will not lead to uncontrollable reexperiencing of symptoms and fear. Stress management techniques are also useful to the child outside of the therapeutic context, if and when reexperiencing symptoms occur.

• Faulty beliefs about the trauma (e.g., "It was my fault," "I'm not safe anywhere") should be explored and challenged, beyond mere assurances. Challenging is most often accomplished through step-by-step logical analysis of the child's cognitive distortions within therapy sessions.

• Other issues, such as survivor guilt, should also be addressed.

• The inclusion in treatment of significant others such as parents is important. Parental emotional reactions to the traumatic event and parental support of the child can influence the child's PTSD symptoms. Including parents in treatment also helps the parent monitor the child's symptoms and learn appropriate behavior management techniques. Helping parents resolve their own emotional distress related to the trauma, to which the parent usually has had either direct or vicarious exposure, can help the parent be more perceptive of, and responsive to, the child's emotional needs. Many parents benefit from direct psychoeducation about their child's PTSD symptoms and how to manage them.

• Children exposed to a known trauma who are asymptomatic may not require treatment but may need monitoring for emergence of delayed symptoms.

The Elderly

There have been no controlled trials of the use of CBT in treating PTSD in the elderly (defined as people 65 years and older). Case reports suggest that it can be useful (Hyer & Sohnle, 2001; Weintraub & Ruskin, 1999). Imaginal exposure can be included as part of a broader review of the positive and negative aspects of a patient's life (Maercker, 2002). This may help place the traumatic events in context, that is, as events that are simply episodes of a long and varied series of life experiences.

Very little is known about the best way to treat PTSD in people who are dementing. On the basis of clinical experience, Flannery (2002) suggested a number of interventions that could be implemented by long-term care staff. Ensuring the physical safety of demented individuals is the first consideration, including the prevention of abuse by significant others (i.e., elder abuse), which could exacerbate preexisting PTSD. Flannery suggested that some form of exposure therapy may reduce PTSD, even though the patient is dementing. However, it is also cautioned that "long-term care staff need to decide whether the patient is better served by addressing the traumatic incident directly or by containing the memories of the event and providing symptomatic relief" (p. 282). Simple strategies for targeting hyperarousal symptoms are also suggested, such as physical exercises and other diverting activities (e.g., walking, gardening, aerobic exercise, music, dance, or other hobbies) or calming activities (e.g., relaxation exercises, meditation, or prayer). Facilitating mastery, within limits of the person's cognitive capabilities, is also recommended, such as allowing patients to select their own meals and allowing them to be responsible for personal grooming to the extent it is possible. Flannery also recommended grounding exercises (Chapter 9) for managing flashbacks. These interventions make good clinical sense, although research is needed to determine whether they are truly helpful in managing PTSD in people who are dementing.

Refugees

Many refugees have experienced traumatic events, such as violence, torture, or other forms of suffering (e.g., humiliation, starvation, illness). Preliminary research indicates that CBT can successfully reduce PTSD in refugees settled in other countries (e.g., Hinton et al., 2004, 2005; Paunovic & Öst, 2001). However, many refugees are interred in camps, rather than being resettled in safe havens. In addition to experiencing trauma in their country of exodus, refugees may experience trauma in the refugee camps, such as physical and sexual assault, along with malnourishment and persecution because of religious or political beliefs. Research by Neuner, Schauer, Klaschik, Karunakara, and Elbert (2004) provides important information about the treatment of PTSD in refugees in such settings. They compared four sessions of either narrative exposure therapy (NET), supportive counseling, or a session of psychoeducation for treating PTSD in an African refugee settlement. Each intervention commenced with a session of psychoeducation. Counseling involved problem solving about current concerns.

In NET, the therapist helped the patient construct a detailed chronological account of his or her biography. The biography was recorded by the therapist and corrected by the patient with each subsequent reading. A special focus of therapy was on constructing a coherent narrative report of the patient's traumatic experiences. During the discussion of traumatic experiences, the therapist asked about current emotional, physiological, cognitive, and behavioral reactions. The patient was encouraged to relive distressing emotions while reporting the events. The discussion of the traumatic event proceeded in much more detail than the narrative of other aspects of the patient's life and was not terminated until a reduction in distress had occurred (sessions were approximately 90 minutes). In the final session, the patient received a written report of his or her biography. An advantage of this method over conventional exposure therapy is that NET tackled multiple traumas in the course of one exposure session (via the biographical narrative), rather than trying to expose patients to one traumatic experience at a time. The NET approach is efficient because many refugees with PTSD (and many other patients with PTSD for that matter) have had numerous traumatic experiences.

At the beginning of treatment all refugee participants had PTSD. One year after treatment, PTSD rates were 29% (NET), 79% (counseling), and 80% (psychoeducation). The NET results are noteworthy, given that patients continued to live in hazardous conditions (i.e., refugee camps). NET appeared to be quite acceptable because most refugees were quite willing to enter treatment and very few dropped out (Neuner et al., 2004). Subsequent research provides further support for the efficacy of NET, including the treatment of traumatized children (Schauer, Neuner, & Elbert, 2005).

The NET approach may prove to be a very useful format for treating other types of multiply traumatized patients. The advantage of this approach is that instead of defining a single event as the target in therapy, the patient constructs a narration about his or her entire life, from birth to the present situation, while focusing on the detailed report of the traumatic experiences. In this way the therapist can address multiple traumatic events within a single session of exposure therapy.

Combat Veterans

Research suggests that PTSD treatments are less effective for combat veterans than for nonveteran patients (Creamer & Forbes, 2004). This could be partially a result of compensation benefits tied to the diagnosis of combat-related PTSD, which may entice some veterans to overreport trauma exposure and symptoms and underreport treatment benefits (Frueh et al., 2003, 2005). In other cases CBT protocols in veterans programs may be insufficient; exposure interventions used in many Veterans Administration programs are based on the method of trauma focus group therapy, which involves very limited (single-session) trauma-related exposure and has been associated with weak treatment effects (Ruzek et al., 2001; Schnurr et al., 2003).

For trauma patients treated in the theater of combat, preliminary evidence supports the old clinical principle of "proximity, immediacy, and expectancy" (Solomon & Benbenishty, 1986), that is, the idea that afflicted soldiers should be treated in close proximity to the combat zone, as soon as possible after the onset of symptoms, and with the expectation of a quick return to combat. This procedure has been adopted by several armies. Treatment focuses on replenishing depleted physiological needs by satisfying the need for sleep, food, and drink for a few days in relative safety. During this period minimal psychiatric intervention is carried out. Soldiers whose symptoms persist or worsen are evacuated for more intensive assessment and treatment (Lamberg, 2004).

There are several reasons for supposing that this method is effective (Solomon & Benbenishty, 1986). Treatment provided in close proximity to the front facilitates continuing contact with comrades and commanders, thereby strengthening the soldier's commitment to one's peers and reinforcing one's military identity. This is further strengthened by the fact that patients are required to wear their military uniforms. Frontline treatment also implies that the soldier's problem is merely a temporary crisis, and that he or she should be capable of resolving the problem and resuming military duties. Immediate treatment on or near the battlefield conveys the expectation that patients will maintain their role as soldiers, and that they are still perceived as an integral part of the unit. This presumably reduces the stigma associated with having PTSD. Treatment near the front also prevents social support from comrades from being disrupted, which would happen if the soldier was shipped off to a hospital.

According to a retrospective chart study by Solomon and Benbenishty (1986), all three treatment principles—proximity, immediacy, and expectancy—were correlated with a higher rate of return to the military unit and lower rates of PTSD. The effects were linear; more of each principle (e.g., the greater the degree of expectancy) and the use of more principles were associated with better outcomes. Despite these promising findings, some clinicians have expressed skepticism, claiming that the benefits have been exaggerated (Jones & Wessely, 2003).

Battered Women

Domestic violence typically involves chronic victimization via multiple types of trauma (e.g., physical or sexual assault, stalking, psychological abuse), and survivors may be exposed to ongoing threats of violence by the batterer (Kaysen, Resick, & Wise, 2003). Survivors of domestic violence may have complex relationships with their abusive partner, such as intense, ambivalent feelings (e.g., love combined with guilt or fear). It may be difficult to detach completely from the abusive spouse if the couple has children. Safety considerations are important before deciding whether to treat battered women with PTSD.

Kubany and Watson (2002) formulated a CBT program designed for treating battered women with PTSD. It involves treating PTSD and associated features (e.g., trauma-related anger, guilt, and shame), along with cognitive and interpersonal interventions for dealing with encounters with the abusive spouse (e.g., assertiveness training). Research indicates that this form of CBT is effective (Kubany et al., 2004).

People Involved in Work-Related Accidents

Treatment of PTSD for people involved in work-related (e.g., industrial) accidents can be facilitated by integrating a return-to-work program into treatment. This is illustrated in a study of PTSD associated with work-related hand injuries (Grunert et al., 1990). Hand injuries, particularly the loss of the hand or upper limb, tend to be more traumatizing than the loss of a lower limb, because hands play a vital role in self-care (e.g., eating and grooming), self-expression (e.g., hand gestures), communication with others (e.g., shaking hands), one's occupation (e.g., operating machinery), and in one's self-image and social acceptance (Cheung, Alvaro, & Colotla, 2003; Meyer, 2003).

Grunert et al. (1990) compared the rates of return to work for four different forms of CBT: (1) imaginal exposure and coping skills training, (2) situational exposure that involved returning to the worksite, (3) graded work exposure that involved increasing hours of work each week, and (4) worksite evaluation that involved teaching the individual how to apply and practice learned skills "on the job." All treatments were associated with reductions in PTSD symptoms. Graded work exposure produced the highest rate of return to work among the four approaches. At a 6-month follow-up, 61% of the workers (74 of 122) remained successfully employed with their preinjury employer. More treatment studies are needed to replicate, extend, and improve on these promising findings.

Complex PTSD in Adult Survivors of Childhood Abuse

Adult survivors of childhood physical or sexual abuse may have complex PTSD (Chapter 1). Accordingly, it has been suggested that these people would best benefit from a two-stage approach (Cloitre, Koenen, Cohen, & Han, 2002). The first involves training in skills to address problems that are typically associated with personality disorder traits arising from chronic childhood abuse (training in emotion regulation and interpersonal skills training). The second involves conventional trauma-related exposure therapy. This treatment has been shown to be effective, compared to no treatment at all, although it remains to be shown that it is better than conventional CBT. Studies of conventional CBT for PTSD (e.g., cognitive restructuring, exposure, relaxation training) suggests that simple and complex PTSD respond equally to short-term CBT (Resick, Nishith, & Griffin, 2003; Taylor et al., 2006), although the personality disorder traits that characterize complex PTSD do not appear to respond to such PTSD-focused interventions (Taylor et al., 2006). The latter finding raises the possibility that Cloitre's two-stage treatment may be a particularly promising treatment for complex PTSD.

Clinical Exotica

A special population that requires further investigation consists of those patients presenting with "clinical exotica," that is, patients presenting with unusual problems, such as (1) PTSD associated with recovered memories of abuse, (2) PTSD associated with claims of being subjected to unusual traumas (e.g., purportedly witnessing human sacrifice by members of satanic cults), (3) atypical presentations such as posttraumatic conversion disorder, and (4) PTSD with concurrent psychotic symptoms, such as hallucinations (usually visual or auditory) or delusions.

Case studies suggest that cognitive-behavioral interventions can reduce PTSD associated with recovered memories and can also reduce posttraumatic conversion disorder (Rothbaum & Foa, 1991; Taylor & Thordarson, 2002; Wald et al., 2004b). Treatment studies of coexisting psychotic symptoms in PTSD, or of people with PTSD comorbid with either schizophrenia or bipolar disorder, have been limited to case reports and pilot studies. Such studies have generally found that these clinical presentations tend to be largely treatment resistant to both pharmacological and psychosocial interventions (Bleich & Moskowits, 2000; Chan & Silove, 2000). However, a recent pilot study suggests that a 12- to 16-week individual CBT package—consisting of psychoeducation, breathing retraining, and cognitive restructuring, with treatment closely coordinated with the patient's community support treatment teams— may be effective (Rosenberg, Mueser, Jankowski, Salyers, & Acker, 2004)

Treatment decisions about how to best manage clinical exotica must be made on a case-by-case basis. In some cases traditional CBT for PTSD may be contraindicated; treatment could do more harm than good. For example, repeated imaginal exposure for a patently false memory may strengthen or enhance the person's belief that the event actually occurred (Taylor & Thordarson, 2002). Similarly, exposure therapy for psychotic patients, even those in remission, could aggravate their psychoses. Emotion regulation strategies (Chapter 9) may be the safest and most useful intervention in such cases.

Cultural Issues

There have been few studies of the role of cultural factors in treating PTSD. For the Veterans Administration PTSD treatment programs, there are, on average, no major effects of ethnicity on treatment outcome (Rosenheck, Fontana, & Cottrol, 1995; Rosenheck & Fontana, 1996). Case reports (Cooke & Shear, 2001; Feske, 2001) and a controlled trial (Zoellner et al., 1999) further suggest that cognitive-behavioral interventions can be effectively used to treat African American survivors of sexual assault or physical abuse. No differences in attrition or outcome were found between African

American and Caucasian patients (Zoellner et al., 1999). However, all currently available PTSD treatments are far from universally effective. Greater attention to cultural issues might improve treatment outcome.

USING BASIC SCIENCE
TO GUIDE FUTURE DEVELOPMENTS

CBT in a Biological Context

Although we are far from having an integrated biopsychosocial theory of PTSD, great strides have been made in recent years. On a psychological level, PTSD can be regarded as a disorder in which trauma memories and associated dysfunctional beliefs are hyperaccessible (i.e., readily activated by environmental and other cues) and emotionally charged. The neural correlates of trauma memories include a host of brain structures (e.g., the amygdala, hippocampus, medial frontal cortex), interconnected through a complex network of circuits. Trauma memories can be established through fear conditioning, which is mediated through sensory inputs reaching the amygdala. As we saw in Chapter 4, the amygdala appears to play a role in assigning emotional significance to events, and extinction of conditioned fear responses appears to involve inhibition of amygdala activity by frontal cortical regions, especially the orbital frontal cortex. These findings suggest that PTSD can be treated by targeting the neurotransmitter systems that modulate the structures and circuits involved in PTSD (e.g., modulation of amygdala activity), and by psychosocial interventions aimed at either deconditioning emotional reactions that were conditioned by trauma exposure (imaginal and situational exposure), or by altering the meaning of the traumatic event (cognitive restructuring).

A strength of CBT has been its links with basic science, particularly cognitive psychology and the animal learning literature. In recent years, however, it seems that CBT has overemphasized cognitive psychology to the neglect of other important fields of basic science, particularly neuroscience. Important developments in CBT may arise by considering how the findings from neuroscience and related fields can be used to refine or modify CBT for PTSD. In the following sections the potential for using basic science to develop new CBT protocols will be illustrated by two important examples: animal research on the role of context in extinction and research on the pharmacological enhancement of fear extinction.

Context and Extinction

The animal learning literature suggests that extinction of emotional responses, such as the reduction of emotional reactions to trauma cues, involves new learning that is stored along with the old (Bouton, 2002; LeDoux, 2000). Consider, for example, a person who develops PTSD after being in a building that nearly collapsed during an earthquake. Exposure therapy does not undo the old learned associations (e.g., the associations between buildings and danger); rather, it involves the strengthening of new associations (e.g., the association between buildings and safety). Over the course of exposure exercises, such as repeated trips into tall buildings, the person learns to associate buildings with safety, and this memory representation increasingly inhibits the activation of the memory representation in which buildings are associated with danger.

A consequence is that a given stimulus (e.g., the interior of an office) has two available "meanings" (e.g., dangerous vs. safe) and so is just like an ambiguous word; its current meaning depends on its context (Bouton, 2002). Contexts can be provided by a variety of background stimuli, including the physical environment, one's internal physical state, and time. The animal learning literature indicates that fear reduction tends to be most complete and enduring if exposure is conducted across multiple contexts (e.g., in different environments and at different times of day; Bouton, 2002). This suggests that treatment for PTSD would be most effective if the person were exposed to many different contexts (e.g., different buildings and different locations within each building, and at different times of day). Similarly, imaginal exposure may be most effective when it is practiced in many different locations and times of day, and under different internal states (e.g., under different baseline emotional or physical states). Cognitive-behavioral practitioners have typically not paid much attention to the contexts in which imaginal exposure occurs. Such exercises are typically practiced either in the therapist's office or in some quiet place in the patient's home. By varying the context of imaginal and situational exposure, we may improve the durability of CBT for PTSD.

Pharmacologically Enhanced CBT

Adding Psychotropic Medications

Research on the effects of combining CBT with medications may lead to advances in treatment outcome. Expert consensus recommendations are that combined CBT and medication should be considered when PTSD is comorbid with other severe disorders (Foa et al., 1999b). Randomized, controlled trials are needed to empirically evaluate this proposal. According to research on other anxiety disorders, particularly panic disorder (Taylor, 2000), the effects of CBT may be compromised if it is combined with benzodiazepines. This may be because benzodiazepines dampen the level of emotion evoked by exposure exercises, thereby interfering with fear extinction. A further concern is that the sedating effects of benzodiazepines are readily detected by patients, especially if they take short-acting medications such as lorazepam on an as-needed basis. Under these conditions, the patients may be likely to attribute their therapeutic gains to the drug rather than to their efforts in therapy and therefore cease to practice CBT exercises that would otherwise have reduced their symptoms and given the person a sense of mastery and self-control. Accordingly, more treatment (CBT plus medications) may not necessarily be better than CBT alone in the treatment of PTSD.

A further caveat in adding medication involves the recent concerns about prescribing SSRIs to children and adolescents. Research on these populations suggests that SSRIs have limited efficacy and may have untoward side effects such as increased suicidal ideation and aggression (Garland, 2004). More conservative (i.e., largely psychosocial) interventions may be optimal for treating traumatized children and adolescents.

Cognitive Enhancers

Another approach to enhancing the reduction of PTSD symptoms involves the search for pharmacological agents than facilitate the extinction of emotional responses by strengthening the inhibition of trauma memories. Recall from Chapter 4 that evidence suggests that amygdala NMDA receptors play an important role in conditioned fear extinction. This has prompted studies of whether NMDA agonists, administered before exposure therapy, facilitate extinction. One such compound is D-cycloserine, which has been used for years in humans to treat tuberculosis and is not associated with significant side effects. Animal research has shown that this compound facilitates extinction (Walker, Ressler, Lu, & Davis, 2002). It or similar agents might be usefully combined with exposure therapy in the treatment of clinical fear. Findings so far suggest that this compound may facilitate exposure-related fear reduction and could be useful as a pharmacological adjunct to exposure therapy for PTSD (Davis et al., 2005; Heresco-Levy et al., 2002; Ressler et al., 2004). The compound could be administered shortly before an imaginal or situational exposure exercise in order to facilitate the reduction (extinction) of trauma-related distress. Other pharmacological agents, such as oxytocin or oral cortisone, may also facilitate CBT for PTSD (Ginsberg, 2004; Soravia et al., 2006).

SUMMARY

From the perspective of patient preference, psychosocial interventions and medications are equally acceptable options (Roy-Byrne, Berliner, Russo,

Zatzick, & Pitman, 2003), and the evidence suggests that CBT is one of the most effective PTSD treatments. But like all currently available treatments, CBT is far from universally efficacious, so various efforts have been made to enhance or modify treatment protocols. Treatment may be improved by matching particular interventions to particular clinical problems (e.g., using cognitive restructuring for trauma-related guilt) and by integrating CBT with other interventions.

PART II

TREATMENT METHODS AND PROTOCOLS

CHAPTER 6

Assessment

The selection of assessment instruments is shaped by several consider ations, including the goals of the assessment, the model the therapist uses to conceptualize the patient's problems, and the types of treatments being considered. The goals of assessment discussed in this chapter are focused largely on identifying causal factors—preexisting, precipitating, perpetuating, and protective factors—as formulated from the perspective of the emotional processing model described in Chapter 3. Thus, issues such as the patient's learning history and the nature and strength of dysfunctional beliefs are relevant here. The focus of this chapter is on the most clinically useful assessment methods, rather than on the plethora of tools used primarily in PTSD research. Clinically important tools include gold standard interview measures (available commercially or through research centers) and important new self-report measures, such as instruments for measuring dysfunctional beliefs associated with PTSD (including the one reproduced in Handout 6.1 at the end of this chapter).

The targets of a comprehensive assessment of patients referred for treatment of PTSD are listed in Table 6.1. A detailed initial assessment is required for a good treatment plan. Assessment then continues throughout CBT to monitor treatment progress and to collect further information to evaluate and, if necessary, revise the case formulation. To facilitate the collection of relevant information, the clinician can ask the patient's permission to interview one of the patient's significant others in order to get another perspective on the patient's symptoms and functioning. For example, a significant other who shares a bed with the patient can be a good source of information about nightmare frequency and severity, including vocalizations, movements, sweating, and sleepwalking (Wilson, 2001).

TABLE 6.1. Assessment Targets and Suggested Methods of Assessment

Assessment domain	Assessment method
General medical evaluation to rule out medical mimics of anxiety symptoms (e.g., general medical conditions causing hyperarousal symptoms) and to identify medical contraindications to CBT interventions (e.g., to identify patients who are physically too frail to endure the arousal associated with exposure exercises).	Background information from referral sources, including assessment reports and medical records (as appropriate). If this information is insufficient, then the therapist can gather information from the patient and request further information from the referral source.
Current and past Axis I and II diagnoses.	Clinical interview, such as the Structured Clinical Interview for DSM-IV (SCID-IV).
Detailed assessment of PTSD symptoms, including symptom severity and associated features such as trauma-related guilt or dissociative symptoms.	Clinical interview, combined if necessary with questionnaire measures, such as measures of dissociation, guilt, or anger.
Patient safety, including risk of subsequent trauma exposure and risk of suicide or homicide.	Clinical interview.
General history (e.g., developmental history) and trauma-related history.	Clinical interview.
Trauma-relevant dysfunctional beliefs.	Posttraumatic Cognitions Inventory, the Anxiety Sensitivity Index, clinical interview, and prospective monitoring.
Maladaptive safety signals and safety behaviors.	Clinical interview, along with prospective monitoring using Handout 6.2.
Living conditions, including (1) social functioning and relationships with important others (e.g., are they a source of hostility?), (2) occupational functioning, (3) ongoing stressors, large and small, and (4) coping resources, such as opportunities to extricate oneself from stressful circumstances (e.g., housing options to move to a less dangerous neighborhood).	Clinical interview.
Past history of treatment and reasons for seeking treatment at the present time.	Clinical interview.
Patient goals for therapy.	Clinical interview. The therapist needs to ensure that the patient's goals are realistic. For example, "Never thinking about the trauma again" is not a realistic goal.
Prognostic indicators, including variables indicating that the treatment protocol needs to be modified to overcome the poor prognostic factors.	Clinical interview.

(continued)

TABLE 6.1. (continued)

Assessment domain	Assessment method
Monitoring of symptoms and beliefs over the course of treatment.	Weekly or other periodic monitoring using questionnaires and brief interview questions. Useful questionnaires include the symptom section of the Posttraumatic Diagnostic Questionnaire and the Beck Depression Inventory-II. Prospective monitoring can also be used to assess whether dysfunctional beliefs are changing over the course of treatment.
Evaluating treatment outcome.	Posttraumatic Diagnostic Questionnaire, Beck Depression Inventory-II, Posttraumatic Cognitions Inventory, the Anxiety Sensitivity Index. If time permits, the SCID-IV could also be administered.

Note. This is a simplified guideline for assessment and may need to be modified according to particular clinical presentations. For example, if the patient had comorbid chronic pain, then this would need to be assessed in detail and monitored throughout the course of treatment.

INFORMED CONSENT AND MANDATORY REPORTING

Prior to commencing the assessment, it is necessary to advise the patient of the nature and limits of confidentiality. These vary, to some degree, from one jurisdiction to another, but there are many common elements. Confidentiality must be breached if patients are at imminent risk of harming themselves or others. If the patient is involved in litigation, such as suing for damages over the trauma, then it is possible that the intake evaluation and treatment progress notes may be subpoenaed. If the perpetrator of a trauma is still at large and is at risk for committing child abuse, then it also may be legally necessary to breach confidentiality to notify the appropriate authorities. If the patient referred for treatment is a minor, it also may be mandatory to report any maltreatment. Reporting elder abuse is also mandated in some jurisdictions.

Some special ethical or legal issues may be encountered when the clinician encounters PTSD patients suffering from anger problems. It is not uncommon for survivors of interpersonal violence to harbor fantasies of exacting revenge on the perpetrator. Although PTSD patients may experience a good deal of anger about what has happened to them, few ever act on their revenge fantasies. Nevertheless, the therapist should enquire about whether the patient has taken steps toward implementing a plan for retribution, such as purchasing a firearm, or whether he or she has a history of violence.

To illustrate the issues and methods covered in the remainder of this chapter, we begin with a case vignette, which we will revisit during our discussion of the various treatment issues and approaches.

Sarah, a 23-year-old single woman, was referred to a psychologist by her primary care physician. The referral note simply read, "This young woman suffers from depression and anxiety, and has a history of being assaulted. Please assess and treat." During the interview with the psychologist, Sarah provided the following information:

> "I met up with some friends while I was out shopping. They invited me to go with them to a nightclub downtown. I had exams coming up and really should have stayed home and studied, but I was feeling bored so I decided to go. I met my friends at about 10 P.M., where we had a few drinks. We started talking to a group of guys and one guy in particular started flirting with me. I vaguely recognized him from the newspapers; he's a local football player. At first I felt excited that a 'famous' guy would be interested in me but also a bit uneasy because he was coming on so strong. As the night wore on it was time to leave. It was about 2 A.M., I think. The football player offered to give me a ride home, rather than me taking the bus. I felt nervous about this, but he kept pressuring me, so eventually I said, OK. When we got to his car he put his arms around me and started talking really dirty. I said, like, 'no' and started struggling. He got really angry and started shouting, calling me a slut and other names. During the struggle he ripped open my blouse. I started screaming for him to let go. Then he grabbed me by the collar, pulled me up to his face, and head-butted me, twice. The first time, I couldn't believe what was happening; I was shocked, angry, and afraid. I can't recall much of what happened after he hit me the second time. I think I passed out. Next thing I remember I was on the ground with someone trying to help me. My head hurt, my nose was sore, and I was covered in dirt and blood. Someone called the police and an ambulance, and I was taken to hospital. I don't know what happened to the guy."

PATIENT SAFETY

It is essential to determine during the initial assessment whether the patient is physically safe in his or her daily life. Patients may neglect their own safety, which can put them at risk for revictimization. The patient might be suicidal, at risk for HIV or other disease exposure, or at risk for assault (e.g., if the patient is still living with a violent spouse). When the patient is living in hazardous circumstances, it may be necessary to involve a social services agency to arrange the necessary practical assistance. Once the patient's living situation has improved, then it may be appropriate to commence PTSD treatment.

The assessment with Sarah revealed no evidence that she was at risk for future harm. She had no further contact with the perpetrator of the abuse and was too ashamed to go to the police. The therapist expressed respect for her decision but also suggested that Sarah might change her mind in the future. The therapist made a mental note to explore the issue of trauma-related shame during therapy.

INTERVIEW STYLE
AND THE THERAPEUTIC NATURE OF ASSESSMENT

The assessment should provide the therapist with a good deal of relevant information, while also helping the patient gain a better understanding of the nature and potential solutions to his or her problems. A good assessment provides the beginnings of a sound therapeutic relationship.

Although formal cognitive-behavioral interventions are not implemented during the assessment phase, the clinician can offer reassuring comments, especially for patients who blame themselves for their actions, for example, "You must have done the right thing, since you are here to tell about it," or "Even if you feel you did something to encourage him, that did not give him the right to rape you" (Foa & Rothbaum, 1998). A version of the latter phrase was used with Sarah, who severely castigated herself for being assaulted.

If the patient becomes very distressed or dissociates during the assessment, then the clinician could suggest a short emotion regulation exercise (Chapter 9). After the assessment, a debriefing between the patient and clinician can take place, where the patient shares his or her experience with the assessment and describes what was helpful and what parts were the most difficult. This provides the clinician with important information. For example, if the patient has a history of substance use disorder, which may have developed in attempts to dampen arousal-related symptoms, then it is possible that drug cravings may have been triggered by the assessment (Coffey et al., 2002).

STRUCTURED AND UNSTRUCTURED
CLINICAL INTERVIEWS

Comparison of Diagnostic Interviews for PTSD

Diagnoses are important for beginning to build a case formulation and treatment plan, although diagnoses are insufficient in themselves for this purpose. For patients with suspected PTSD, there are several structured diagnostic interviews. Given that PTSD is commonly comorbid with other disorders, it is necessary to use an interview that assesses a range of disorders. Commonly used interviews for Axis I disorders include the Structured Clinical Interview for DSM-IV (SCID-IV: First, Spitzer, Gibbon, & Williams, 1996), the Anxiety Disorders Interview Schedule for DSM-IV (ADIS-IV: DiNardo, Brown, & Barlow, 1994), and the Composite International Diagnostic Interview (CIDI: Kessler & Ustun, 2004). The SCID-IV and CIDI, compared to the ADIS-IV are broader in the range of disorders they assess, as well as being more efficient. The ADIS-IV contains a number of questions and rating scales that may be useful for research purposes but are not needed for diagnostic purposes. The SCID-IV can be combined with a complementary measure for personality disorder, the SCID-II (First et al., 1994). The latter has the same structure and format of interview questions as the SCID-IV, thereby making them easy to combine. An advantage of combining the SCID-IV and SCID-II is that it encourages the clinician to look beyond the patient's most salient problems to identify psychiatric problems that might otherwise be missed (Wittchen, 1996). The SCID-IV and SCID-II have adequate reliability for the diagnosis of most of the disorders they assess (Taylor, 2000; Williams et al., 1992).

A limitation of the SCID-IV is that it was not designed to assess symptom severity, so other measures must be used to monitor the change in symptoms over the course of treatment. There are several interviews that have been developed specifically for the assessment of the frequency and intensity of PTSD symptoms, with the most popular being the Clinician Administered PTSD Scale (CAPS; Blake et al., 1995). The CAPS is widely used in research as a measure of treatment outcome, although it is insufficient for diagnostic purposes because it does not assess other Axis I disorders. In routine clinical practice, where there may not be sufficient time to use a lengthy interview to monitor treatment progress and outcome, the CAPS can be replaced with a shorter self-report measure of PTSD symptoms.

Sarah's SCID-IV interview indicated a diagnosis of chronic PTSD and current major depressive disorder, with a history of childhood separation anxiety. The following were examples of her PTSD avoidance symptoms: Sarah strived to avoid stimuli that triggered recollections of the trauma, including anything to do with football, tall tattooed men, drinking alcohol, nightclubs, the sound of people arguing, the sound of sirens, hospitals, and the sight of her nose in the mirror (it was slightly crooked as a result of being broken). She also avoided wearing "sexy" clothes for fear that they would attract the attention of men, and avoided socializing with friends. The interview revealed that she avoided these things because they made her anxious and aroused upsetting recollections of the trauma. In other words, these forms of avoidance were features of PTSD, rather than features of withdrawal and isolation commonly associated with major depressive disorder.

Extending the Clinical Interview

Eliciting Important Details of the Trauma and Its Context

Structured interviews such as the SCID-IV elicit the basic details of the patient's trauma history, required for diagnostic purposes. But further interview questions are needed to obtain a detailed picture of the trauma and its context. This is important for the purpose of fully understanding the patient's trauma-related experiences and for planning imaginal exposure and other interventions. When assessing the patient's trauma history, the clinician should enquire about the aftermath. Often the aftermath is just as distressing, and sometimes even more so.

"It's strange," Sarah reported, "but the assault wasn't the worst of it. Maybe because I was drunk and don't remember it all that clearly. The worst part was what happened afterwards. While I was sitting in the waiting area of the hospital emergency room I started to sober up and began to realize what a mess I was in. I tried to cover myself with my torn blouse. I felt dirty, scared, and ashamed. I couldn't find my purse and I worried about my credit cards and how I was going to get home. A bunch of drunken guys were sitting nearby with a friend who looked like he'd been hurt in a fight. I guess they were waiting for a doctor. They were leering at me. I went to clean up in the washroom. I looked a real mess. I had two black eyes and my nose was squished to one side. I felt horrible, like a slut and a loser. Things got worse when a lady cop interviewed me in the waiting room. The way she was questioning me made me feel like it was my fault for getting into this mess. The doctor who saw me also seemed cold and uncaring."

As part of assessing the trauma and its context, one should also assess other stressors that may have occurred around about the time of the trauma, such as minor hardships that might add to the impact of the trauma (e.g., family conflict or a marital breakup occurring shortly before the trauma), or developmental milestones (e.g., leaving home for college).

When assessing details of trauma exposure in military veterans, it is important to remember that deployment in a war zone does not necessarily mean that the person was exposed to trauma. Moreover, people in the military can experience traumatic stressors that do not necessarily involve combat exposure (Keane, Street, & Stafford, 2004). To illustrate, in a study of over 3,000 veterans applying for PTSD-related disability benefits from the Department of Veterans Affairs, 71% of women and 4% of men reported being sexually assaulted during their military service (Murdoch, Polusny, Hodges, & O'Brien, 2004). Sexual harassment and racial discrimination are also important problems in the military, which can compound the effects of traumatic stress (Fontana, Litz, & Rosenheck, 2000; Loo et al., 2001).

Functional Analysis of Symptoms and Behaviors

During the clinical interview, one should attempt to obtain information about the temporal or causal relationships among variables. For example, are there stimuli that regularly trigger flashbacks or other dissociative reactions in the patient? Under which circumstances are ruminative thoughts about the trauma most likely to occur? Prospective monitoring, discussed later in this chapter, can add to the information derived from the clinical interview.

Posttrauma Social Support

The aftermath includes reactions by significant others, friends, and other people. Were they supportive of the patient, or were they critical, implicitly or even explicitly blaming the patient for being exposed to trauma?

"I stayed in my apartment for the rest of the week after the assault. I missed my exam and was too ashamed to tell the professor why I didn't take it. Eventually I had to leave the apartment to get groceries. I still looked horrible. I had a bandage on my nose and the bruises around my eyes had turned a sickly yellowish color. From the way my friends looked at me I could tell that they thought it was my fault. My mother even came out and said so. That made me even more ashamed and depressed."

When assessing social support, the clinician can inquire about the number and quality of friendships and family contacts, and whether these are perceived as supportive (Briere, 2004). The clinician can investigate whether any of the social contacts are characterized by high expressed emotion (i.e., criticism, hostility, and overinvolvement from significant others), which can exacerbate PTSD and interfere with treatment efficacy (Chapter 5).

Another important pattern to assess is whether there has been the gradual deterioration of social contacts. This could occur in a variety of ways. For example, the patient could be gradually withdrawing from social contacts, or other people could be increasingly avoiding the patient because it can be aversive to be with someone who is frequently dysphoric and irritable. It is also important to assess the availability, and use of, community resources. For example, are there community support groups or government assistance programs that the patient could draw on?

Personal and Family History

Information about the patient's personal and family history of psychopathology is typically obtained by clinical interview. This includes an assessment of the patient's pretrauma functioning, such as the presence of preexisting emotional or personality disorders. Knowledge about such factors can help the clinician estimate the patient's risk for problems in the future. If the patient had a pretrauma history of antisocial personality traits, for example, then he or she might be at risk for future trauma exposure.

Sarah suffered from separation anxiety as a young child, although this later abated. Aside from her recent assault, she had not had any other traumatic experiences. In fact, she reported having led a sheltered, privileged life in which she had never had to deal with any major stressors. During the interview she wondered whether her sheltered life had left her unprepared to deal with her current problems. Sarah believed that her mother had suffered from anxiety and depression but was not aware of any other family history of psychopathology.

Understanding the person's pretrauma level of functioning can also provide an indication of the maximum likely benefits of PTSD treatment, and whether other interventions might be required. If the person's pretrauma level of function was not very high, then the best that PTSD treatment might accomplish is to return the person to that modest level of functioning. This might be the case if, for example, PTSD arose in a person with a severe, preexisting personality disorder. To improve the person's level of functioning it would be necessary to treat the personality pathology.

A review of the patient's personal history also provides an opportunity to assess whether there are interactions between PTSD and other disorders or problems (Newman, Kaloupek, & Keane, 1996). This can reveal, for example, interrelations between PTSD and substance use disorders.

Malcolm was an oil-rig maintenance worker who was working on the scaffolding when he lost his footing and fell 30 feet onto the iron crossbeams below. He eventually recovered from his physical injuries but developed PTSD. Malcolm had always been a heavy drinker prior to his injury, but it never interfered with his social or occupational functioning. However, from the assessment it was clear that he relied on alcohol as his primary means of coping with stress. After he developed PTSD his alcohol consumption escalated to the point that he became severely alcohol dependent.

One should also assess the patient's history of previous treatment. If the patient has received partial or temporary benefit from previous behavioral or cognitive-behavioral therapy, information on why the response was incomplete can guide planning of the current course of treatment.

Interview Methods for Cognitive Assessment

The clinician can listen for themes in the patient's narrative, such as themes concerning safety, trust, power, esteem, intimacy, and danger, which can be explored with specific questioning (McCann & Pearlman, 1990). In addition, the clinician can directly ask questions to identify dysfunctional beliefs: What does the trauma mean to you? Does it say anything about the world, other people, or yourself? Why do you think it happened?

In response to such questions, Sarah expressed the following strongly held beliefs: "Life will never be the same," "People can't be trusted," "I'm a dirty, worthless person," "I have to stay on guard," "No one cares about what happens to you," "I can't trust my own judgment," "Danger is everywhere."

These beliefs may be summary statements of more basic, underlying beliefs. To identify the latter, the clinician can ask the patient to explain, in greater detail, the implications of the belief (e.g., what does it mean to the patient, or what would happen if the belief was true?). This is the downward arrow method (Burns, 1980). Such additional detail is important to elicit because cognitive restructuring is more effective when the therapist and patient are working with highly specific beliefs. Vague beliefs are difficult to challenge. The following is an example of this assessment concerning one of Sarah's beliefs.

THERAPIST (who was also the assessing clinician): You mentioned that you believe you're a dirty, worthless person. That must be a very painful thing to believe. And it sounds like something that would be important to work on in treatment. In order to do this, I need to get some more information about that belief, if that's all right with you.

SARAH: OK.

THERAPIST: Thanks. Please tell me, what do you mean when you call yourself dirty and worthless?

SARAH: I feel like I've become one of "those people," you know, like a tramp or a slut, who everybody looks down on. Somebody everyone sees as being a piece of trash.

THERAPIST: I don't think that way about you. I see you as a worthwhile person who happened to be in the wrong place at the wrong time. But to help me understand things, if it was true that you were trash, what would that mean to you?

SARAH: It would mean I would never be happy. My life would be ruined. I'd never have a family or career, and I'd probably wind up living on the streets.

THERAPIST: If that was true, what would happen?

SARAH: I'd probably be murdered.

THERAPIST: OK, to summarize, it sounds like you believe that the assault has been kind of like a death sentence; it's changed you into an unworthy person who is now doomed to a miserable life and early death.

SARAH: I guess when you spell it out, I do think all those things about myself. It's funny, but when all these things are spelled out, they don't seem all that believable. I mean, like you said, I was in the wrong place at the wrong time. That doesn't mean that my life will be ruined forever.

When this line of questioning is conducted with empathy and sensitivity, it yields important information and also can form the beginning of cognitive restructuring. In using this method, the clinician needs to ensure that the patient doesn't feel demeaned or ridiculed for expressing extreme or catastrophic beliefs.

Interview questions can also be used to assess patients' beliefs about their symptoms. For example, do they think that their reexperiencing symptoms will have harmful consequences, such as death or insanity? People who hold such beliefs tend to have elevated anxiety sensitivity, which appears to play an important role in PTSD (Chapter 2).

Cognitive assessment should not simply focus on negative beliefs, it should also assess whether patients hold any positive beliefs about themselves, the world, and other people, which could be strengthened in therapy. Similarly, there are questions that can be asked to assess whether the patient has developed any adaptive beliefs about the meaning of the trauma and its consequences (Schiraldi, 2000): Why did you survive? For what purpose? Why have you kept going? What is it that makes life worth living? What matters to you in life?

Assessing Maladaptive Coping Behaviors

Interview measures, combined with prospective monitoring, can be used to identify safety behaviors (e.g., avoidance, escape, checking, reassurance seeking) and safety signals. The latter are stimuli that the person believes will be associated with the absence of feared outcomes (e.g., carrying a concealed weapon in a shopping mall, or carrying a good-luck charm while driving). These are important to identify because they may perpetuate PTSD (Chapter 3). Attempts to suppress (avoid) trauma-related thoughts (e.g., by distraction) are other important safety behaviors to identify because thought suppression can contribute to the persistence of reexperiencing symptoms (Chapter 2). Maladaptive coping behaviors may also include reckless attempts at self-exposure, such as deliberate attempts to go into dangerous situations in order to overcome one's fears, or excessive acts of contrition (e.g., excessively donating or "overgiving" one's money or resources to others) in an attempt to assuage strong feelings of guilt (Matsakis, 1998). Here, persons may go to great lengths to perform acts of kindness, such as giving away their prized possessions or money, or overindulging their children or other family members. They may spend so much time helping others that they neglect their own well-being. For example, a survivor of spousal abuse may overgive to her children because of feeling guilty that her children were abused.

Maladaptive coping behaviors can be identified by asking questions contained in the SCID-IV to assess PTSD avoidance symptoms. Other useful questions include the following: Do you do anything to try to avoid your unwanted thoughts, images, or memories of the trauma? How about other symptoms: do you do anything to try to avoid feeling numb or anxious? Do you consume drugs or alcohol to cope with symptoms, for example, to cope with bad thoughts or feelings, or to get to sleep at night? Do you do anything harmful or risky to cope with bad feelings, like binge eating, cutting yourself, going on spending sprees, or engaging in unsafe sex? How do you keep yourself safe at home? How about when you go out? Is there anything you do or bring with you to protect yourself from harm? Do you have any checking routines that you use to feel safe, such as checking and rechecking that the doors and windows are locked at night? Do you ask other people for reassurance in order to feel safe, such as reassurance that it's safe to do a particular thing or go to a particular place? Please give me some examples.

Sarah's maladaptive coping behaviors included the following: staying home as much as possible, checking (three times) the locks of her front door and windows before retiring at night, sleeping with lights on, and trying to be with someone she trusted, such as her sister, whenever she had to leave the apartment.

SELF-REPORT INVENTORIES

Uses and Limitations

Structured clinical interviews are the gold standard for PTSD assessment. Self-report questionnaires are inappropriate for diagnosing PTSD, but they do play a useful role. Self-report inventories provide an efficient way of assessing a wide range of clinical variables, such as the strength of dysfunctional beliefs and commonly associated features like dissociation, depression, anger, and guilt. Self-report measures also can be used to assess response sets, such as symptom exaggeration or minimization. Finally, many self-report measures are short enough to be used at the beginning of each treatment session to monitor treatment progress.

Symptom Measures

There are three main classes of symptom measures used in the assessment of PTSD: (1) measures of trauma exposure and PTSD symptom severity (i.e., PTSD checklists), (2) measures of features that are commonly associated with PTSD (e.g., a measure of trauma-related guilt), and (3) multiscale inventories that assess PTSD and associated features and contain validity indices.

There are many PTSD checklists available, and only some of the better measures will be reviewed here. For clinicians wanting to use a psychometrically sound PTSD checklist to gauge symptom severity and monitor treatment progress for the full range of PTSD symptoms, the following are among the best measures:

- The Posttraumatic Diagnostic Scale (PDS; Foa, 1995). The scale contains a detailed trauma checklist, a full assessment of Criterion A, and items assessing the severity of each of the DSM-IV-TR PTSD symptoms. The scale has good reliability and validity and can detect treatment-related changes in PTSD (Foa, 1995; Taylor et al., 2003).
- The Davidson Trauma Scale (Davidson, 1996) is similar to the PDS in its coverage of PTSD symptoms. There are encouraging data on its reliability and validity, and the scale is sensitive to treatment effects (Davidson, 1996).
- The PTSD Checklist (Weathers, Litz, Huska, & Keane, 1994) similarly assesses each of the PTSD symptoms, and initial studies suggest that it has good psychometric properties (Ruggiero, Del Ben, Scotti, & Rabalais, 2003).

There is little to distinguish among these scales. Each takes about 5–10 minutes to complete. Details of their psychometric properties (norms, reliability, and validity), along with information on where to obtain the scales, are discussed elsewhere (e.g., Foa, 1995; Norris & Hamblen, 2004; Ruggiero et al., 2003). For clinicians assessing refugees, the Harvard Trauma Questionnaire can be useful because it has been translated into many different languages, including several Asian and Eastern European languages (Mollica et al., 1992, 2001).

Useful, psychometrically sound measures of features commonly associated with PTSD include the following. With the exception of the questionnaire measure of personality pathology, each of the following measures requires about 5 minutes to complete.

• The Trauma-Related Guilt Inventory (Kubany et al., 1996) is a useful measure to include in an assessment battery because guilt is easily overlooked in the clinical interview.
• The tendency to become angry, regardless of whether it is trauma related, can be assessed with the trait version of State–Trait Anger Expression Inventory (Spielberger, 1988).
• The Dissociative Experiences Scale (Bernstein & Putnam, 1986) is the most widely used questionnaire for assessing dissociative symptoms and has good psychometric properties. One study suggests that it can be broken down into two subscales, pathological dissociation (a putative categorical or present–absent entity) and nonpathological dissociation (Waller, Putnam, & Carlson, 1996). Subsequent research has found that this distinction is unreliable (Watson, 2003). Accordingly, the Dissociative Experiences Scale is typically scored according to the total sum of the items. As with all questionnaires, the clinician can scan the patient's responses to each of the items and ask follow-up questions to clarify high item scores.
• The most widely used self-report measure of depressive symptoms is the Beck Depression Inventory, which is now available in a second edition (BDI-II; Beck, Steer, & Brown, 1996).
• If there is insufficient time to conduct a structured clinical interview, then either the SCID-II screening questionnaire or the Personality Diagnostic Interview–4 (Hyler, 1994) could be used as a screen for DSM-IV-TR personality disorders.
• Additional measures can be added as needed, depending on the nature of the patient's presenting problems. These might include measures of chronic pain, substance use disorders, eating disorder symptoms, and so forth. Reviews of these various measures can be found in a number of sources. A particularly good source is Corcoran and Fischer (2000).

Some of the most widely used multiscale inventories include the Minnesota Multiphasic Personality Inventory–2 (MMPI-2; Butcher, Dahlstrom, Graham, Tellegen, & Kaemmer, 1989) and the Trauma Symptom Inventory (TSI; Briere, 1995). The TSI assesses PTSD symptoms along with other symptoms and associated personality traits (e.g., traits similar to borderline personality traits). The TSI contains validity scales, although recent research raises concerns about their adequacy (Elhai et al., 2005). A further problem is that the TSI contains a lot of items assessing sexual behavior, which are not relevant to patients who have not experienced sexual trauma and do not have sexual difficulties. For these patients, the items are irrelevant and needlessly intrusive.

The MMPI-2 is broader in scope than the TSI and offers a more detailed assessment of response sets via its many validity scales. The MMPI-2 clinical and validity scales have good psychometric properties. A good deal of research suggests that the MMPI-2 is useful in assessing PTSD malingering (e.g., Bury & Bagby, 2002; Elhai et al., 2002; Moyer, Burkhardt, & Gordon, 2002). A drawback of the MMPI-2 is the time required to complete the scale (60–90 minutes). Clinically, it is most useful when malingering or significant symptom exaggeration is suspected.

Dysfunctional Beliefs

Several measures have been developed to assess beliefs in trauma survivors. Most of these instruments are unpublished research tools that have not been psychometrically evaluated. Two of the best-known exceptions are the World Assumptions Scale (WAS; Janoff-Bulman, 1989) and the Posttraumatic Cognitions Inventory (PTCI; Foa et al., 1999c). The latter is reproduced in Handout 6.1 (pp. 115–116). An advantage of the PTCI over the WAS is that it draws on constructs and items from the WAS and similar scales, along with other findings about dysfunctional beliefs in PTSD, in order to develop a more comprehensive measure. The PTCI subscales were factor-analytically derived. Although the scale was designed to be comprehensive, the items can be parsimoniously combined to form three factor-analytically derived subscales: (1) negative cognitions about the self (mean of items 2–6, 9, 12, 14, 16, 17, 20, 21, 24–26, 28–30, 33, 35, and 36 in Handout 6.1); (2) negative cognitions about world (mean of items 7, 8, 10, 11, 18, 23, and 27); and (3) self-blame (mean of items 1, 15, 19, 22, and 31). Items 13, 32, and 34 are not included in subscales but can provide clinically useful information.

The PTCI is sensitive to treatment-related change (Foa & Rauch, 2004). For no trauma controls, the median (and SD) scores on each of the subscales (self, world, and self-blame) are as follows: 1.1 (0.8), 2.1 (1.4), and 1.0 (1.5). For PTSD patients assessed prior to treatment, the corresponding median (and SD) scores are: 3.6 (1.5), 5.0 (1.3), and 3.2 (1.7) (Foa et al., 1999c). Higher scores correspond to stronger beliefs. As with other scales, the clinician should scan all of the responses to the PTCI items to look for high scores, which may reveal particularly strongly held dysfunctional beliefs that need to be addressed in therapy.

A domain of dysfunctional beliefs not assessed by the PTCI concerns the patient's beliefs about the meaning of his or her arousal-related symptoms (i.e., anxiety sensitivity). Recall from Chapter 2 that PTSD patients often believe that arousal-related reactions—such as uncontrollable thoughts, rapid heartbeat, or shaking and trembling—have catastrophic consequences, such as insanity, death, or social rejection. The most widely used method for assessing such beliefs is the Anxiety Sensitivity Index (Peterson & Reiss, 1992).

PROSPECTIVE MONITORING

Prospective (ongoing) monitoring—during a baseline period of 1 or 2 weeks after the intake assessment but before commencing treatment, and throughout the course of treatment—can provide useful information about the patient's symptoms, beliefs, behaviors, and triggering stimuli. Such information can be used to better understand the patient's problems and to plan interventions such as exposure or cognitive restructuring exercises.

A form for prospectively monitoring these variables, along with two of Sarah's entries, appears in Handout 6.2 (pp. 117–118). The handout contains an "insights" column, in which patients can record what they learned from each monitoring episode. This can enhance the therapeutic value of assessment by promoting adaptive belief change, as illustrated in the first example listed in the handout. Monitoring can also help the patient identify stimuli that trigger intrusive memories and distressing emotions. Thus, the upsetting memories and emotions can become more predictable and less mysterious and frightening.

The insights column can also reveal maladaptive cognitive processes. The second example entry in the handout shows that Sarah was not able to learn anything new from the monitoring exercise but instead returned to unanswered "why" questions. This indicates that she was ruminating about the trauma and its implications. Recall from Chapter 2 that rumination is associated with the persistence of PTSD. Thus, the "insights" column can reveal clinically important information about maladaptive thoughts or thought processes. In other words, what the patient lists as insights might be insightful but not necessarily beneficial. But they nevertheless can provide the therapist with information relevant to treatment planning (e.g., planning to use interventions for reducing rumination).

SPECIAL POPULATIONS

Children and Adolescents

Interview measures of both the patient and caregiver are used for younger children (especially those age 7 and younger), whereas interviews and questionnaires for the patient alone can be used for older children and adolescents. Regardless of age, the diagnostic method of choice remains the structured interview. Useful diagnostic measures include the Clinician Administered PTSD Scale for Children and Adolescents (CAPS-CA; Nader et al., 2004) and the children's version of the Anxiety Disorders Interview Schedule (Silverman & Albano, 1996). The latter is particularly useful for providing an assessment of PTSD and any comorbid disorders, such as behavioral problems that may arise as a result of trauma exposure (e.g., oppositional behaviors or separation anxiety).

As part of these assessments, one should examine family factors that may facilitate or impede the resolution of the child's PTSD, such as the caregiver's emotional response to the trauma, the caregiver's ability to talk with and support the child, the caregiver's reinforcement of appropriate coping strategies, and the impact of the trauma on family functioning (Salmon & Bryant, 2002).

There are several challenges in assessing PTSD in children and adolescents, particularly in young children. Children may have difficulty understanding complex concepts such as emotional numbing, and their failure to recall important aspects of the trauma may simply be due to their failure to appreciate its significance at the time rather than to psychogenic amnesia. To facilitate the ratings of symptoms, the CAPS-CA includes pictorial scales and cartoons to facilitate the assessment of symptoms.

A further problem is the consistently poor correspondence between parent and child reports of the child's symptoms of anxiety and depression. Some evidence suggests that children provide more reliable information concerning their internal states than that which others provide, especially after trauma. Caregivers' reports of children's PTSD symptoms tend to indicate less distress than children's self-reports, possibly because children disclose less trauma-related distress to caregivers in order not to upset them (Lonigan, Phillips, & Richey, 2003).

For children ages 3–9 years, the clinician can ask them to draw the traumatic event, which can help the child provide a more detailed verbal description of what happened, while reminding the child to draw only what actually happened. Drawing may facilitate memory retrieval, and it may reduce the social and emotional demands inherent in the interview context by providing a focus other than the interviewer (Salmon & Bryant, 2002). The merits of using anatomically correct dolls for helping children describe episodes of abuse remains controversial because of debates about the validity of the assessment information (Dickinson, Poole, & Bruck, 2005; Hungerford, 2005).

The Elderly

With some exceptions, assessment in the elderly is much the same as assessment in younger adults. Age-related changes need to be considered in the assessment of symptoms. Age-related reductions in the duration and quality of sleep should not be confused with PTSD-related insomnia. Sleep difficulties are likely to be PTSD related rather than age related if they (1) arise shortly after trauma exposure, (2) arise in concert with other PTSD symptoms (particularly other hyperarousal symptoms), or (3) fluctuate over time in concert with fluctuations in other PTSD symptoms.

One needs to be careful not to confuse trauma-related avoidance with avoidance due to physical limitations. For example, an elderly assault survivor might be reluctant to venture out of the house, but this may be due to fear of falling and breaking a hip rather than fear of being assaulted. Similarly, difficulty remembering important aspects of a trauma need not indicate psychogenic amnesia; it could be due to age-related deterioration in memory function.

Cultural Considerations

Cultural factors are important concerning the way in which people describe their distress, and in terms of their willingness to discuss emotional problems. In some cases the person may describe his or her problems entirely in somatic terms (e.g., headaches or generalized malaise) rather than in terms of reexperiencing and hyperarousal symptoms. Thus, it is important for the clinician to have background knowledge of the patient's culture. In some cases it may be necessary to use a translator to conduct the assessment interview. Ideally, the translator will have at least a basic understanding of PTSD and DSM-IV-TR, and will not become emotionally overwhelmed by the patient's discussion of his or her traumatic experiences.

For therapists to have credibility with their patients, it may even be important for them to display familiarity with the subcultures of patients belonging to the mainstream culture. For example, the therapist can gain credibility with Vietnam combat-era veterans if the therapist understands acronyms like FNG or REMF. These terms are described in many sites on the Internet and need not be defined here.

TROUBLESHOOTING

The initial assessment can be stressful because the patient is asked to describe emotionally painful experiences. One needs to be sensitive to the patient's current level of functioning. Therapist skill is required to help the patient through this process. To avoid problems, the clinician could say, at the outset of the interview, something like the following:

> "In order for me to understand your problems and plan for treatment, I
> need to ask some questions about your trauma experiences and about
> the problems you've been having. Sometimes, these sorts of questions

can stir up unpleasant memories and emotions. I want you to know that you're in charge of the assessment process. If the assessment is getting too painful we can stop at any time, or if you need to take a break, please let me know. Remember, this assessment is for you, and you're in charge. OK?"

Sometimes patients are unable to reveal all of their traumatic experiences in a single interview. Typically, they are able to reveal enough detail for the purposes of assessment and treatment planning, although the therapist should not be surprised if the patient reveals other traumas, or particularly painful details of a given trauma, during the course of therapy.

Another challenge in the assessment of PTSD is nonadherence, especially nonadherence with prospective monitoring. If the patient is unable to complete the intake assessment, then it is doubtful that he or she will be able to complete treatment (Foa & Rothbaum, 1998). The reasons for assessment nonadherence need to be evaluated in an effort to solve the problem. Nonadherence may occur if the patient does not understand the rationale and importance of a thorough assessment. Other reasons for nonadherence should also be investigated and addressed, such as patients' fears that they will become uncontrollably upset if they think about or monitor their symptoms. In such cases a gradual approach could be used, where the patient monitors symptoms for a short period of time (e.g., half a day) and reviews the outcome. Patients typically overestimate the degree of distress associated with discussing or monitoring their symptoms. Other methods of improving adherence with prospective monitoring include the following:

- Emphasize that treatment has the greatest change of success if it is based on accurate information.
- Elicit an agreement from the patient to complete the assessment measures.
- Identify beforehand any obstacles to completing the assessment, such as obstacles to prospective monitoring, and develop strategies for circumventing these difficulties.
- Ensure that the patient is adequately trained in using the prospective monitoring forms.
- Review the results of any prospective monitoring during each session and ensure that you acknowledge or praise the patient's efforts at monitoring his or her symptoms.

During the clinical interview, if the clinician suspects that the patient is either underreporting symptoms (sometimes due to the desire to avoid painful memories) or overreporting symptoms (due, for example, to a "cry for help" or symptom exaggeration driven by financial incentives), then the MMPI-2 could be administered to gauge the seriousness of under- or overreporting. The use of this instrument for these purposes is described in detail elsewhere (e.g., Butcher, 2005; Graham, 1999; Pope, Butcher, & Seelen, 2000).

SUMMARY

For patients presenting for treatment of PTSD, a comprehensive assessment is required in order to make an accurate diagnosis, to develop a case formulation and treatment plan, and to monitor treatment progress. Although assessment should be tailored to the specifics of the patient, there are several measures that can be usefully administered to all patients. A comprehensive package is presented in Table 6.1. Most of the measures described in this chapter are available from commercial distributors; an exception is the Posttraumatic Cognitions Inventory, presented in Handout 6.1.

HANDOUT 6.1. Posttraumatic Cognitions Inventory

Instructions: We are interested in the kind of thoughts that you may have had after a traumatic experience. Below are a number of statements that may or may not be representative of your thinking. Please read each statement carefully and tell us how much you AGREE or DISAGREE with each statement. People react to traumatic events in many different ways. There are no right or wrong answers to these statements.

	Totally disagree	Disagree very much	Disagree slightly	Neutral	Agree slightly	Agree very much	Totally agree
1. The event happened because of the way I acted	1	2	3	4	5	6	7
2. I can't trust that I will do the right thing	1	2	3	4	5	6	7
3. I am a weak person	1	2	3	4	5	6	7
4. I will not be able to control my anger and will do something terrible	1	2	3	4	5	6	7
5. I can't deal with even the slightest upset	1	2	3	4	5	6	7
6. I used to be a happy person but now I am always miserable	1	2	3	4	5	6	7
7. People can't be trusted	1	2	3	4	5	6	7
8. I have to be on guard all the time	1	2	3	4	5	6	7
9. I feel dead inside	1	2	3	4	5	6	7
10. You can never know who will harm you	1	2	3	4	5	6	7
11. I have to be especially careful because you never know what can happen next	1	2	3	4	5	6	7
12. I am inadequate	1	2	3	4	5	6	7
13. I will not be able to control my emotions, and something terrible will happen	1	2	3	4	5	6	7
14. If I think about the event, I will not be able to handle it	1	2	3	4	5	6	7
15. The event happened to me because of the sort of person I am	1	2	3	4	5	6	7
16. My reactions since the event mean that I am going crazy	1	2	3	4	5	6	7
17. I will never be able to feel normal emotions again	1	2	3	4	5	6	7
18. The world is a dangerous place	1	2	3	4	5	6	7
19. Somebody else would have stopped the event from happening	1	2	3	4	5	6	7
20. I have permanently changed for the worse	1	2	3	4	5	6	7
21. I feel like an object, not like a person	1	2	3	4	5	6	7
22. Somebody else would not have gotten into this situation	1	2	3	4	5	6	7
23. I can't rely on other people	1	2	3	4	5	6	7

(continued)

	Totally disagree	Disagree very much	Disagree slightly	Neutral	Agree slightly	Agree very much	Totally agree
24. I feel isolated and set apart from others	1	2	3	4	5	6	7
25. I have no future	1	2	3	4	5	6	7
26. I can't stop bad things from happening to me	1	2	3	4	5	6	7
27. People are not what they seem	1	2	3	4	5	6	7
28. My life has been destroyed by the trauma	1	2	3	4	5	6	7
29. There is something wrong with me as a person	1	2	3	4	5	6	7
30. My reactions since the event show that I am a lousy coper	1	2	3	4	5	6	7
31. There is something about me that made the event happen	1	2	3	4	5	6	7
32. I will not be able to tolerate my thoughts about the event, and I will fall apart	1	2	3	4	5	6	7
33. I feel like I don't know myself anymore	1	2	3	4	5	6	7
34. You never know when something terrible will happen	1	2	3	4	5	6	7
35. I can't rely on myself	1	2	3	4	5	6	7
36. Nothing good can happen to me anymore	1	2	3	4	5	6	7

HANDOUT 6.2. Prospective Monitoring Form and Example Entries

Instructions: The purpose of this form is to collect information about your symptoms and the situations in which they occur. Please carry this form with you (e.g., in your wallet or purse) and record details of upsetting experiences after they occur, or as soon as possible afterwards. Use extra sheets as needed.

Day and date	Situation: Situation in which upsetting thoughts or emotions occurred.	Specific trigger: Specific things that triggered unpleasant thoughts or emotions. These could be a particular thing, person, or even a bodily sensation. If you are unable to identify a trigger, please leave this column blank.	Thoughts, memories, or mental images: Thoughts, memories, or mental images that occurred when you were exposed to the trigger.	Emotional reactions: Emotions that occurred when you were exposed to the trigger. Rate the intensity of the emotions on a 0 to 100 scale, where 0 = none and 100 = the maximum intensity.	Behaviors: What did you do after you were exposed to the trigger? For example, did you escape from the situation or use some sort of coping behavior, or did you simply stay in the situation until the unpleasant emotions passed?	Insights: List any insights that occur to you as a result of collecting information on upsetting experiences. These could include insights about the sorts of triggers that bother you, or insights about the way your mind works.
EXAMPLE	Eating lunch in the food court.	A friend came up behind me and tapped me on the shoulder.	I had the thought that I'm in danger, associated with an image of being assaulted.	Momentarily startled and frightened (100%), and then felt anxious for a while afterwards (40%).	I jumped up from the table. When I saw it was my friend I calmed down and sat down. After my friend left, I went home to be by myself, away from people.	I'm afraid of people. I tend to assume the worst when someone touches me. I need to feel more comfortable with people. I need to be able to trust people while also being able to protect myself.
EXAMPLE	Watching the news on TV.	Saw a news report on terrorist attacks.	Even though the news report had nothing to do with my traumatic experience, it made me think about how dangerous it is to live in the world.	Anxious (40%), sad (50%), and angry about how other people behave (50%).	Turned off the TV and told myself that I wasn't going to watch the news anymore.	No particular insights, but some unanswered questions came to mind: Why are people so cruel? Why is there so much evil in the world? Why is life so unfair?

(continued)

117

HANDOUT 6.2. *(page 2 of 2)*

Day and date	Situation	Specific trigger	Thoughts, memories, or mental images	Emotional reactions	Behaviors	Insights

CHAPTER 7

Cognitive-Behavioral Therapy
An Overview

In Chapter 3 we saw that the emotional processing model offers one of the best accounts of PTSD. This model suggests that a key ingredient of effective treatment is to provide patients with corrective learning experiences, which can occur in the form of cognitive restructuring or exposure exercises. These interventions are facilitated by including other interventions, such as psychoeducation and emotion regulation skills. There are many ways in which the various interventions can be assembled into a treatment protocol. One of the challenges in devising a treatment plan is to select, among the many treatment protocols, an empirically supported treatment package that can be adapted to the needs of a given patient. To help the therapist navigate through this welter of treatment packages, the present chapter offers an overview of treatment packages, along with guidelines for selecting among them.

In this chapter we review the various elements of CBT and consider the ways in which the elements can be combined. Generic PTSD protocols will be discussed along with protocols for special populations, such as those for PTSD in children and for PTSD comorbid with substance use disorders. Issues in selecting and sequencing interventions will be considered, along with guidelines concerning therapist self-care. The latter is an important component of good therapy. This is because CBT is more than just a collection of techniques; treatment efficacy critically depends on the interpersonal skills and emotional well-being of the person delivering the treatment. If the therapist is highly distressed by listening to patients describing their traumatic experiences, the quality of therapy could be compromised.

TREATMENT ELEMENTS

Therapist Characteristics

The style of PTSD therapy is much the same as those of cognitive-behavioral treatments for other disorders (e.g., Beck et al., 1979; Taylor, 2000; Taylor & Asmundson, 2004). Therapist warmth, genuineness, acceptance, accurate empathy, and reflective listening are used to build a trusting therapeutic relationship. It is important to create a nonjudgmental atmosphere so the patient can discuss emotionally painful topics.

The therapist strives to avoid any implication that the patient should be blamed for what happened to him or her. Regardless of whether the patient's actions contributed to the trauma, nobody deserves to be traumatized (Resick & Schnicke, 1993). Being blamed by others simply contributes to the self-denigration commonly seen in people with PTSD.

Most trauma patients, including survivors of sexual assault, work equally well with male or female therapists (Resick & Schnicke, 1993). However, some patients express strong preferences either way. Sometimes preference for, say, a female therapist can be a form of avoidance, but it may be necessary to permit this avoidance in order for the patient to enter treatment.

Interventions

The methods used in treating PTSD can be grouped into two classes: those commonly used (core interventions) and those implemented on an as-needed basis. Both are listed in Table 7.1. Although the core interventions focus on the patient's traumatic experiences and PTSD symptoms, these interventions—particularly cognitive restructuring and emotion regulation exercises—can help patients better cope with daily stressors in their lives. Emotion regulation exercises are also used to help patients tolerate and complete exposure exercises. If the patient has particularly low tolerance for distress, or has a tendency to engage in self-destructive behaviors when distressed (e.g., drug abuse, wrist cutting, or impulsive appetitive behaviors such as binge eating), then exposure exercises would not be implemented until emotion regulation exercises have enabled the patient to better cope with aversive emotions. Mastery and pleasure exercises and interpersonal interventions (e.g., couple therapy) can bolster the patient's level of social support, which is also important for coping with stress in general, and with the distress associated with exposure therapy. The general applicability of CBT interventions for dealing with daily stressors is important because people with PTSD tend to be more reactive to minor stressors than people without the disorder; that is, PTSD is associated with a greater and longer-lasting emotional and physiological arousal in response stressors

TABLE 7.1. Cognitive-Behavioral Interventions for PTSD

	Chapter
Core interventions	
• Psychoeducation. This includes information about PTSD and its treatment, along with the case formulation, which is shared with the patient.	9
• Treatment engagement strategies.	9
• Emotion regulation exercises, such as breathing retraining, relaxation exercises, and mastery and pleasure exercises. These can help patients reduce negative emotions and promote positive emotions.	9
• Some mix of cognitive restructuring and exposure, that is, either exposure alone, cognitive restructuring alone, or a combination of the two. Exposure can include imaginal, interoceptive, and situational exposure exercises.	10–13
• Preparation of a posttreatment program for maintaining and improving gains, and for preventing relapse.	14
Interventions implemented on an as-needed basis	
• Grounding exercises for managing dissociative symptoms.	9
• Anger management exercises.	13
• Interventions for treating comorbid disorders, particularly disorders that may interfere with PTSD treatment or disorders that may worsen as a result of PTSD treatment. Examples include substance use disorders and chronic pain disorders.	14
• Interpersonal skills training, such as assertiveness training.	14
• Couple or family interventions.	14

(Chapter 4). Interpersonal skills training is also used to reduce the risk of revictimization.

When the patient is ready for exposure therapy, it is implemented gradually, and typically only one type of exposure exercise (imaginal, interoceptive, or situational) is conducted per session. However, more than one form of exposure may be implemented during a given week as a homework assignment (e.g., a combination of imaginal and situational exposure exercises). When planning exposure therapy, it is important to address any misconceptions that the patient or his or her significant others or referring clinician may have about the treatment. The patient and relevant others should be advised that (1) exposure is one of the most effective interventions for PTSD, (2) exposure is implemented gradually, usually with the aid of coping strategies, and only when the patient is ready, (3) exposure is generally quite safe and does not involve exposure to objectively risky situations, and (4) exposure, like all potent treatments, has side effects, but they tend to be short-lived (e.g., transient increases in anxiety and nightmare frequency). Clinically, most patients who are suitable for exposure are willing to undergo this form of therapy. The rate of treatment dropout for exposure (used as the sole intervention) is no different from the dropout rates of PTSD treatments that don't use exposure, and exposure can be effective even for patients who have been multiply traumatized (Chapter 5).

If the patient suffers from prominent anger, guilt, shame, or mental defeat, then cognitive restructuring would be used in addition to, or instead of, exposure. Foa and Rothbaum (1998) recommended using cognitive restructuring and emotion regulation skills for patients with severe hyperarousal symptoms. Although these interventions are useful, extreme hyperarousal does not mean that exposure can't be a component of treatment. Severity of hyperarousal does not predict the outcome of exposure therapy (Taylor, 2004; see also Chapter 5). However, cognitive restructuring alone might be used if the patient is unwilling or unable to tolerate exposure, or if there is concern that exposure might worsen a comorbid problem, such as a substance use disorder.

Problems with treatment nonadherence are addressed by the therapist and patient jointly discussing and analyzing the problems to identify possible solutions. Treatment engagement strategies can be used to enhance the patient's motivation for completing treatment. Treatment sessions are tapered toward the end of treatment (i.e., sessions are increasingly spaced apart, so the patient can become increasingly self-reliant), and the therapist and patient devise a plan for maintaining and extending treatment gains, and for preventing relapse.

Therapy Structure

The goals of the early stages of treatment are to establish a sound therapeutic relationship, to formulate a treatment plan and discuss it with the patient, and to implement psychoeducation and emotion regulation strategies. Throughout the entire course of treatment, the therapy is educational, interactive, and collaborative. Beliefs are framed as hypotheses to be tested, and the therapist and patient work together to identify evidence for and against the beliefs. The therapist encourages the patient to ask questions and express any doubts about what is discussed during treatment. For example, the therapist might ask, "Does the cognitive-behavioral model of PTSD fit with your experience?" This helps the therapist identify any misconceptions about treatment and other problems.

Sessions tend to be highly structured, particularly at the beginning of therapy. Sessions typically start with a review of the patient's symptoms over the past week and a review of any assigned homework. This gives the therapist an idea of what is important to cover during the session. As part of the check-in at the beginning of each session, patients can be asked to name at least one brief example of good coping since the last session (e.g., "What went well for you this week? Were there any good things that happened?"). This encourages patients to respect their strengths and positively reinforces efforts at overcoming their problems (Najavits, 2002). Then an agenda is set for the remainder of the session. The agenda typically includes a discussion of specific problems along with plans for interventions. Some interventions are implemented during the session, whereas others are assigned as homework. Sessions typically end with the patient and therapist producing a verbal summary of the session (e.g., "What was today's session like for you? What was the main take-home message for you?"). The importance of homework and continued practice of the various exercises is emphasized.

Throughout each session feedback is elicited to check the patient's understanding of the material, for example, "Can I ask you to summarize what we've just discussed so I can check that we're on the same track?" During each session the therapist provides periodic capsule summaries of important topics that have been discussed and asks whether the patient agrees with the summaries. Capsule summaries help educate the patient, help the therapist check the accuracy of his or her understanding of the patient's problems, and help the patient and therapist focus on the most important issues. Sessions are often audiotaped and the patient is asked to listen to the tape in between sessions. This is to consolidate learning. Learning is further facilitated if the patient writes out a summary of the most important things learned from the tape.

SELECTING A TREATMENT PROTOCOL

There are many empirically supported protocols (e.g., Foa & Rothbaum, 1998; Marks, Lovell, Noshirvani, Livanou, & Thrasher, 1998; Resick & Schnicke, 1993). These protocols, even the ones initially developed for a specific trauma population such as rape- or combat-related PTSD, can be used, sometimes with some modification, with a range of trauma populations and symptom profiles. The protocols can be selected and adapted to the needs of a given patient, based on information contained in the case formulation and treatment plan.

Group versus Individual Treatment

CBT protocols can be used in either individual or group format. On average, both formats are equally effective (van Etten & Taylor, 1998). Group therapy is most useful for patients who have all experienced the same trauma and have much the same level of symptom severity and adaptive functioning. An advantage of group therapy is that many patients can be treated at once, and patients can gain emotional support from one another. Being in a group of people who have experienced similar traumatic events can reduce the patient's sense of isolation and estrangement from others, and can reduce the stigma associated with having an emotional disorder.

Some cognitive-behavioral interventions are readily implemented in groups. Psychoeducation and emotion regulation exercises are readily conducted in groups. Group-based cognitive structuring can be used to address general themes in the dysfunctional beliefs held by most patients. However, if cognitive restructuring is a prominent part of therapy, then individual treatment may be preferable because it can be difficult to devote a sufficient amount of time in the treatment group to the patients' particular beliefs. Similarly, imaginal exposure may be more successful if implemented individually (Turner, Beidel, & Frueh, 2005). A further problem with group therapy is that some patients may become highly disturbed by listening to the traumatic experiences of other patients. Also, trauma-related anger or irritability can disrupt the smooth running of groups. For practitioners in private practice or working in small clinics, it can be difficult to recruit enough patients suffering from the same sort of trauma to form a treatment group. Including patients with mixed trauma (e.g., patients with PTSD associated with combat and those with rape-related PTSD) may lead patients to feel embarrassed about discussing their particular trauma (e.g., sexual assault) in front of other patients who have not experienced such trauma. Thus, despite the advantages of group treatment, there are several important disadvantages. The selection of group or individual format depends on weighing these factors as they apply to a given clinical setting. If the therapist is planning to treat a large number of disaster survivors, for example, then one might opt for group treatment. For complex cases requiring highly individualized treatment protocols, individual treatment may be preferable. The treatment methods described throughout this volume can be used in both treatment formats, although for illustrative purposes the individual treatment format is used to demonstrate how the methods are applied.

Empirically Supported Protocols

Generic protocols, which have been used to treat a range of trauma populations, usually involve 8–20 sessions, typically weekly, of 60–90 minutes each for individual treatment or 120 minutes for group treatment. Commonly used generic protocols are composed of the following: (1) intake assessment and case formulation (1–2 sessions), (2) developing a mutually agreeable treatment plan, providing psychoeducation, and commencing practice of emotion regulation skills such as breathing retraining (1–2 sessions), (3) cognitive restructuring or commencement of imaginal exposure

(4 sessions), (4) continuation of cognitive restructuring and imaginal exposure or a gradual shift to include other types of exposure, particularly situational exposure (4 sessions), and (5) continuation of interventions (e.g., for 4 sessions), with sessions spaced increasingly further apart, and the development of a treatment maintenance plan in the final two sessions.

Within these generic protocols there is a great deal of latitude, determined by patients' goals and the nature of their problems. Such flexibility is even built into treatment protocols used in treatment-outcome studies (Feeny, Hembree, & Zoellner, 2003; Taylor et al., 2003). This includes flexibility about the types of cognitive interventions and their targets, and the timing and pacing of exposure exercises. The latter is determined by the patient, in consultation with therapist. For protocols combining exposure and cognitive restructuring, there is also a great deal of latitude about how these interventions are combined. Restructuring can be implemented before, during, and after exposure. If stressors unexpectedly arise during the course of treatment, then it is sometimes necessary to suspend exposure therapy and focus on generic stress management (e.g., an increased focus on emotion regulation exercises and problem solving) until the crisis has passed.

Other interventions can be added to the generic protocols on an as-needed basis. For example, interpersonal skills training might be included for a rape survivor who has trauma-induced assertiveness difficulties. Grounding exercises would be added for patients with prominent dissociative symptoms. Interoceptive exposure would be added for patients who have high anxiety sensitivity. This form of exposure is especially useful for patients with comorbid PTSD and panic attacks (Taylor, 2004).

For PTSD patients with comorbid substance use disorders, the most promising protocol is the Seeking Safety program, as described in the treatment manual by Najavits (2002). Patients receive 20 or more sessions of treatment for substance use problems combined with stress management training. The latter involves cognitive restructuring and training in emotion regulation skills. Once the substance use disorder is in stable remission (for at least 6 months—the window within which the risk for relapse is highest; Brecht, von Mayrhauser, & Anglin, 2000; Marlatt & Donovan, 2005), then trauma-focused exposure exercises can be implemented. Treatment of PTSD comorbid with psychotic disorders can take the same approach; treatment could consist of generic stress management along with pharmacological and other interventions for psychosis. Once the psychosis is in stable remission (for at least 12 months), then specific treatments for PTSD, such as exposure therapy, could be considered.

A similar approach can be used with patients with PTSD combined with severe chronic pain (Wald et al., 2004a). Treatment involves stress management plus pain management strategies. The latter may be multidisciplinary in nature (e.g., medication and CBT) and includes cognitive restructuring to address dysfunctional beliefs about pain, such as the belief that "If physical activity causes pain, then that means the activity is damaging to my body." Such "hurt equals harm" beliefs can promote a sedentary lifestyle, which is associated with muscle deconditioning and persistent pain (for further details, see Thorn's [2004] chronic pain treatment manual). Once the patient's pain is sufficiently under control, then exposure exercises can be gradually introduced, in combination with relaxation exercises to reduce the risk of exposure-induced pain exacerbation (e.g., due to tension-related muscle spasms).

Cloitre's protocol, called "Skills training in affect and interpersonal regulation plus prolonged imaginal exposure" (Cloitre et al., 2002; Levitt & Cloitre, 2005) also takes a two-stage approach. The first set of sessions (e.g., eight sessions) focuses on emotion regulation skills, cognitive restructuring, and interpersonal skills training. The second set of sessions (e.g., eight sessions) focuses on imaginal and situational exposure. This protocol can be used for people with marked problems with emotion regulation and interpersonal skills (i.e., so-called complex PTSD; see Chapter 1). Exposure alone is also effective in treating PTSD for such patients, although it does not modify maladaptive personality traits associated with emotional dysregulation and interpersonal problems (Taylor et al., 2006).

For other types of comorbidity, such as PTSD combined with mild to moderate major depression, it may not be necessary to modify a generic PTSD protocol, because associated problems like depression often abate when the PTSD is treated (Taylor et al., 2001, 2003). The case formulation and associated treatment plan can provide guidance as to whether comorbid disorders are likely to require specific treatment.

In some cases the patient may desire only to improve his or her ability to cope with daily stressors rather than work on trauma-related concerns. Here, stress management procedures could be used, such as emotion coping exercises and cognitive restructuring focused on beliefs or appraisals concerning daily stressors. Training in time management and problem-solving skills could also be added (see Taylor & Asmundson, 2004, for details on generic stress management). At a later date, when the patient is ready, he or she may wish to work directly on the traumatic experiences and PTSD.

Treatment protocols for children and for the elderly are broadly similar to the generic PTSD protocols discussed above, with the exception that the protocols are adapted to match the level of cognitive development or functioning of the child or elderly person. For example, cognitive restructuring would not be used, or used in a highly simplified form, for young children. Emotion regulation skills and exposure exercises can be implemented, for children ages 4–12, by using play therapy techniques (e.g., Kaduson & Schaefer, 1997, 2001), which are engaging and enjoyable for many children. These are illustrated in later chapters. In the case of sexually abused children, it can be valuable to include the nonoffending parent in therapy, as described in Deblinger and Heflin's (1996) treatment manual.

The selection of the various treatment options is summarized in the decision tree in Figure 7.1. Patients who fail to benefit substantially from 12 sessions of CBT are unlikely to profit from additional sessions (Foa & Rothbaum, 1998), that is, unless the source of the problem is identified and the treatment protocol is adjusted accordingly.

WORKBOOKS AND OTHER INSTRUCTIONAL MATERIALS

There are many patient guides and workbooks available for PTSD (e.g., Matsakis, 1996, 2003; Williams & Poijula, 2002). For most people suffering from PTSD, these books are unlikely to be sufficient, but they could be used as supplements for face-to-face therapy. The main problem with these books is that they tend to be long and detailed, which is off-putting for some patients. People with PTSD typically have concentration and memory problems, which makes it additionally difficult for them to benefit from self-help books. Short patient handouts, such as the ones presented in the later chapters in this volume, are clinically more useful. Such handouts are supplemented by additional information provided by the therapist.

If the patient desires further information or specifically requests a book that the patient or significant others could read, then one of the best choices is Matsakis's (1996) book titled *I Can't Get Over It* (2nd ed.). Although the book is over a decade old, and some of the research findings are outdated, it has several strengths that make up for these limitations The book is comprehensive and well written and provides good descriptions and illustrations of the many clinical problems associated with PTSD. The treatment advice is also generally consistent with a cognitive-behavioral approach. If patients express interest in reading this book, then it is suggested that the patient and therapist briefly review the material covered at the beginning of each treatment session. Patients should be encouraged to read each of the early chapters and then pick later chapters that are most relevant for them. For example, survivors of natural disasters may want to read the chapter on that topic and skip chapters on traumas that are not relevant.

If patients plan to search the Internet for information on PTSD, they should be warned that the quality is highly variable, ranging from websites providing scientifically informed advice to websites touting quackery. One of the best Internet resources for empirically supported consumer information is the website of the National Center for PTSD (www.ncptsd.va.gov). To ensure that patients are not being misled by what they find on the

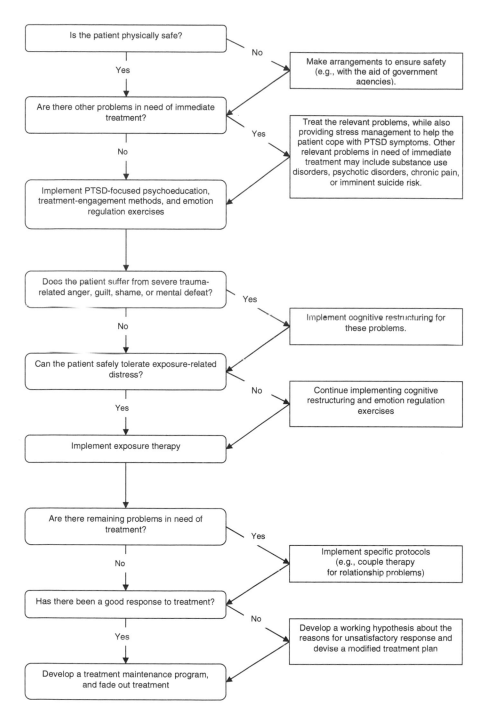

FIGURE 7.1. Decision tree for selecting and sequencing cognitive-behavioral interventions.

Internet, the therapist should periodically inquire about whether they are searching the Web (or other sources) for information, and what they have found.

CULTURAL CONSIDERATIONS

A small number of treatment programs have been specifically developed to cater to the needs of particular cultural groups. An example is Kataoka et al.'s (2003) school-based CBT in Los Angeles for traumatized Latino immigrant children who have been exposed to community violence. The program was developed by a team of school clinicians, educators, and researchers. It consists of eight sessions of group CBT delivered in Spanish by bilingual, bicultural school social workers. Parents and teachers are offered psychoeducation about trauma and PTSD, as well as support services. Compared to a wait-list control, the program was found to be effective in reducing symptoms of PTSD and depression, although the magnitude of symptom reduction was modest (Kataoka et al., 2003). Nevertheless, the program is a promising one that could be improved by, for example, increasing the number of treatment sessions. Anecdotal comments from participants suggested that stigma usually associated with mental health services was minimized in this program because it was administered in schools.

Another example of a treatment program that emphasizes cultural factors is Jones et al.'s (2000) Veterans Center group therapy for African Americans with PTSD. The benefits of this program have yet to be empirically evaluated. However, it looks promising for two reasons. First, linguistic style, speech structure, slang, metaphors, and nonverbal communication that are clearly understood among African Americans are sometimes misinterpreted by Caucasians. Participants in Jones et al.'s African American group reported that their communications usually were accurately understood by other members, whereas they often felt misunderstood in previous, Caucasian-majority groups they had attended (Jones, Griffiths, & Humphris, 2000).

Second, racism can occur in the context of traumatic stressors (e.g., while the person is in the combat theater). Racism adds to the burden of stress experienced by trauma survivors (Loo et al., 2001). In some cases the traumatic stressor consists entirely of life-threatening racial abuse, either in the military or in civilian life (Jones et al., 2000). Accordingly, attention to cultural issues in treatment, including racism-related stress, may facilitate treatment engagement and treatment outcome. Veterans in the African American group felt more comfortable discussing racism in that group than in Caucasian-majority groups. Attempts to discuss racism in the latter groups had frequently elicited embarrassed silence, a change of topic, or the implication that the African American veteran was paranoid or exaggerating (Jones et al., 2000).

Although Jones et al. focused on group treatment, there are reasons to expect that the efficacy of individual (one-to-one) CBT also might be improved by greater attention to cultural factors. If the therapist is able to demonstrate to the patient that he or she is sensitive to, and familiar with, the patient's particular cultural background, then patient–therapist communication may be improved (e.g., misunderstandings will be reduced), and the patient may feel more comfortable about discussing any effects of racism or other cultural factors on his or her presenting problems. Thus, understanding the patient's cultural background is important for developing a sound working relationship. For a start, the therapist should be familiar with culturally appropriate greetings. For example, people from South American cultures often prefer to be called by their title and last name, or by Don or Doña and the first name if the person is older (Nieves-Grafals, 2001).

Culture is also important for understanding why the patient holds particular beliefs. To illustrate, some Southeast Asian trauma survivors are extremely frightened of flashbacks because they believe that the soul leaves the body during a flashback and is transported back to the site of the trauma. This is terrifying because some patients believe that the soul may become trapped at the trauma site, leading to insanity or death (Hinton et al., 2005). These beliefs arise in the cultural context of beliefs about the nature of the soul. If a Western therapist did not understand this cultural context, then the therapist might mistakenly conclude that the patient was psychotic.

Language and cultural barriers can pose serious problems in work with refugees. Treatment may need to be conducted through an interpreter, which makes communication with the patient a difficult and time-consuming task. This problem often makes cognitive interventions difficult because, compared with exposure exercises, they require more lengthy communications and discussions about the details of the traumatic event and beliefs about them. Exposure therapy, on the other hand, requires relatively less verbal communication with the patient once the treatment rationale has been explained and understood by the patient (Başoğlu, Ekblad, Baarnhielm, & Livanou, 2004).

SELF-CARE FOR TRAUMA THERAPISTS

Treating PTSD patients can be taxing on the trauma therapist, not only in terms of listening to the patient's descriptions of their often horrific experiences but also in terms of being with, and trying to help, patients who are highly distressed. This can be highly distressing to therapists, and they may become emotionally exhausted and try to find ways of avoiding the worst of the patient's trauma experiences (e.g., by encouraging patients to skip over the worst parts of their trauma during imaginal exposure exercises). Therapist burnout and avoidance is bad for therapists and patients. It impairs the therapist's ability to respond empathically to the patient, and can also reinforce the patient's maladaptive avoidance of trauma memories and can strengthen maladaptive beliefs (e.g., "Even my therapist seems to believe that my experiences are too horrible to discuss; I'm a hopeless case").

Treating trauma patients is not for everyone. On the one hand the therapist needs to become desensitized, to some degree, to the horrors of trauma narrations and to patient displays of emotional distress. But on the other hand, therapists do not want to lose their empathy and compassion. A challenge for the therapist is to find a balance between (1) tolerating the patient's distress and account of horror without becoming highly upset, and (2) remaining in tune with the patient's thoughts and feelings. With sufficient training and supervised experience, many clinicians are able to become competent trauma therapists. But emotional self-care remains an important issue for all of us. Regardless of how many PTSD patients a therapist has treated, there will always be patients who present with traumatic experiences that the therapist finds especially upsetting. Sometimes this has to do with what is happening in the therapist's life at the time. Therapists who have newly become parents, for example, may suddenly find themselves becoming distressed when patients talk about childhood physical or sexual abuse.

There are several useful strategies for therapist self-care. The most important first step is for therapists to remind themselves that emotional self-care is important; if you don't take care of yourself emotionally, this may seriously undermine your ability to take care of your patients. It's easy for us to offer advice about self-care to our patients, but it can require more work to implement these important strategies on ourselves. Fortunately, there are several effective therapist self-care methods available, including the following.

• Maintain a healthy balance in your life (e.g., a balance between work and recreation) and a balance in your patient load. If you find that PTSD patients are especially taxing, make sure that you are not spending all of your clinical hours with trauma patients. Keep your "dose" of trauma to a manageable amount. Some clinics specializing in torture survivors have a policy that therapists should spend no more than three days per week in direct clinical work with trauma survivors. To prevent burnout, therapists are encouraged to diversify their clinical practice, for example, by treating other types of patients or by engaging in other sorts of important activities, such as teaching, research, or clinical administrative duties.

• If you are concerned that a patient may behave violently toward you, then take all appropriate precautions. This would include a thorough assessment of the patient's risk of violence, anger management interventions, and a contractual agreement between the patient and therapist about violence (e.g., "If you start to feel angry, then you need to tell me, so we prevent the anger from escalating"). If the patient's risk of aggression is high, then PTSD treatment may need to be deferred until the aggression problems have been addressed.

• Ensure that you have professional support, either in the form of supervision from mentors or peer supervision. This is important for two reasons. First, it provides a form of social support, which is important for coping with stress. For example, discussing distressing clinical cases in peer supervision can help you understand that you're not alone in feeling stressed by challenging cases. Second, supervision can provide you with ideas about interventions for particular cases.

• If you find yourself becoming upset about the degree of distress displayed by patients with PTSD during treatment, such as during cognitive restructuring or during exposure exercises, then remind yourself of the treatment rationale (Hembree et al., 2003). Remind yourself that there is a sound theoretical foundation for cognitive-behavioral interventions, that these treatments have a good deal of empirical support, and that the strong emotions that patients experience during therapy are not dangerous. Remember, CBT for PTSD is similar to dentistry for root canal problems (endodontics); both are empirically supported and generally effective, but both involve some degree of pain.

• Take a break from your PTSD practice if you're feeling burned out or overwhelmed. This is a sign of wisdom and self-knowledge. You don't need to be a supertherapist. If you're stressed out with PTSD work, then take a break and try something new. If you eventually return to working with trauma patients, then that's all well and good. Or if you move on to another area of clinical endeavor, then that's fine too. There are plenty of other important areas for clinical work.

SUMMARY

There are many considerations in devising a CBT package for a given patient. Important considerations include the patient's treatment goals and the case formulation, which guide the selection and sequencing of interventions. In this chapter we reviewed the many different elements of CBT, which can be combined into various types of empirically supported treatment packages. The case formulation for a given patient, along with the information reviewed in this chapter, is used to develop a treatment plan. The viability of treatment depends not only on the techniques that are used but also on the way that they are used. Thus, the skills and interpersonal qualities of the therapist are an essential part of the equation. A good goal for therapists in training is to aim to be safe and competent in the basics of CBT, and mindful of managing their own emotional reactions to listening to the often horrific experiences reported by PTSD patients. Details of the various interventions included in the treatment plan are the focus of the remaining chapters of this volume.

CHAPTER 8

Developing a Case Formulation and Treatment Plan

Much has been written about the importance of developing a case formulation in order to devise an effective treatment plan (e.g., see the seminal work of Persons, 1989). Yet, comparatively little has been written about how to develop a formulation and treatment plan for PTSD. Accordingly, this is the topic of the present chapter.

The case formulation is a working hypothesis of the four *P*s of clinical causation: the predisposing, precipitating, perpetuating, and protective factors in the patient's problems. The formulation is used to develop an individualized treatment plan. The approach used in this volume is based on my previous work (Taylor, 2000; Taylor & Asmundson, 2004) and the work of Persons (1989; Persons & Tompkins, 1997). The case formulation depends critically on an adequate assessment of the patient's problems. If the assessment has overlooked some important factor, then the formulation and associated treatment plan may fail to be useful.

The therapist shares the formulation with the patient, elicits feedback, and makes any necessary adjustments. Once a formulation is agreed upon, then the patient and therapist can decide on a treatment plan derived from the formulation. Thus, the sharing of the case formulation helps the therapist to identify any errors in his or her conceptualization. The formulation also helps the patient understand how his or her problems may have arisen, along with possible solutions to the problems. The formulation can therefore counter any feelings of shame or guilt that the patient may harbor. Instead of believing, for example, "I'm to blame for being a weak person for developing emotional problems," the formulation can encourage the person to consider a more adaptive interpretation; for example, "Anyone would have developed these problems if they'd had my family history and learning experiences—you can't choose your genes or what your parents do to you as a kid." The case formulation and associated treatment plan can also foster optimism in the patient about overcoming the problems and facilitate treatment adherence (e.g., "Now that I better understand my problems, I can see why it would be useful to try this form of therapy").

Why develop a case formulation and individualized treatment plan? Why not simply follow the steps laid out in a treatment manual? Formulations play an important role even in protocol-driven treatment. For example, formulations can help the therapist determine the timing of interventions (e.g., when to use exposure and when to refrain from or defer the use of exposure), along with the targets of treatment (e.g., the types of beliefs selected for cognitive restructuring) and the pacing or difficulty level of treatment (e.g., whether to start with a challenging exposure assignment or whether to begin more gradually, with a less distressing assignment). Case formulations also encourage the therapist to spot potential treatment obstacles and to devise plans for circumventing or dealing with problems if they arise. Case formulations are particularly useful for complicated cases (e.g., PTSD associated with multiple traumatic experiences, or PTSD comorbid with one or more other disorders), for which there may be no empirically validated treatment protocol. The treatment plan is most likely to be successful if it draws from the pool of empirically supported interventions. Treatment manuals provide useful templates for developing treatment plans, which can be adapted in light of the case formulation for a given patient.

ELEMENTS OF A CASE FORMULATION AND TREATMENT PLAN

One useful way of devising a formulation is to divide the process into the series of steps shown in Table 8.1. Details from the assessment are used to compile information for each step until a formulation and treatment plan has been assembled. The following sections describe and illustrate each of these elements.

Presenting Problems and Problem History

Presenting problems can include symptoms, current stressors (including occupational, financial, interpersonal, legal, housing, or general medical problems), and difficulties in adaptive functioning (e.g., inability to work or to enjoy leisure activities because of disabling symptoms). Some problems might not be ones that can be addressed by CBT (e.g., financial difficulties). Even so, a full list of problems is important for understanding the

TABLE 8.1. Elements of a Cognitive-Behavioral Case Formulation and Treatment Plan

Element	Description
1. Presenting problems and problem history	A list of the patient's traumatic experiences and current difficulties, beginning with the chief problem. This includes problems specified by the patient and other problems identified by the clinician.
2. Functional and dysfunctional beliefs	Includes maladaptive beliefs about the self, one's symptoms, other people, or the world. Some of these beliefs may be causing the patient's current difficulties.
3. Triggers and problem context—aggravating and ameliorating factors	Objects, people, events, or situations associated with the worsening or amelioration of the patient's problems. For example, a high expressed-emotion social environment can worsen a patient's problems, whereas a socially supportive environment may promote recovery or prevent problems from getting worse.
4. Coping strategies—adaptive and maladaptive	Ways that the patient copes with stressful life events and with emotional arousal. Includes behaviors that worsen or perpetuate the patient's problems (e.g., excessive avoidance or needless reliance on safety signals).
5. Salient learning experiences	Learning experiences that may have contributed to the patient's dysfunctional beliefs, including events occurring before and after the trauma. Salient learning experiences may have shattered assumptions or strengthened dysfunctional beliefs.
6. Working hypothesis	A model specifying links among the above-mentioned components, which describes the predisposing, precipitating, and perpetuating factors for all the problems on the problem list. Protective factors (if any) are also described. The working hypothesis emphasizes cognitive and behavioral mechanisms, although other factors can also be included.
7. Treatment goals and interventions	A statement of specific and measurable treatment goals and plans for attaining these goals.
8. Treatment obstacles and potential solutions	A list of predicted or actual obstacles to successful treatment and strategies for overcoming them. Strategies for overcoming the obstacles are based on either the working hypothesis or, if the obstacles arise unexpectedly, a specific formulation of these new difficulties.

patient's current life context, including the way in which the problems are interrelated. For example, hyperarousal symptoms may be influenced by the patient's financial stressors, which would suggest that it may be useful to implement some form of stress management, as well as recommending a referral to someone who might be able to help solve the financial problems (e.g., a social services worker or financial officer at the patient's bank).

The problem list should include problems identified during the assessment, regardless of whether the patient recognizes them as issues of concern. For example, the patient may be heavily using cannabis. The patient might not recognize this as a problem, but the assessment might reveal social and occupational impairment, hazardous behaviors (e.g., operating machinery while intoxicated), and potential legal problems associated with the patient's drug use. Accordingly, this would be placed on the problem list for discussion with the patient.

The problems should be described specifically (e.g., in terms of beliefs, emotions, and behaviors) and, if possible, broken down into their components. This is done in order to (1) identify relationships among problems and thereby shed light on underlying mechanisms, (2) plan how to treat the sub-problems, and (3) mobilize the patient's hope by showing how overwhelming problems can be broken down into manageable units (Persons, 1989).

Details regarding the history of the patient's problems should provide important information on the possible causes of the problems, along with clues about how the problems are interrelated. The history of a patient with PTSD and cannabis abuse, for example, might reveal that PTSD initially arose from an accident while operating heavy machinery due to cannabis intoxication, and cannabis abuse worsened thereafter, as a form of self-administered sedation.

Not all of the identified problems will necessarily be the targets of treatment. If treatment is time limited, the patient and therapist might decide to focus on only, say, the three most debilitating problems, or on the problem that seems to worsen the other problems. The working hypothesis, along with the patient's goals, will determine which problems to address and the order in which to address them.

The following is a summary of the presenting problems and problem history of Margot, a patient we will follow throughout this chapter.

Margot, a 40 year old Canadian journalist, was referred by her family doctor for treatment of PTSD and major depression. Margot had a history of childhood physical abuse and had been exposed to violence and bloodshed while she was working on a newspaper assignment in the Middle East. Margot, an only child, was physically abused by her father—a chronically depressed and irritable man—from age 8 until she left home at age 17. At least weekly, her father would hit, slap, or punch her, particularly when he had been drinking. On some occasions she was so frightened she wet herself, which only fueled her father's rage. The school nurse questioned Margot on a number of occasions because of bruises on her face. Terrified of what might happen if her father learned that she had reported on him, Margot always made excuses to explain the bruises (e.g., "I fell off my bike" or "I slipped on the icy pavement"). Margot's mother died of cancer when she was 7 years old.

As an adult, while on a newspaper assignment in the Middle East, Margot was required to "seek out the action." She and her cameraman roamed dangerous regions, attempting to be first on the scene of newsworthy events. As a result, she witnessed much horror, such as the bloody and mutilated victims of bombings, and child amputees who had stepped on land mines. Margot also vividly recalled when she saw a group of men, suspected of being rebels, being rounded up, beaten, and dragged off by soldiers. While this was happening the wives and children of the men were screaming and crying. Margot and the cameraman were grabbed by the soldiers and briefly detained and questioned because they had attempted to document the event.

Upon returning to Canada, Margot was acutely aware of the relative affluence and safety enjoyed there. She felt distant and alienated because she had witnessed and experienced the brutality that people are capable of, while the citizens of her home community lived in "blissful ignorance." When she presented for treatment, Margot's major problems included the following:

- Severe, chronic anxiety associated with feelings of dread that something bad could happen at any time. Whenever she got into arguments with people, she had vivid, intrusive recollections of the abuse experienced from her father and from the soldiers in the Middle East.
- Inability to work because of her psychological problems. She was currently subsisting on government disability assistance.
- Fear of sleeping because of recurrent, terrifying nightmares.
- Recurrent intrusive images of the events she witnessed in the Middle East, along with occasional recollections of the abuse she had suffered at the hands of her father.
- Depressed mood and loss of enjoyment in life, associated with passive suicidal ideation. Margot felt that life was not worth living, but she denied any intention, plan, or urge to harm herself.
- Irritability and bouts of anger (e.g., when driving, when standing in lines and when dealing with "stupid people," such as unhelpful sales clerks).
- Social isolation and difficulty trusting people. Margot spent most of her waking hours alone in her apartment. She had few friends and was not in a relationship. She had been briefly married and divorced when she was in her 30s. She had no children and had no contact with her relatives. Her father was killed in a road traffic collision when Margot was in her 20s.

A diagnostic interview confirmed the referring physician's diagnosis of chronic PTSD. Some of Margot's problems—such as difficulty trusting people, nightmares, hypervigilance, and intermittent bouts of depressed mood—developed in her early teens. However, she did not develop full-blown PTSD and major depression until after her experiences in the Middle East. No other psychological problems were identified. There was some suggestion of features of paranoid personality disorder (e.g., pervasive mistrust of others), although these may have been associated features of her PTSD. Margot was in good physical health. The only treatment she had received for her problems was pharmacotherapy (initially lorazepam on an as-needed basis to manage particularly intense bouts of anxiety, along with sertraline for depression and PTSD). These agents had been moderately effective during the first year of drug treatment, but Margot reported that the effects gradually wore off over time. She had been unresponsive to other pharmacotherapies. Her current medications were paroxetine and as-needed lorazepam.

Functional and Dysfunctional Beliefs

A goal of treatment is to reinforce or strengthen adaptive beliefs (e.g., "I can become a survivor rather than a victim") and to weaken maladaptive ones (e.g., "I don't belong in human society"). Accordingly, both types of beliefs are important to identify. Dysfunctional beliefs about the self, one's symptoms, other people, and the world appear to play an important role in PTSD (see Chapters 2 and 3). Dysfunctional beliefs also have been implicated in other disorders; for example, negative beliefs about the self and world and pessimistic beliefs about one's future have been implicated in depression (Beck et al., 1979). Accordingly, such beliefs are typically an important component of the cognitive-behavioral case formulation. Functional beliefs can be important to the extent that they play a protective role, in keeping the patient's problems from getting worse (e.g., functional or adaptive beliefs can motivate hope and encourage the patient to persist at trying to overcome his or her problems).

Margot's assessment indicated that she had some positive beliefs about herself, although she did not place much credence in them. Such beliefs included "I've overcome bad stuff before, so I can overcome this" and "There must be a solution somewhere to my problems." However, she also harbored many strongly held negative beliefs. These beliefs, along with associated clinical problems (in parentheses), were as follows:

- "I can't trust anyone. I have to rely on myself." (anxiety, hypervigilance, loneliness, suspiciousness)
- "Something terrible will happen again; I'm not safe anywhere." (anxiety, hypervigilance, and efforts to avoid public places whenever possible)
- "In this world, horrible things are more likely to happen than good things." (anxiety, depression)
- "People, especially men, can easily turn into cruel, violent animals. It just takes the right situation to bring out their aggressive instincts." (anxiety, hypervigilance, and anger)
- "Most people haven't got a clue about all the evil in the world." (resentment and feelings of alienation from others)

- "I'm a damaged person. I'll never be able to return to work." (depression, hopelessness)
- "I'll never get over my problems; they're only going to get worse." (depression, hopelessness)

Triggers and Problem Contexts: Aggravating and Ameliorating Factors

Aggravating factors include stimuli or conditions that trigger or exacerbate the patient's problems, such as things that induce reexperiencing symptoms. They also include nonspecific environmental conditions that exacerbate symptoms. Being in crowded, noisy situations, for example, may be particularly disturbing to some people with PTSD. Similarly, being in a high expressed-emotion home environment in which the patient is frequently criticized by hostile, overinvolved significant others can worsen the patient's symptoms. Such contexts may play a role in perpetuating the patient's problems.

Contexts or resources associated with the amelioration of problems—such as a socially supportive milieu—are also important to identify for the purpose of constructing a case formulation. Sometimes, contexts that are associated with the reduction of some symptoms are also associated with the worsening of others, as in the case of Margot.

Margot experienced distress and vivid recollections of her traumatic experiences when she was exposed to the following stimuli or situations:

- Men acting aggressively, speaking in loud voices, wearing uniforms, drinking alcohol, or touching her, and disheveled men who looked like "alcoholics" and men of Middle Eastern descent.
- Television programs, newspaper or magazine articles, or movies dealing with violence of any kind (e.g., family violence, combat, riots).
- Skinny, poorly dressed children, which reminded her of her own childhood and of the children she had seen in the Middle East.
- The gravesites of her mother and father and the site where her family home used to stand.
- Colleagues from her former newspaper, especially foreign correspondents.
- Stray cats and dogs, which reminded her of her Middle East experiences.
- Sudden loud noises, such as cars backfiring or plates being dropped, which reminded her of both her abusive upbringing and her Middle East experiences.
- Particular smells, such as body odor, cheap cologne, the smell of alcohol, and the smell of raw sewage. Body odor and sewage reminded Margot of her Middle East experiences and body odor, cologne, and alcohol triggered memories of her father.

Exposure to these stimuli triggered reexperiencing symptoms, so she attempted to avoid exposure by remaining in her apartment. However, when she stayed in her apartment she tended to ruminate over her problems, which thereby worsened her irritability and depression. Few situations ameliorated all her symptoms. Margot had marked concentration difficulties, so she had given up trying to read books or magazine articles. She had two supportive female friends with whom she had occasional contact. Margot tended to feel better on days that she got together with her friends, but she often avoided them because she didn't want to burden them with her troubles.

Coping Strategies: Adaptive and Maladaptive

Treatment involves the strengthening of adaptive coping behaviors (e.g., getting regular exercise and maintaining a regular "diet" of pleasurable activities), as well as encouraging patients to drop maladaptive coping strategies. The latter include safety behaviors (e.g., avoidance and escape from objectively harmless situations), as well as overreliance on needless safety signals. Maladaptive coping strategies can perpetuate the patient's problems, whereas adaptive strategies can help the patient overcome his or her problems. Accordingly, both are important for the purpose of developing a case formulation.

Margot's repertoire of coping strategies was rather limited, consisting mostly of avoidance and distraction. She attempted, whenever possible, to avoid reminders of her traumatic experiences. When she was alone in her apartment, she constantly had the television turned on, tuned to a soap opera or other innocuous program, for distraction. When Margot was unable to avoid triggers, such as when she had to leave the apartment on errands, she reportedly did a number of things to "protect" herself. She carried pepper spray in her handbag and was considering buying a small handgun. She also deliberately scanned her environment, so she "wouldn't be caught unprepared" if something bad should happen. When traveling on a bus, Margot would try to sit up front near the driver and the exit and would keep her handbag on her lap, with the pepper spray close at hand.

Salient Learning Experiences

Salient learning experiences include those that contribute to the formation or strengthening of dysfunctional beliefs and those that shape the patient's choice of coping strategies. Such learning experiences can include traumatic events, as well as experiences before or after the trauma. A review of the patient's important learning experiences is not only important for developing a case formulation; it also can help patients understand why they currently think, feel, and behave in particular ways today.

For Margot, the assessment suggested that relevant learning experiences commenced at about the time her mother was hospitalized with terminal cancer when she was 7 years old. At that time she had to largely fend for herself after school because her father was working the night shift at a nearby factory. The situation worsened when her mother died. Her father became depressed and irritable, began drinking heavily, and became increasingly abusive to Margot. It appeared that these early learning experiences led Margot to develop the belief that she had to be self-reliant because other people were either unavailable or couldn't be trusted.

Margot's life was also characterized by unpredictable, uncontrollable exposure to her father's violence, which likely led her to believe that bad things are more likely to happen than good things, and that terrible things could strike at any time. As she witnessed the effects of alcohol on her father, she acquired the view that people could easily turn cruel and violent under the right circumstances. These beliefs were seemingly strengthened by her encounters in the Middle East. These experiences, combined with a childhood marked by loss and violence, led Margot to believe that she had experienced and witnessed things that most people had never seen. This likely led her to feel distant from others and contributed to her belief that most people don't understand the extent of evil in the world.

As Margot's PTSD and depression worsened, her work performance became impaired, to the point that she had to go on medical leave. At times her thinking seemed "slowed down," while at other times her mind was filled with a jumble of thoughts and images of traumatic experiences. Margot's cognitive problems, along with a largely unsuccessful history of treatment with various pharmacological agents, led her to conclude that she was psychologically damaged and would never recover.

Working Hypothesis

The working hypothesis is a synthesis of all the available information into a model of the predisposing, precipitating, perpetuating, and protective factors involved in the patient's major problems. The working model is guided by cognitive-behavioral research and the emotional processing model (Chapters 2 and 3), along with cognitive-behavioral models of other disorders (e.g., Beck et al., 1979; Beck, Freeman, Davis, & Associates, 2003; Taylor, 2000; Taylor & Asmundson, 2004; Wells, 1997). Mechanisms in the working hypothesis include dysfunctional beliefs, maladaptive coping strategies (e.g., avoidance or reliance on safety signals or safety behaviors), reinforcement contingencies, problems with interpersonal skills, stressors, and other factors (e.g., relevant genetic or other biological factors).

Predisposing factors can be identified by reviewing the patient's developmental history, including important learning experiences that led the patient to interpret stressors and symptoms in particular ways (e.g., high anxiety sensitivity can be a predisposing factor for PTSD and other disorders). Maladaptive beliefs, which may be predisposing and perpetuating factors, may be acquired by verbal instruction, observational learning, or direct experience. A host of other factors may also predispose the person to develop PTSD (e.g., genetic factors) or to encounter traumatic events that increase the risk of PTSD (e.g., a tendency to engage in impulsive, sensation-seeking behaviors).

Precipitating factors for PTSD are typically traumatic events, although other precipitants may be involved in PTSD and associated features. Precipitants for particular symptoms (e.g., episodes of heightened anxiety or dissociation) may be particular stressors or trauma cues. There may be a cascade of precipitating factors involved in the development of PTSD and associated problems. For example, combat exposure, interacting with predisposing factors, may precipitate PTSD and associated irritability and anger. In turn, irritability and anger may lead to job loss and the dissolution of the patient's marriage, which in turn may precipitate a depressive episode.

Perpetuating factors are involved in the maintenance of the patient's problems. Maladaptive coping strategies such as avoidance of trauma cues can also perpetuate PTSD symptoms such as trauma-related fears and reexperiencing symptoms. Rumination may also perpetuate PTSD (Chapter 2). Interpersonal factors also may be relevant to be maintenance of PTSD (e.g., high expressed emotion) or reinforcement contingencies that dissuade the patient from actively attempting to overcome his or her problems (e.g., the threat of losing one's disability benefits if the person overcomes his or her PTSD).

Protective factors either prevent the occurrence of symptoms or prevent them from getting worse. Posttrauma social support, for example, may dampen the severity of symptoms. Social support exerts its effects in many ways; it lessens isolation and feelings of stigmatization that may arise from having a psychiatric disorder, it involves emotional support (e.g., feelings of protection, safety, and comfort), and it may facilitate exposure to corrective information (e.g., information that all men aren't potentially violent animals). Pretrauma training for dealing with disasters can protect emergency response personnel from developing PTSD. Sometimes the emergence of PTSD or other problems is linked to the erosion or loss of protective factors. A police officer, for example, may be resilient in the face of job-related stressors until transferred to another city, away from his or her social group. The sudden loss of social support may put the person at increased risk for PTSD, should a traumatic event be experienced.

The working hypothesis should be as parsimonious as reasonably possible. An initial evaluation of the formulation involves sharing it with the patient to see if it fits with his or her experience. Over the course of treatment the therapist can evaluate new information to check whether it is consistent with the formulation. If inconsistent information is obtained, the formulation may need to be revised.

The following working hypothesis was developed on the basis of the available information collected about Margot's history and her problems.

- *Predisposing factors.* Margot's father had a history of depression and alcohol abuse, and her mother reportedly suffered from postpartum depression for several months after Margot was born. Margot reported that she had a cousin who was a "shut in" (i.e., rarely left the house) and appeared to have suffered from panic disorder with agoraphobia. Another cousin was also said to be taking tranquilizers because he was "high strung." Thus, there was evidence of a family history of anxiety and mood disorders, even among family members who lived apart and in very different environmental circumstances. These findings raised the possibility that Margot possessed a genetic predisposition to develop an anxiety or mood disorder, with the type of disorder depending on the types of environmental events she encountered.
- *Precipitating factors.* Childhood adversity—in the form of maternal loss, paternal abuse, and social isolation—appeared to have precipitated subclinical PTSD along with intermittent bouts of depression (of insufficient severity or duration to meet criteria for major depression or dysthymic disorder). Her later traumatic experiences in the Middle East served as a secondary set of precipitants, which markedly increased the severity of her symptoms. Margot had a learning history whereby some circumstances led to the development of maladaptive beliefs (i.e., childhood adversity), and other events contributed to the strengthening of these beliefs (Middle Eastern experiences). These beliefs appeared to have contributed to her PTSD symptoms and to her depressive symptoms.
- *Perpetuating factors.* Margot's main coping behaviors involved avoidance and distraction. When avoidance was not an option, she relied on safety signals (e.g., pepper spray) and safety behaviors (e.g., sitting at the front of the bus, near the bus driver and the exit). These factors prevented her from learning that she did not need to take these measures to protect herself. Margot's social isolation and limited social support appeared to contribute to her problems in four ways: (1) the lack of support strengthened her feelings of vulnerability, (2) social isolation provided her with more opportunity to ruminate about her problems, thereby perpetuating her sense of hopelessness and depression, (3) the relative lack of contact with others prevented her maladaptive beliefs from being challenged (e.g., isolation prevented the disconfirmation of her belief that the world is largely filled with evil), and (4) social isolation involved a lack of fulfilling, meaningful, and diverting activities and relationships, which might otherwise have ameliorated her depression.

• *Protective factors*. Protective factors, which prevented Margot's emotional problems from becoming worse in her teenage years, included the fact that she was bright, articulate, and conscientious. This meant that she did well in school, obtained a scholarship, and was able to escape her abusive father by moving into a college dormitory. Later in life, her intellectual abilities appeared to play less of a protective role, possibly because her symptoms of PTSD and depression had become so severe that Margot's cognitive functioning (concentration and memory) was compromised, thereby making it more difficult for her to think of effective ways of dealing with her problems.

Treatment Goals and Interventions

The treatment plan, derived from the working hypothesis, consists of a statement of the goals of therapy and an outline of how to attain these goals. Broad goals (e.g., to overcome PTSD) can be broken down into subgoals. The best subgoals are those that are realistic, safe, and clearly defined. They also should be measurable, so the patient and therapist can assess progress toward achieving the goals. The treatment plan can include short-term goals to be achieved during the course of treatment (e.g., to be able to walk in safe, crowded public places without feeling highly anxious) and longer-term goals that would be achieved if the patient continued to implement the treatment exercises after the formal course of treatment ended (e.g., to be able to return to full-time employment).

Goals and subgoals are determined by both the patient and therapist. The following is a sampling of goals from patients in my PTSD treatment studies (e.g., Taylor et al., 2001, 2003). Most of these goals were broken down into specific subgoals, which were pursued in a step-by-step fashion.

- To be able to sleep throughout most of the night.
- To be able to go for a walk in my neighborhood without worrying about being mugged.
- To feel comfortable and confident when talking to male business colleagues.
- To have fewer panic attacks when I encounter reminders of the trauma.
- To be able to resume dating.
- To be able to visit the war memorial without being overwhelmed with fear and rage.
- To feel good about myself and not feel so guilty about not having left my husband sooner.
- To be able to become absorbed in the "here and now" of life without always thinking about the trauma.

- To be able to resume driving without feeling highly anxious and nauseated.
- To improve my concentration and memory so that I don't zone out all the time during conversations with people.
- To feel less afraid and less hateful of men.
- To be able to make more friends instead of hiding away in my house.
- To be able to better cope with my feelings.
- To be able to forgive, in my own mind, my deceased grandfather for what he did to me.

The treatment plan typically draws on an appropriate empirically validated treatment protocol, which is used as a foundation or starting point. The components and indications for various protocols are discussed in Chapter 7. For particular forms of comorbidity (e.g., PTSD comorbid with hypochondriasis) it may be necessary to combine particular protocols (e.g., one for PTSD and one for hypochondriasis, as described in Taylor & Asmundson, 2004). The treatment of complex PTSD may require specific interventions for personality disorder or interpersonal problems (e.g., Beck et al., 2003; Cloitre et al., 2002; Linehan, 1993) in addition to PTSD interventions. The case formulation is used to adapt the selected protocol(s) to the individual patient.

The formulation would include a statement of the patient's tolerance for distress, which is relevant for the selection, timing, and pacing of exposure exercises. If the patient has a history of a substance use disorder, the formulation would also include a statement of the likely risk of relapse, which also would be relevant for treatment planning. If the risk of relapse is judged to be quite low (e.g., if the patient has been abstinent for some years), then exposure exercises might be implemented relatively early in treatment (e.g., after a couple of sessions of training in emotion regulation skills). If the patient is judged to have a high risk for relapse, then the Seeking Safety protocol (Najavits, 2002) might be implemented first, with exposure exercises deferred until the risk of relapse has been sufficiently reduced (see Chapter 7). If the formulation indicated that anger, shame, guilt, or mental defeat played an important role in the patient's problems, then cognitive restructuring would be used prior to the implementation of exposure exercises.

The goals of Margot's treatment, in broad terms, were to help her overcome her PTSD and depression so that she could return to work. Subgoals involved working on the various issues in her problem list (e.g., reducing the frequency of nightmares, increasing her ability to trust people). Given her limited social resources and passive suicidal ideation, the therapist and Margot decided to first work on improving her social network, alleviating her depression, and improving her coping skills before conducting any exposure-related treatment for PTSD. Treatment initially involved Margot purchasing a day planner, in which she would try to schedule each day at least one activity that had formerly brought her a sense of enjoyment or accomplishment (i.e., mastery and pleasure exercises; Chapter 9). Concomitantly, treatment engagement strategies and cognitive restructuring were introduced, primarily in order to improve her hopefulness about recovering and to lessen her suicidal ideation. Other targets of cognitive restructuring also involved her PTSD- and depression-related dysfunctional beliefs (e.g., beliefs concerning the pervasiveness of danger and evil and guidelines for distinguishing safety from danger).

It was planned that imaginal and situational exposure would be introduced later, focusing first on her Middle Eastern experiences and then on her childhood experiences. This was because she experienced greater distress about the former. There was some similarity between her childhood and adulthood traumas (e.g., both involved violence committed by men, and both were associated with fears and dysfunctional beliefs related to men). Accordingly, it was predicted that treatment focused on Margot's Middle Eastern experiences would have some therapeutic impact on the distress associated with her childhood memories.

The pretreatment assessment revealed that Margot's anxiety sensitivity was not clinically elevated, so interoceptive exposure was not included in the treatment plan. As part of situational exposure therapy, it was planned that she would gradually wean herself from her safety signals and safety behaviors. It was initially unclear whether Margot had interpersonal skills problems. Accordingly, prospective monitoring would be used to collect information on the nature of her interpersonal relationships, to determine whether any form of skills training (e.g., assertiveness training for dealing with men) would be useful. The plan included the gradual tapering of treatment sessions toward the end of the course of therapy, along with relapse prevention interventions.

Margot's use of psychotropic medication was also included in the treatment plan; she was encouraged to continue taking her paroxetine (at a stable dose, so the effects of CBT could be evaluated, distinct from the effects of the mediation). Margot was encouraged to use relaxation exercises (as part of applied relaxation) rather than continue taking lorazepam. This was because it was important for Margot to learn that she could enter harmless but feared situations (as part of her situational exposure exercises) without needing to rely on lorazepam. That way she could learn that her fear naturally abated over time, without medication. The treatment plan was discussed with her prescribing physician, who was in agreement with the proposed interventions.

Treatment Obstacles and Potential Solutions

Information from the initial assessment and the resulting case formulation can be used to anticipate potential problems that can arise during treatment. These could stem from the patient's beliefs (e.g., "I don't deserve to feel good about myself"), issues concerning the therapeutic relationship (e.g., difficulty trusting the therapist), or logistic problems concerning treatment attendance and homework completion. An example of the latter is difficulty arranging child care in order to attend treatment, arising from financial difficulties combined with low social support (i.e., few or no people to call on for child care and inability to pay for a babysitter).

Validation of the patient's distress is a widely used method of building a good therapeutic relationship; "validation communicates to the patient in a nonambiguous way that her [or his] behavior makes sense and is understandable in the current context" (Linehan, 1993, p. 221). But the case formulation may suggest conditions in which validation is likely to be counterproductive.

> Validation means different things to different people. Individuals who value autonomy may place a low value on validation: they want a set of tools with which they can solve their problems and, in fact, they may view validation as condescending or too intrusive. However, many patients may believe empathy and validation are essential components of getting help. (Leahy, 2001, p. 86)

Some patients may, as a result of their trauma history, be highly sensitive to invalidation. This can occur in patients who were disbelieved when they reported the trauma to others (e.g., a patient who is told by her parents or police that she was lying about being raped). Here, the case formulation would suggest that difficulties could be encountered in the use of cognitive restructuring because patients may feel that the therapist is invalidating them by challenging beliefs. In such cases, the therapist would rely extensively on Socratic dialogue, so that it is the patient, not the therapist, who is challenging the dysfunctional beliefs.

The case formulation can be used to identify environmental contingencies that might dissuade patients from successfully completing therapy (Persons, 1989). This could involve, for example, a significant other who criticizes the patient for attending therapy ("You should be able to overcome your problems by yourself, without seeing a therapist") or reinforces the patient's maladaptive beliefs. In such cases the case formulation would suggest that couple therapy may be useful. The case formulation can also be used to anticipate the conditions in which relapse is likely to occur. The therapist can implement relapse prevention strategies to address this problem (see Chapter 14) or suggest other interventions. For example, if the patient lives in a dangerous neighborhood or has a high-risk occupation, then a change in these circumstances may be necessary in order to reduce the risk for retraumatization and subsequent relapse. When problems in treatment arise unexpectedly, the therapist can attempt to develop a formulation of the causes of the problems and use this to devise a remedy.

Three main potential problems were identified for Margot's treatment plan. First, her difficulty trusting people could interfere with her participation in therapy. Accordingly, it was important for the therapist to devote more time than usual to establishing rapport and building a solid working relationship. This was done partly by the therapist conveying an understanding of how Margot came to hold particular beliefs. She had had many aversive experiences that had not been encountered by the average person, so it was understandable that she might feel alienated from others. The therapist was careful to validate Margot's experiences and her distress without endorsing her dysfunctional beliefs. The therapist also took time to share the assessment findings and treatment plan, and to fully address any questions or concerns raised by Margot. It was emphasized to her that she would be in complete control of how treatment would proceed.

The second possible problem was that her depression and associated suicidal ideation could worsen, especially if she suffered some sort of loss or setback during treatment (e.g., if her financial situation deteriorated any further). Accordingly, Margot and the therapist agreed that they would assess her mood at the beginning of each session. Margot and the therapist also agreed on a treatment contract, in which she would either notify the therapist, call 911, or go to the nearest emergency room if she felt she was at risk for self-harm. In addition, the therapist assessed whether Margot had the means for harming herself at home. Although she had entertained the idea of purchasing a handgun to protect herself, she was persuaded that such an acquisition would not be in her best interest.

The third potential problem concerned her irritability, suspiciousness, and occasional anger when interacting with people. Such reactions could render any social exercises, such as mastery and pleasure exercises or situational exposure exercises, ineffective or even counterproductive. Accordingly, when such exercises were planned, it was necessary to either select exercises that would be successful or prepare Margot to deal with potential problems (e.g., via cognitive restructuring for managing anger).

SUMMARY

The case formulation approach described in this chapter emphasizes the role of dysfunctional beliefs and maladaptive behaviors, although other factors are also considered. The formulation draws on the empirical literature and on the cognitive models of PTSD (Chapters 2 and 3). The process of developing the formulation is a collaborative process, in which the therapist and patient work together to arrive at a shared understanding of the patient's problems. The formulation can be presented to the patient verbally and in writing. The latter is more likely to be remembered by the patient. For all practical purposes, the value of a case formulation approach lies in whether it leads to a successful treatment. There are several methods for devising a formulation, with no single approach predominating. One approach is described in this chapter.

Regardless of whether one chooses to largely follow the steps laid out in a treatment manual, case formulations play an important role in the selection, timing, and pacing of interventions—and in determining whether it is even appropriate to simply follow a treatment manual. Throughout the course of treatment the therapist should look for evidence for and against the formulation. If the formulation requires revision, then the treatment plan may need to be changed accordingly. If obstacles are encountered during treatment, then a formulation of the causes is devised, and a remedy is derived. Thus, formulation-driven treatment is a self-correcting process.

CHAPTER 9

Psychoeducation, Treatment Engagement, and Emotion Regulation Strategies

The interventions in this chapter are grouped together because they are typically implemented in an integrated fashion in the early stages of treatment. Psychoeducation involves teaching patients about PTSD and its treatment. Treatment engagement strategies also have an educational component, although their primary aim is to enhance the patient's motivation for trying a course of CBT. Emotional regulation skills are also, in a sense, educational and motivational in nature; they involve training patients in exercises that can help them to regulate unpleasant emotions. The emotion regulation skills discussed in this chapter also include strategies for managing some of the consequences of emotional distress, such as grounding exercises for stress-induced dissociation. Early success with emotion regulation exercises can increase the patient's optimism about treatment efficacy and thereby enhance the patient's motivation for completing a course of treatment.

Psychoeducation, treatment engagement strategies, and emotion regulation exercises are important but not sufficient for treating PTSD. However, they are often essential to prepare the way for implementing other, more powerful interventions, such as cognitive restructuring and exposure exercises. That is, psychoeducation, treatment engagement strategies, and emotion regulation exercises can reduce the risk of premature treatment dropout and enhance adherence to other cognitive-behavioral interventions. This is done by enhancing the perceived credibility of treatment (which reduces treatment dropout; Taylor, 2004) and, in the case of emotion regulation exercises, making it easier for the patient to complete distressing exercises such as exposure assignments.

PSYCHOEDUCATION

Rationale

Psychoeducation is essential for informed consent, for correcting any patient misconceptions about PTSD and its treatment and for ensuring treatment adherence. If patients are not given a good explanation of their disorder and its treatment, then they may be reluctant to pursue a course of CBT. If the patient is a child, psychoeducation should be provided to the caregiver and, in developmentally appropriate language, to the child as well.

Methods and Materials

Patient information describing the nature and treatment of PTSD is presented in Handout 9.1 (pp. 170–171). This handout was designed to be relevant for CBT patients even if they are concomitantly receiving pharmacotherapy. Thus, the handout describes the core disturbance in PTSD (the brain's stress response system) in a matter that is consistent with the rationales for both CBT and pharmacotherapy. A consistent rationale is important so as not to confuse patients who are receiving both types of treatments, and for patients who are referred for CBT even though their referring physicians have told them that they are suffering from a "biochemical imbalance." Patients should be informed about what they are *not* suffering from: they are not becoming psychotic or "going crazy."

The therapist can add other explanations or metaphors to explain PTSD, such as the "psychological digestion" metaphor (Foa & Rothbaum, 1998); for example, "Thoughts and memories of the trauma keep coming to mind because the trauma has not been psychologically digested by the brain; the goal of treatment is to help you work through what has happened so that you can put it behind you."

Patients may have the misconception that CBT has no side effects, because it is psychotherapy rather than medication. Patients should be educated that all effective treatments have their side effects, including CBT. The side effects of this treatment include transient increases in reexperiencing and hyperarousal symptoms, especially during exposure exercises and particularly for highly avoidant patients. Patients should be informed that side effects are not signs that treatment is going awry. They are indications that therapy is working in the expected fashion.

For children, CBT can be framed as a method for helping them successfully resist or "boss back" PTSD. The latter is framed as a something that is "bossing" them around (March, Amaya-Jackson, Murray, & Schulte, 1998).

TROUBLESHOOTING

There are two main problems associated with psychoeducation: (1) reluctance, on the patient's part, to engage in treatment because the treatment rationale seems unconvincing, and (2) treatment adherence problems because the patient has not understood or has forgotten the treatment rationale. Patients may find the treatment rationale to be unconvincing if they strongly believe in some other model of PTSD (e.g., strict biological determinism). When providing psychoeducation, the therapist should elicit patients' beliefs about the causes and treatment of their problems. The therapist can attempt to reconcile the cognitive-behavioral model with the patient's beliefs (e.g., beliefs are rooted in the brain, and psychotherapy can change brain function; see Chapter 4). The therapist can also use cognitive restructuring to correct any misconceptions. If patients strongly believe that only one treatment is "right" for them (such as some other form of psychotherapy or pharmacotherapy), then the therapist has several options. The therapist can discuss, in a nondefensive manner, the treatment outcome research on CBT and other interventions (Chapter 5) to educate the patient about the relative efficacy of treatments. A trial of CBT can be presented as a "no lose" option. If it is beneficial, then the patient has profited from the experience. If treatment is not effective, then the patient has many other treatment options. If the patient insists on some other form of treatment, then the therapist can offer to make arrangements for the suitable referral. The patient can also be invited to return for CBT if, in the future, he or she decides to pursue that option.

The treatment rationale may seem unconvincing to the patient if it is not clear how the interventions are relevant to his or her symptoms. When exposure exercises are described, patients sometimes object that they are "already" doing exposure because they can't stop thinking about the trauma. The therapist can review the nature of reexperiencing symptoms and contrast them with exposure therapy. Reexperiencing symptoms are typically brief, intense, and difficult to control. The patient may resort to distraction or avoidance to escape them. This is different from exposure exercises, which are prolonged and typically begin with relatively mild stimuli, in which the patient retains complete control over the exercises. Exposure exercises also differ from reexperiencing symptoms in that treatment aims to incorporate corrective information with the trauma memory, which may come in the form of information provided by distress reduction (extinction of emotional responses), and information about the meaning of trauma-related stimuli (e.g., learning that trauma memories are not dangerous). Such corrective information typically does not arise from naturally occurring reexperiencing symptoms (Rothbaum & Mellman, 2001).

TREATMENT ENGAGEMENT STRATEGIES

Rationale

My approach to treatment engagement draws on the methods of motivational interviewing (Miller & Rollnick, 2002), which are used for enhancing the odds that the patient will enter and actively pursue treatment. Treatment engagement strategies may be implemented in the first session and used, as needed, throughout treatment.

People are often ambivalent about important issues in their lives. People with PTSD, for example, may be highly distressed and want to get over their problems, but also be reluctant to engage in treatment because therapy involves talking about distressing things that the patient would sooner avoid. It can be useful for the therapist to *amplify* the patient's ambivalence (Miller & Rollnick, 2002). This induces a form of cognitive dissonance, which the person seeks to resolve. The state of ambivalence motivates efforts to change. The therapist can, therefore, strengthen ambivalence to motivate PTSD patients to engage in therapy.

Attempts to force resolution of ambivalence in a particular direction, such as by forcefully telling a person that they need to try a course of CBT, can sometimes lead to a paradoxical response, even strengthening the very beliefs or behaviors that the therapist is seeking to diminish (Miller & Rollnick, 2002). This phenomenon is known as *reactance* (Brehm, 1962). When the therapist forcefully presents one side of an issue ("You need to confront your fears"), the ambivalent patient may respond by thinking of counterarguments ("Yes, but that will make my nightmares worse"). Rather than forcefully trying to convince patients to change their attitudes, therapists are more effective when they elicit arguments for change from the patients themselves (Emmons & Rollnick, 2001). This can be done by means of open questions, reflective listening, summary statements, and differential reinforcement of the patient's utterances in order to elicit self-motivating statements.

Methods

Open-Ended Questions and Reflective Listening

Open questions are those that do not involve yes/no or similarly circumscribed sets of responses. Such questioning is useful in helping patients identify self-defeating beliefs and actions. Open questioning can be followed by reflective listening. In reflective listening the therapist reflects what the patient has said, but often in a slightly modified or reframed fashion. The reflection may include the patient's expressed or implied emotions. There are several advantages of reflective listening (Miller, 1995):

- It is unlikely to evoke resistance ("Yes, but . . . " responses) to what the therapist says.
- Reflective listening communicates the therapist's respect and caring for the patient, thereby contributing to a good working relationship.
- It clarifies for the therapist exactly what the patient means.
- It can be used to reinforce self-motivating statements. Patients hear themselves making self-motivating statements and then hear the therapist reflect them back (e.g., Therapist: "You're saying that it's important for you to stop avoiding things that remind you of the trauma").
- Reflective listening can be used to selectively reinforce ideas expressed by the patient (e.g., Therapist: "I hear you saying that trying to suppress thoughts of the trauma has not worked, and in some ways has made you even more preoccupied with the trauma").
- Open-ended questions and reflective listening can also increase awareness of ambivalence and move patients toward more adaptive thinking (e.g., Therapist: "You mentioned that, on the one hand, all this avoidance is ruining your life, but on the other hand, it's been hard for you to confront your fears, and so you sort of want to avoid. I wonder how this dilemma could be solved").
- Open questioning and reflective listening are also useful tools for exploring the patient's skepticism about the value of CBT. This can help to correct any misconceptions. (e.g., Therapist: "I appreciate you telling me that you're skeptical. I'd be happy to answer any questions. But first, tell me, what made you decide to come to this appointment in the first place?")
- Open questions can also be used to build motivation for change. The patient can be asked, for example, whether there is anyone in their life, their spouse or children, whose life would improve if the patient got better (Najavits, 2002).

Eliciting Self-Motivating Statements and Strengthening Self-Efficacy for Change

An important goal of treatment is to have the patient voice adaptive responses, because self-generated responses are more likely to be remembered and believed by the patient, compared to responses provided by the therapist ("If I said it, and nobody forced me to say it, then I must believe it"; Miller, 1995). The therapist therefore assists patients in talking themselves into changing (Moyers & Rollnick, 2002).

Self-motivating statements are useful for initially encouraging patients to try a course of CBT and, later in treatment, encouraging them to persist at homework assignments, such as exposure exercises. The following illustrates one useful strategy for eliciting self-motivating statements, and for identifying motivational barriers (Miller & Rollnick, 2002), as applied to PTSD.

> THERAPIST: To help me understand your reasons for seeking help, I'd like to ask you a couple of things. On a scale of 1 to 10, with 10 being the highest, how motivated or interested are you in trying some CBT sessions to help you with your PTSD?
>
> PATIENT: My rating would be 3.
>
> THERAPIST: OK, 3 out of 10. Thanks for being frank with me. What made you choose 3? Why not choose a lower number like 2 or 1?
>
> PATIENT: People keep telling me that I need to see you, and I've heard that CBT can help people.
>
> THERAPIST: They sound like good reasons. And why choose 3 instead of a higher number, like 9 or 10?
>
> PATIENT: Nothing has helped me so far, so I'm not optimistic about CBT.
>
> THERAPIST: What would it take to get you to a 9 or 10?
>
> PATIENT: I'd need to see some proof that treatment is starting to work.
>
> THERAPIST: So, are you willing to give it a try?
>
> PATIENT: Yes, I need to do something to get over my problems.
>
> THERAPIST: So, to summarize, you're saying that CBT might be worthwhile because other people have been helped, and because other people think you need this sort of help. But for you to get really interested in CBT, we first need to see if we can do something that might help even just a little bit.
>
> PATIENT: Yes, that's right.
>
> THERAPIST: OK, good. Let's talk about where we could start . . .

TROUBLESHOOTING

Resistance to CBT can take many forms, such as the patient arguing with the therapist, repeatedly interrupting, and rejecting or ignoring the therapist's suggestions. A general guideline is to avoid confronting resistance directly, because that can escalate rather than reduce resistance (Moyers & Rollnick, 2002). There are three useful strategies for dealing with resistance, early and throughout treatment (Miller, 1995; Miller & Rollnick, 2002; Moyers & Rollnick, 2002): amplified reflection, double-sided reflection, and strategic responses to resistance.

Amplified Reflection

With this method the therapist slightly overstates the patient's resistance, in a sincere, nonaccusatory fashion. This capitalizes on the natural tendency of patients to speak against either side of an issue about which they are ambivalent. This induces the patient, rather than the therapist, to advance arguments for the desired change (Moyers & Rollnick, 2002).

> PATIENT: I thought about using a day planner to schedule things that would get me out of the house, but then I thought, "What's the point?"
>
> THERAPIST: I appreciate you telling me that. Do you think that there's absolutely no way that these sorts of activities could help you with your feelings of being emotionally numb and cut off from people?
>
> PATIENT: Well, I wouldn't take it that far.
>
> THERAPIST: OK. So, what effects would these exercises have on the way you feel?
>
> PATIENT: I guess I don't know yet.
>
> THERAPIST: Do you think it's worth finding out?
>
> PATIENT: I think I should give it another try.

Double-Sided Reflection

When offering a double-sided reflection, the therapist voices arguments for and against a given issue, using the linking words "and" or "but." Such questions encourage the patient to examine the discrepancies between beliefs or between behaviors.

> THERAPIST: You'd like to start dating again because it's lonely and boring doing everything by yourself, *but* you're also reluctant to go on dates because you have a lot of trouble trusting men because of what happened to you.
>
> PATIENT: Yes, I feel like I'm stuck between a rock and a hard place.
>
> THERAPIST: Right. So, what are some ways of solving this problem? For example, how might you figure out who you can trust?

Strategic Responses to Resistance

These involve shifting the direction of the discussion. To illustrate, the therapist might overtly shift focus by declining to argue about whether the patient's PTSD is caused by a "biochemical imbalance." This can involve "agreeing with a twist," where the therapist offers initial agreement but with a slight twist or change of direction (Miller & Rollnick, 2002).

> THERAPIST: Thanks for being open with me. It's important for me to know that you don't see how talking about the trauma can help, because you've heard that PTSD may involve a biochemical imbalance. I agree that biochemistry certainly plays some role in PTSD. By the way, has the medication helped so far?
>
> PATIENT: It's helped a little bit, but the effects seem to be wearing off.
>
> THERAPIST: Was that why your psychiatrist suggested that you come and see me?
>
> PATIENT: Yes, I suppose so.
>
> THERAPIST: OK. If you like, we can discuss how talk therapy can work, even if the person's problems are associated with changes in brain chemistry. Would that be a useful way to spend our time today?
>
> PATIENT: Yes, that's a good idea. I need to understand how talk therapy could help.

EMOTION REGULATION EXERCISES

Emotion regulation exercises can be used in the patient's daily life in order to manage distressing emotions, and to manage high levels of emotion during treatment, such as before and after exposure exercises or if the patient otherwise becomes very distressed while discussing the trauma or other stressful experiences. The following sections describe the most effective emotion regulation exercises: breathing retraining, applied relaxation, grounding exercises, and mastery and pleasure exercises.

The key challenge in using these exercises is to discourage the patient from using them as a means of avoiding feared consequences (e.g., "If I let myself get too anxious I'll go crazy"). In such cases the patient should be encouraged to gradually test the fear consequences, which may involve fading out the use of emotion regulation exercises. Misuse of the exercises is less likely to occur if they are employed simply to reduce unpleasant emotions (e.g., "I know that anxiety won't hurt me, but it feels really unpleasant, so it would be good to reduce it"). In such cases the use of these exercises can improve the patient's sense of control over his or her ability to manage stressors.

Breathing Retraining

Rationale

When some people become distressed they tend to hyperventilate, which is defined as oxygen intake that is in excess of metabolic needs. Hyperventilation is harmless but induces bodily sensations such as dizziness, shortness of breath, palpitations, and chest tightness or pain. Chest discomfort is caused by breathing with the chest muscles, which commonly occurs during hyperventilation, rather than with the diaphragm. Breathing retraining exercises, which involve slow, diaphragmatic breathing, can be used to reduce hyperventilation. With repeated practice, slow, diaphragmatic breathing becomes habitual. Patients can be taught to identify stimuli that might trigger hyperventilation (e.g., stressful events) and to implement slow, diaphragmatic breathing at these times. Even if the person does not hyperventilate when distressed, he or she can benefit from breathing retraining because it induces a state of calm and relaxation.

Exercises

Breathing retraining consists of a number of simple exercises that can be taught in a couple of sessions. The procedures, based on those described in Taylor (2000), are as follows.

- Patients are first educated about the distinction between "chest breathing" and "diaphragm breathing." Patients are told that chest breathing can produce harmless but uncomfortable sensations such as chest tightness or pain and is associated with hyperventilation. The therapist emphasizes that chest breathing and hyperventilation are harmless but can cause unpleasant sensations, such as chest pain, dizziness, or shortness of breath
- The therapist demonstrates the two types of breathing and shows how to best observe the difference between the two. Placing one hand on the chest and one on the stomach (in order to show differences in movement), the therapist demonstrates how the rib cage moves upward and outward during chest breathing. Then, the therapist demonstrates how the stomach but not the chest moves in and out during diaphragmatic breathing. Patients then perform the exercise, placing their hands over their own chest and stomach, practicing the two types of breathing and observing the differences.
- Patients are then asked to practice diaphragmatic breathing for 10 minutes in the therapist's office. Respiration should be at a comfortable rate, with breathing through the nose rather than the mouth. The goal is to achieve a slow, smooth, shallow pattern of breathing.

- The patient should observe the abdomen rising and falling with each breath, while breathing with the diaphragm and keeping the chest still. Patients are instructed to notice the cool air slowly coming in through the nostrils as they inhale, then pause for 1–2 seconds, and then notice the warm air slowly flowing out as they exhale. As they exhale, patients should try to relax their bodies, including the muscles in the jaw and face (which are often sites of tension). A coping statement can also be added, such as saying to oneself the word "calm" or "serene" while breathing out. Initially, the target respiration rate is about 12 breaths per minute (i.e., inhaling for 2 seconds, pausing for 1 second, and exhaling for 2 seconds).

- For homework, the patient is requested to sit or lie down in a quite place at home, free from distractions, and practice the diaphragmatic breathing 2–3 times per day for 10 minutes each time. Breathing should be at a comfortable rate. The importance of regular practice is emphasized.

- Application training usually commences in the next treatment session. To train patients to abort episodes of hyperventilation, they are asked to hyperventilate for 1–2 minutes and then practice controlling their respiration by implementing slow diaphragmatic breathing. This is practiced several times during the therapy session. Patients should be advised that their breathing rate should always feel comfortable.

- For homework, the patient continues practicing slow diaphragmatic breathing while sitting at home for 10 minutes 2–3 times per day. The respiration rate can be slowed down to 8–10 breaths per minute.

- Patients are also asked to complete application training homework. This consists of practicing slow diaphragmatic breathing in a variety of everyday situations: while watching TV, waiting in lines in stores, sitting in the car at traffic lights, and so forth. Patients gradually practice in increasingly challenging situations. Various stimuli can be used as cues or reminders to practice a breathing exercise, including particular situations (e.g., stressful circumstances).

- For children, ages 4–12 years, breathing retraining (and other emotion regulation exercises) can be taught by using engaging, developmentally appropriate play therapy techniques, as illustrated in the following case example.

Six-year-old Mathew was taught how to calm himself in stressful situations by using the "Bubble Breaths" method (Cabe, 2001). The session began with the therapist explaining how he was going to show Mathew how blowing bubbles can make you feel calm. A bottle of "Mr. Bubbles" liquid and a bubble wand was produced, and for a few minutes the therapist blew bubbles while Mathew popped them. Mathew was then asked to blow some bubbles. The therapist next instructed Mathew how to blow special bubbles by using diaphragmatic breathing:

"Now, Mathew, I'd like to show you a special kind of breathing that can help you feel calm. The best way to learn this method is to practice blowing only one big bubble at a time. I'd like you to take a slow, deep breath from your tummy. That is, push your tummy out as you breathe in. Then, slowly blow the air out so you can blow one big bubble."

Several minutes were spent practicing this method, and Mathew was also given the same type of information that adults receive about the rationale and use of breathing retraining. This information was presented in terms that Mathew could readily comprehend. For example, "When you feel anxious or upset, you can practice the breathing exercise by taking some long, slow, deep breaths, and imagine that you're slowly blowing great big bubbles."

TROUBLESHOOTING

It is not uncommon for anxious patients, whether they are adults or children, to have trouble slowing down their breathing. Patients should be reminded that their breathing rate should be slowed to a rate that remains comfortable. The therapist can assure patients that they're doing the exercise properly even if they're only able to slow their breathing to a small degree. With time and practice patients are typically able to slow their breathing even more, to a rate that remains comfortable.

Applied Relaxation

Rationale

Applied relaxation (Öst, 1987) consists of exercises to help the patient rapidly relax in a variety of situations, particularly stressful circumstances. It typically requires some weeks of practice for patients to become proficient at all the components of the program. Applied relaxation can be used if breathing retraining is insufficient to relax the patient. Applied relaxation would be used, for example, if the patient suffered from intense, persistent hyperarousal sensations. Here, breathing retraining can be included as a component of applied relaxation.

Exercises

This version of applied relaxation, which is abbreviated from Öst's (1987) original version, consists of three exercises, taught in three sessions: tense–release relaxation, release-only relaxation, and rapid relaxation. The therapist begins by educating patients about the purpose of applied relaxation: to teach a coping skill that will enable them to recognize the early signs of arousal and relax rapidly in order to reduce harmless but unpleasant stress-related bodily reactions. The goal is to relax within 20–30 seconds. The protocol is summarized in Handout 9.2 (pp. 172–173). The handout is supplemented by an audiotape, recorded by the therapist specifically for a given patient, in which the therapist goes through each of the exercises.

The patient listens to the tape as a homework assignment. The audiotape is particularly useful in guiding the patient through the early stages of practicing tense–release and release-only relaxation. The tape is gradually discontinued in order to encourage the patient to implement self-directed relaxation. Patients then practice the exercises for several weeks until they become proficient at relaxing. Then the exercises are used as needed. Details of the relaxation procedures are as follows.

TENSE–RELEASE RELAXATION

This exercise, described in Handout 9.2, can be practiced in a comfortable chair. Each muscle group is tensed for 5 seconds and then relaxed for 5–15 seconds. Muscle tensing and releasing is used to deepen relaxation and to sharpen the patient's ability to identify the difference between tension and relaxation. The better the ability to detect tension, the greater the chances of implementing relaxation when tension develops. The goal of the tense–release relaxation is not to tense the muscles until they hurt. If pain or cramps occur—or if the patient has a history of some sort of recurrent pain (e.g., low back pain)—then the affected muscles should be weakly tensed or not tensed at all. Tense–release relaxation begins by having the patient work through the muscle groups in the handout during the therapy session. Homework consists of practicing for 15–30 minutes twice per day, for at least 2 weeks. The exercise can be audiotaped to facilitate practice. The audiotape is then faded out as the patient learns to relax without the tape.

When such relaxation exercises are used with children, it is helpful to include concrete metaphors to facilitate relaxation. For example, for the "tense" portion of tense–release relaxation, children can be asked to imagine that they are a robot, and for the "release" portion they can be asked to imagine that they are a wet noodle or rag doll (Vernberg & Johnston, 2001).

RELEASE-ONLY RELAXATION

The next step is to repeat the protocol for tense–release relaxation, but this time omitting the tensing portion of the exercise. Patients are simply asked to focus on releasing tension from the various muscle groups, starting at the top of the head and working down to the toes. If patients notice tension in a particular muscle group, then they can briefly tense and release those muscles. As before, the exercise is practiced in the session and as home-work. The latter should be done twice per day for at least a week. The exercise can be audiotaped to facilitate practice, and then the tape is faded out. The following is a sample script of release-only relaxation, in which the therapist guides the patient through the exercise. This script pairs the cue "relax" with the relaxation of each muscle group.

"Breathe with calm, regular breaths and feel how you relax more and more with every breath . . . Just let go . . . And as you relax, say to yourself, under your breath, the word "relax" each time you breathe out . . . Imagining the word "relax" each time you breathe out . . . Relax your forehead . . . eyebrows . . . eyelids . . . jaws . . . tongue and throat . . . lips . . . your entire face . . . Imagining the word "relax" each time you breathe out . . . Relax your neck . . . shoulders . . . arms . . . hands . . . and all the way out to your fingertips . . . Imagining the word "relax" each time you breathe out . . . Breathe calmly and regularly with your stomach all the time . . . Let the relaxation spread to your stomach . . . waist and back . . . Relax the lower part of your body, your behind . . . thighs . . . knees . . . calves . . . feet . . . and all the way down to the tips of your toes . . . Imagining the word "relax" each time you breathe out . . . Breathe calmly and regularly and feel how you relax more and more by each breath . . . Take a deep breath and hold your breath a couple of seconds . . . and let the air out slowly . . . slowly . . . Notice how you relax more and more."

RAPID RELAXATION

This exercise teaches patients to quickly relax in everyday situations. Rapid relaxation consists of (1) taking 1–3 deep breaths and slowly exhaling; (2) thinking "relax" before each exhalation; and (3) scanning one's body for tension and trying to relax as much as possible as one breathes out. In-session practice begins with a few trials of relaxation in a comfortable chair. Then the patient practices relaxing under increasingly active circumstances. Patients are asked to perform a series of exercises in which activities are performed in which only the essential muscles are tensed. Examples include: (1) opening one's eyes and looking around while relaxing all the muscles except those required to sit upright and look about; (2) lifting one arm, and then the other, lifting one foot, one leg and then the other, while relaxing all the muscles that are not needed for those activities; and (3) tensing the biceps while keeping the hands relaxed. Patients then practice relaxing under increasingly active circumstances, such as walking about while relaxing all the muscles except those required for ambulation. For homework, the exercises are practiced in various settings at least 20 times per day. Colored dots or other salient stimuli are used as reminders to practice relaxation. A blue dot, for example, might be stuck on a patient's cell phone as a reminder to use the relaxation exercise.

TROUBLESHOOTING

The therapist should check whether the patient has any unpleasant associations to the words used as relaxation cues ("calm," "relax," etc.), and use alternative cues (e.g., "serenity" or "peace"). Sometimes words like "calm" or "relax" are counterproductive as relaxation cues because they remind the patient of the trauma (Meadows & Foa, 1998; Najavits, 2002). For example, the patient may have been previously told by an abusive parent or spouse to "Calm down, or I'll give you something to cry about!" A rapist may have told his victim to "relax, and you won't get hurt."

Relaxation exercises sometimes trigger anxiety, panic, or dissociation (Taylor, 2000). This can happen if patients harbor catastrophic beliefs about relaxation sensations. Such sensations include warmth, numbness, falling or floating feelings, depersonalization, and slowed heart rate. Beliefs about relaxation sensations include misconceptions that the sensations will lead to insanity ("Unreal feelings will become so strong that I lose touch with reality") or beliefs about loss of control ("If I let go of muscle tension then I won't be able to protect myself"). Relaxation-induced anxiety and panic can be treated by providing corrective information about the harmlessness of the sensations, for example, the information that increased peripheral blood flow and reduction in muscle tension produces many of the sensations. If problems persist then relaxation can be used as a form of interoceptive exposure (Chapter 12). Another option is to have the patient relax with eyes open if he or she tends to dissociate while relaxing with eyes closed.

It is important to identify the misuse of relaxation as an avoidance strategy in patients who are frightened of their hyperarousal and other PTSD symptoms (i.e., in patients with high anxiety sensitivity). This is illustrated in the following case example in which an oversight in developing the case formulation led to an ineffective treatment plan.

Christie reported that there were so many trauma cues (reminders) and other stressors in her life that she constantly felt anxious and overwhelmed. Based on this information, the therapist assumed that recurrent stressors were fueling Christie's PTSD symptoms and that the symptoms persisted because exposure to the trauma cues was too brief for the extinction of emotional responses to occur. Accordingly, the therapist initiated treatment with a program of applied relaxation to help Christie manage her hyperarousal symptoms. The treatment plan also included gradual situational exposure to harmless but distressing trauma cues. Christie agreed to the treatment plan and assiduously practiced her relaxation exercises. In fact, the therapist was surprised by Christie's diligence. Despite practicing relaxation for nearly two months, however, Christie continued to report that she was troubled by anxiety symptoms and that it was still too difficult for her to attempt any of the exposure exercises. The therapist and Christie agreed to revisit the case formulation and to attempt to identify the source of the problems. The therapist decided to administer the Anxiety Sensitivity Index (see Chapter 6), which had not been administered in the initial assessment because of time constraints. Christie obtained an extremely high score on this scale. The therapist further learned that Christie's main reason for practicing relaxation was that she was frightened that she would lose control and go crazy if she allowed herself to become too anxious. This additional information also seemed to explain her extreme reluctance to engage in situational exposure exercises because they evoked anxiety. The therapist shared this information with Christie, and they agreed on a revised formulation in which elevated anxiety sensitivity was shown to be playing an important role in her problems. The treatment plan was revised accordingly. Instead of continuing with relaxation training, the next three treatment sessions were spent exploring Christie's beliefs about arousal-related sensations and implementing cognitive restructuring exercises (Chapter 11). This was followed by four sessions of interoceptive exposure (Chapter 12). These interventions were sufficient in reducing her anxiety sensitivity, thereby making it easier for Christie to complete her situational exposure exercises. She no longer had a strong urge to practice relaxation because she was better able to tolerate anxiety.

Grounding Exercises

Rationale

Grounding exercises (Benham, 1995; Chu, 1998) can be used for managing two types of dissociation seen in PTSD: stress-induced dissociative alterations in awareness (e.g., depersonalization, derealization) and flashbacks triggered by exposure to trauma cues (i.e., feeling like one is back in the trauma situation).

These exercises can be used to manage dissociation in the patient's everyday life and dissociation induced by exposure therapy exercises. Grounding exercises are emotion regulation exercises in the sense that dissociation is usually (but not always) induced by exposure to distressing stimuli. Grounding exercises can be useful regardless of whether dissociation is an automatic (involuntary) or a controlled (intentional) coping response. Clinically, dissociation is most often described by patients as being an involuntary reaction. If the patient is deliberately dissociating as a means of avoiding awareness of stressful stimuli, then the therapist and patient should explore the efficacy and pitfalls of this coping response, and more adaptive strategies could be considered.

Grounding exercises are typically not needed for mild dissociative reactions. These tend to abate after the patient has had a few minutes to calm down. However, grounding exercises can be used to give the patient a tool for managing more intense dissociative reactions, which are often disturbing and disruptive.

Exercises

Handout 9.3 (pp. 174–175) provides information on the nature and management of dissociative reactions. The first step in managing dissociation is to help the patient identify stimuli or conditions that are likely to give rise to dissociation. This can make dissociative reactions appear less mysterious and more predictable and understandable to the patient.

Patients can be encouraged to come up with their own variations on the grounding strategies described in Handout 9.3, using whatever methods they find most effective. Adaptations of these grounding methods include exercises like the following: Name as many colors in the room as you can; count the number of books or pieces of furniture in the room; look outside and describe the weather; describe your shoes; or name as many different cities, animals, or TV shows as you can (Chu, 1998; Najavits, 2002). Other grounding exercises include running cool or warm water over one's hands, stretching, or eating something and focusing on the texture of the food and the flavors (Najavits, 2002). Najavits provides a particularly good example of therapist dialogue used to help patients ground themselves if they dissociate during the therapy session.

> "Notice your feet on the floor. They are literally grounded, connected to the floor. Wiggle your toes inside your shoes. Dig your heels gently into the floor to ground yourself even more. Good. Now touch your chair: Tell me anything you can about it—what material is it made of? Now touch the table (or desk): What is it made of? Is it colder or warmer than the chair? Good. Now, find any object that's near you—perhaps a pen, or your keys, or something here on the desk. Pick it up and hold it, and say everything you can about it: What it's made of, how heavy it is, whether it's cold or warm, what color it is. Now clench your fists; notice the tension in your hands as you do that. Now release your fists. Good. Now press your palms together, with elbows at the side; press as tightly as you can. Focus all of your attention on your palms. Now let go. Excellent! Now grab onto your chair as tightly as you can; then after a few moments, now let it go. Finally, roll your head around in a circle a few times. Excellent." (2002, pp. 130–131)

The therapist's tone of voice should be matter of fact and reassuring, not hypnotic (Chu, 1998). If the patient has a flashback during the session, the therapist can remind the patient that he or she is safe and that the trauma is in the past. Asking the patient to make eye contact and listen to the therapist's voice can also help end the dissociative state.

Grounding exercises are best used in situations in which there is good ambient lighting (in the clinic or at home) (Chu, 1998), in order to highlight the patient's current (safe) environment and to distract him or her from internally generated scenarios (flashbacks). Outside of the therapeutic setting, patients should be discouraged from sitting or hiding in dark or dimly lit environments when they feel anxious or dissociative. Dark facilitates reexperiencing and dissociation because of the lack of competing external (environmental) cues (Chu, 1998).

TROUBLESHOOTING

If dissociation tends to occur when the patient is in potentially hazardous situations (e.g., while driving), then it may be necessary to avoid those situations until the dissociation has been effectively treated, with grounding or other treatment methods. In rare instances, a patient might dissociate during a treatment session in which his or her trauma is being discussed and not emerge from the dissociative state by the time the session ends. The patient may appear dazed and may be minimally responsive to the therapist. Here, the therapist can tell the patient something like the following.

> "I see that our time for today is up. I'm going to step out of the office now for a few minutes to give you all the time you need to wind down and get grounded. Take all the time you need. It's OK. I'll be in back in few minutes to see how you are. I'll bring a glass of water for you in case you're thirsty."

Mastery and Pleasure Exercises

Rationale

Mastery and pleasure exercises are derived from Beck's cognitive therapy for depression (Beck et al., 1979). They are used in treating PTSD for a variety of reasons, such as to reduce numbing symptoms, to provide distractions in order to reduce ruminative thinking, and to treat comorbid depression and improve quality of life (Blanchard et al., 2003; Jaycox & Foa, 1996; Taylor et al., 2001).

Exercises

Mastery exercises are typically implemented in a graded fashion, starting with relatively simple, low-effort activities and gradually progressing to more effortful ones. For example, a patient who spends most of the day in bed might be encouraged to get out of bed each day, shower, and get dressed. Once these tasks are being routinely done, the patient would progress to other tasks, such as spending 20 minutes each day doing housework. The goal is to gradually progress up the activity hierarchy to a desired level. The choice of mastery exercises depend on what is important to the patient to accomplish. Patients are encouraged to keep a diary or day planner in which they track their progress in completing these exercises.

Pleasure exercises can be conducted in a similar manner, starting with exercises that are low in effort and expense, and are feasible to do. The patient should be encouraged to complete at least one of these exercises each day, in addition to a mastery exercise. The patient should be encouraged to do the pleasure exercises regardless of whether they currently induce a sense of enjoyment. With time, practice, and patience, these exercises can increase the patient's enjoyment in life.

PTSD patients with severe numbing and depressive symptoms often have difficulty thinking of feasible and potentially enjoyable activities. A list of suggestions, such as the one in Handout 9.4 (pp. 176–177), can be useful for providing them with ideas. Using the handout, patients indicate which of the activities they did in the past week. The patient and therapist can then review the checklist to see if there are other enjoyable activities that the patient has not been doing. Patients can then be encouraged to attempt these activities in order to improve their quality of life.

TROUBLESHOOTING

Some patients resist these sorts of exercises, particularly the pleasure exercises, because they strongly believe that they don't deserve good things. In such cases it may be important to do cognitive restructuring on guilt-related beliefs (Chapter 11). If the patient expresses beliefs concerning hopelessness or helplessness about performing the exercises, then cognitive methods for treating these depressogenic beliefs could be implemented (Beck et al., 1979).

When patients are implementing pleasure exercises, the therapist should ensure that these are not self-defeating activities, such as things that bring short-term enjoyment or relief from distress but longer-term problems. Examples include binge eating, substance abuse, spending or gambling beyond one's budget, and unsafe sex.

SUMMARY

Psychoeducation is an essential intervention for PTSD treatment, whereas treatment engagement strategies and emotion regulation exercises are frequently used but are not necessary for every case. Some patients come to treatment with strong treatment motivation and are able to tolerate their emotional distress. Most patients, however, can benefit from treatment engagement interventions and from training in emotion regulation strategies. Despite the importance of the interventions described in this chapter, they are typically insufficient for treating PTSD. Rather, they facilitate the implementation of other, more potent, interventions such as the cognitive restructuring and exposure exercises discussed in the following chapters.

A CONCISE GUIDE TO POSTTRAUMATIC STRESS DISORDER (PTSD)

What Is PTSD?

PTSD can arise after a person has been exposed to a traumatic event. A traumatic event is something in which the person is exposed to actual or threatened harm. Examples include sexual or physical assault, war zone experiences, natural disasters such as severe earthquakes or floods, and serious motor vehicle accidents. PTSD is diagnosed when the person has experienced a traumatic event and then experiences, for a month or more, the following symptoms:

1. *Reexperiencing symptoms, in which the person relives the trauma in at least one of the following ways:*
   - Recurrent, unwanted recollections of the trauma
   - Recurrent distressing dreams of the trauma
   - Acting or feeling as if the trauma was recurring ("flashbacks")
   - Intense bodily reactions when reminded of the trauma (e.g., sweating, pounding heart)
   - Intense emotional distress when reminded of the trauma (e.g., intense anxiety)

2. *Persistent avoidance of things associated with the trauma, and a sense of emotional numbing, as indicated by at least three of the following:*
   - Efforts to avoid thinking about or talking about the trauma
   - Efforts to avoid people, places, or things that are reminders of the trauma
   - Inability to recall important parts of the trauma
   - Markedly diminished interest in things that the person used to enjoy
   - Feeling distant or emotionally detached from other people
   - A restricted range of emotion (e.g., unable to experience loving feelings)
   - A sense of that one's future will be cut short (e.g., the sense that one will not live long enough to have a career, marriage, or family)

3. *Persistent symptoms of increased arousal, as indicated by at least two of the following:*
   - Difficulty falling asleep or staying asleep
   - Irritability or outbursts of anger
   - Difficulty concentrating
   - Feeling hyperalert for danger (e.g., feeling on guard all the time)
   - Exaggerated startle response (e.g., feeling jumpy or easily startled)

The following case example illustrates these symptoms.

> Mike was caught in a severe earthquake while on holiday. He barely escaped the hotel before it collapsed. When Mike returned home he thought that the worst was over, but he was wrong. Each night he was tormented by terrifying nightmares, from which he would awake drenched in sweat. The nightmares were so intense that he dreaded going to sleep at night. During the day he found that every time he closed his eyes he had involuntary recollections of the devastation he had witnessed, as if he was watching a movie. Friends said that Mike seemed to have changed since the earthquake; he rarely smiled, and seemed distant and preoccupied. Family members were puzzled that he would always change the topic whenever they mentioned the quake. They knew something was wrong, but didn't know what to do. Mike avoided phone calls from his fellow travelers, who were also were involved in the quake. Whenever he walked into a building he found himself scanning the walls and ceiling to check for cracks or other signs that the building was not structurally sound. Since the quake Mike had become increasingly irritable and impatient, especially while driving or waiting in line at the grocery store. He was unable to read newspapers or keep track of conversations because he couldn't concentrate.

(continued)

What Causes PTSD?

The brain contains a stress response system, which interprets events, decides whether the events are threatening, and reacts with anxiety or fear if threat is detected. PTSD arises from a hypersensitive stress response system, which leads the person to feel like they're on "red alert" much of the time. The sensitivity of the stress response system is influenced by the beliefs that people hold about themselves, other people, and the world. For example, if a person believes that "all tattooed men are potential murderers" then he or she is likely to be anxious, jumpy, and vigilant in situations in which there are tattooed men.

There are two main things that influence the sensitivity of the stress response system. The first is the person's genetic makeup. Some people inherit a strong disposition to develop PTSD, whereas other people have less of an inherited tendency to develop the disorder. Even people who are well-adjusted, successful, and competent can develop PTSD if they have a genetic predisposition to the disorder.

The second important cause of PTSD is the sorts of events that the person has experienced. There are two important types of events: the actual traumatic stressor, and the things the person experienced in the past, such as experiences that happened years before the traumatic event. The experience of past trauma can sensitize the stress response system, thereby increasing the chances that the person will develop PTSD in the future if he or she experiences a traumatic event.

The severity of the traumatic event is another important cause of PTSD; severe stressors, such as being caught in a hurricane, are more likely to lead to PTSD than comparatively less severe events. Everyone has a breaking point; even elite soldiers develop PTSD if the stressor is sufficiently severe. The person's breaking point is determined, in part, by genetic makeup. A person who has little or no genetic predisposition to develop PTSD may develop this disorder only after experiencing a severely traumatic event (such as being tortured). A person with a strong genetic predisposition will develop PTSD in response to less severe stressors, such as being mugged.

Once people develop PTSD they find that they are sensitive to things in their world that trigger memories of the trauma. Triggers may include reminders of the trauma (e.g., the sight of black hoodies, if that was what the assailant wore, or the sight of people in uniforms if you were involved in combat). Triggers can also be things that were only part of the trauma, such as certain smells (e.g., cologne) or sounds (e.g., honking horns) that were associated with the trauma.

What Are the Effective Treatments?

The good news is that there are a number of scientifically proven treatments for PTSD. If a person does not benefit from one treatment, then the other treatments can be helpful. The two main groups of treatments are (1) a psychological (non-drug) treatment known as cognitive-behavioral therapy, and (2) various types of medications, such as medications known as selective serotonin reuptake inhibitors (e.g., Prozac, Zoloft, Paxil). Cognitive-behavioral therapy involves a number of treatment sessions in which the patient and therapist explore the meaning of the traumatic event, to help the patient make sense of experience, along with exercises to help *desensitize* the patient to distressing but harmless reminders to the traumatic event. For example, Mike was asked to write out his experience in the earthquake, and to read his description each day. At first, Mike found this to be distressing. With time, however, he could read the description without becoming upset, and became less worried about earthquakes in general. Cognitive-behavioral therapy and medications are equally effective. Only qualified healthcare professionals can provide these treatments, such as a psychologist or psychiatrist.

HANDOUT 9.2. Relaxation and Breathing Exercises

APPLIED RELAXATION

What Is Applied Relaxation?

Applied relaxation (AR) is a portable skill that helps you recognize and overcome the effects of stress, including tension, pain, and a host of other bodily reactions. Just like any other skill, such as learning to play the piano or drive a car, AR requires practice in order to become good at implementing the relaxation exercises. Your therapist will help you by making a relaxation tape for you to listen to. With sufficient practice, you will be able to implement the AR exercises rapidly in practically any situation. The goal is to be able to relax in 20–30 seconds. To achieve this goal, follow these steps:

- *Tense–release relaxation*: Practice tensing and relaxing various muscle groups. Each muscle group is tensed for a brief period and then relaxed. The purpose is to increase your awareness of muscle tension, and to enhance relaxation from the inertia built up by tensing then releasing. The entire exercise takes about 15 minutes. After that, we will begin to shorten the procedure to develop more portable relaxation skills. We do this by working through the following exercises:
- *Release-only relaxation*: This is the same as the above but without tensing the muscles first. This takes 10 minutes. During this exercise we teach you to connect the self-instruction "relax" to the bodily state of relaxation.
- *Rapid relaxation*: Here, you practice a quick relaxation exercise many times each day in nonstressful situations. This also involves practicing relaxation while doing various activities, such as walking. You will then be asked to practice rapid relaxation in daily stressful situations.

Please be aware that when you first begin to use AR, you probably won't become very relaxed. Don't give up! With practice you will get better and better at relaxing.

Tense–Release Relaxation

Duration: 15 minutes

Instructions: (1) Sit in a comfortable position, free from distractions. (2) Close your eyes and scan your body, looking for areas of muscle tension. Attempt to "let go" of any tension. (3) Work through each of the following muscle groups, tensing them for 5 seconds and then relaxing for 10–15 seconds. Work through each muscle group twice. This will be easier to do if you follow the relaxation tape recorded by your therapist.

Muscle Group	Activity
Fingers and hands	Clench each hand into a fist, one hand at a time
Wrists and forearms	Bend wrists back toward forearms
Biceps	Tense both biceps ("Strong Man" act)
Shoulders	Hunch shoulders
Forehead	Raise eyebrows and then frown
Eyes	Squint eyes

(continued)

Jaw .... Jut lower jaw outward
Tongue .... Push tongue against roof of mouth
Throat .... Yawn
Neck .... Gently rotate neck left, right, back, and then forward
Chest .... Take a deep breath and then slowly exhale
Chest and upper back .... Pull shoulders back and push chest outward
Abdomen .... Push out stomach and then suck it all the way in
Lower back .... Arch lower back
Thighs and legs–I .... Knees locked, feet pointing upward
Thighs and legs–II .... Knees locked, feet pointing down
Toes and feet–I .... Toes curled down
Toes and feet–II .... Toes curled upward

Release-Only Relaxation

Duration: 10 minutes twice per day.

Instructions: (1) Sit in a comfortable position, free from distractions. (2) Close your eyes and scan your body, looking for areas of muscle tension. Attempt to "let go" of any tension. (3) Go over each of your muscle groups and focus on relaxing them—your face, chest, arms, hands, stomach, legs, feet—while continuing to say "relax" each time you breathe out. Do this for about 5 minutes (4) Say to yourself, under your breath, the word "inhale" each time you breathe in, and the word "relax" each time you breathe out. Continue this for about 5 minutes.

Rapid Relaxation (which includes Breathing Retraining)

Duration: 20–30 seconds, about 20 times each day.

Instructions: (1) Take several slow, deep breaths, thinking to yourself "inhale" as you breathe in, and "relax" as you breathe out. Your breathing should be slow and comfortable, letting the air in and out slowly. Breathe with your diaphragm ("belly breathing"); your stomach should rise as you breathe in, and fall as you breathe out. Don't breathe with your chest. (2) As you breathe out, let go of as much muscle tension as you can. Try, for example, relaxing all of your face and jaw muscles as you breathe out. (3) Practice this form of relaxations in all kinds of safe situations, for example, while sitting in a waiting room or while standing in line. Or, you can try it while doing activities, such as standing or walking, while letting go of all the muscle tension that is not involved in these activities. For example if you are standing, you can relax the muscles in your face, shoulders, and stomach. (4) Practice relaxing in your daily life, initially in calm situations and then in increasingly more challenging circumstances (e.g., while taking a stressful phone call). Use reminders to prompt yourself to practice Rapid Relaxation. For example, a post-it note on the dash of your car or on your computer monitor at work might contain the message "Practice Rapid Relaxation every 30 minutes." Similarly, you could place a colored dot on your wristwatch or telephone. Every time you used the phone or looked at your watch, the dot would remind you to practice Rapid Relaxation. You can also practice this form of relaxation before you try any distressing exercises that may be included in the treatment of your PTSD.

HANDOUT 9.3. Grounding Exercises

STAYING GROUNDED

When people are under stress they sometimes *dissociate*. The purpose of this handout is to provide you with some information about dissociation and how you can manage this harmless but sometimes unpleasant feeling.

What Is Dissociation?

When people are stressed out they sometimes dissociate. There are two main types of dissociation: feeling *spaced out* and having a *flashback*. Spacing out is when your surroundings and your body start to feel strange or unreal. You feel like you're in a fog or in a daze. Flashbacks are when a person suddenly feels like he or she is actually back in the traumatic situation. Flashbacks are not merely thoughts or memories of the trauma—the person feels like the trauma is happening all over again. Feeling spaced out and having flashbacks can be very intense experiences and they can be emotionally unpleasant.

What Causes Dissociation?

It is important to remember that spacing out or having a flashback lasts only a short time and is *harmless* and *does not* mean that you're going crazy or developing schizophrenia. It is simply part of a hypersensitivity of the brain's stress response system. When the stress response system is hypersensitive, then everyday stressful events can cause you to space out. This is a way of psychologically avoiding stress by becoming less aware of your surroundings. Flashbacks are similarly caused by the stress response system, when it is triggered by reminders of the trauma. Here, flashbacks are a way of preparing to deal with, or escape, a stressor. Lots of people who have posttraumatic stress disorder (PTSD) feel spaced out or have flashbacks from time to time. These dissociative reactions tend to stop happening when the person recovers from PTSD.

What Can I Do If I Start to Dissociate?

The first thing to do is learn to recognize the things that trigger dissociative reactions. Marie, for example, noticed that she often started to space out when she was reminded about the time she was raped. Evan sometimes had flashbacks of the bank holdup whenever he saw young guys wearing sweatshirts with hoods. Once Marie and Evan got good at spotting these triggers, they were able to prepare to cope with them.

There are several ways of coping. One is to practice a relaxation exercise, which your therapist can teach you. Another is to become desensitized to the triggers by practicing exposure exercises. Again, these are things that you can discuss with your therapist. A third method, which is the focus of this handout, involves *grounding exercises*.

When you notice that you are starting to space out or it feels like you're back in the traumatic situation, you can *stay grounded in reality* by trying one or more of the following simple, effective exercises:

(continued)

- *Remind yourself where you are.* You might describe to yourself, either mentally or out loud, where you are. For example, "Today is _____ and I am in _____." If you just had a flashback, you can remind yourself that you're not back in the trauma situation: "I am safe; I'm not back in _____."
- *Pay attention to your surroundings.* Look around you and describe what you see. If you're in a room, describe the contents of the room, such as the color of the walls, the color, shape, and type of the furnishings, the decorations, the type of light fixtures, and so forth.
- *Pay attention to your body.* If you're sitting in a chair, notice how the chair feels; is it hard or cushioned? Notice the pressure of the chair on your legs. Pay attention to how the back of the chair feels as you lean back. If the chair has armrests, notice the sensations of your arms. Observe the feeling of pressure of your feet on the floor, and notice what it feels like when you wiggle your toes. Pay attention to your breathing; notice how the cool air slowly flows in through your nostrils, and how the warm air slowly flows out. If you decide to get up, pay attention to the feelings in your muscles as you move around. Have a glass of water; notice what it feels like to sip cold water. Notice the feeling as the water flows down your throat.
- *Don't rush, and don't fight the feelings.* There's no urgent need to push away flashbacks or spacey feelings. Remember, they're harmless. Remind yourself that you're safe. Gradually take your time to get grounded and the feelings will go away. Rushing and fighting the feelings won't hurt you, but it will make you feel more stressed.

HANDOUT 9.4. Pleasant Event Exercises

ACTIVITIES FOR ENHANCING YOUR QUALITY OF LIFE

Instructions: Enjoyable activities are *essential* to one's quality of life. But sometimes people neglect these activities when they are worried or stressed. Please look through the following checklist of activities. Did you do any of them in the past week? If so, did you enjoy the activity? Are there any activities that you haven't done but would like to do? This list of activities might help you think about ways of improving your quality of life. Some of these activities might distract you from your health worries, while others can improve your health and fitness.

	Indicate (√) which of these activities you did in the past week.	For the activities you indicated, were they enjoyable? (yes/no)	Indicate (√) which of these activities you didn't do but would like to do.
Creative activities			
Doing artwork or crafts			
Knitting, needlework, sewing			
Taking a course in something creative (e.g., cooking, photography)			
Decorating or redecorating your house or apartment			
Woodwork, carpentry, or furniture restoration			
Repairing things			
Mechanical hobbies (e.g., fixing gadgets)			
Photography			
Creative writing or doing a journal or blog			
Musical hobbies (e.g., singing, dancing, playing an instrument)			
Games and entertainment			
Watching TV, videos, or DVDs			
Playing video games			
Listening to music or radio programs			
Going to the movies			
Going to a play, concert, opera, or ballet			
Going to a museum, art gallery, or exhibition			
Going to a sporting event			
Educational activities			
Reading books, magazines, or newspapers			
Going to a lecture on a topic that interests you			
Learning a foreign language			
Surfing the Internet			
Learning about computers (e.g., learning to make a Web page)			
Going to the library			

(continued)

Adapted from Taylor and Asmundson (2004). Copyright 2004 by The Guilford Press. Adapted by permission in *Clinician's Guide to PTSD* by Steven Taylor (2006). Permission to photocopy this handout is granted to purchasers of this book for personal use only (see copyright page for details).

	Indicate (√) which of these activities you did in the past week.	For the activities you indicated, were they enjoyable? (yes/no)	Indicate (√) which of these activities you didn't do but would like to do.
Physical activities			
Playing tennis, squash, or racquetball			
Playing golf			
Bowling			
Water activities (e.g., swimming, sailing, canoeing)			
Walking or hiking			
Jogging, aerobics classes, or working out at a fitness center			
Snow sports (skiing, skating, snowboarding)			
Bike riding			
Horseback riding			
Playing team sports (e.g., volleyball, hockey, basketball)			
Fishing or hunting			
Playing billiards or pool			
Social and community activities			
Writing, telephoning, or e-mailing friends			
Visiting a friend or inviting a friend to your place			
Going out to lunch or dinner with a friend			
Giving a party or going to a party			
Going on a date			
Joining a club (e.g., a book club or social club)			
Going to a bar or restaurant			
Involvement in community or political activities			
Involvement in religious or church activities			
Other			
Sitting in the sun			
Going for a scenic drive			
Gardening, caring for houseplants, or arranging flowers			
Visiting fun or interesting places (e.g., park, beach, zoo)			
Caring for or being with pets			
Planning or going on a holiday			
Going to a sauna			
Soaking in the bathtub			
Doing yoga or meditation			
Buying yourself something special			
Hobbies (e.g., stamp collecting, model building, flying a kite)			
List your favorite activities here, if they are not listed above:			

CHAPTER 10

Cognitive Interventions I
General Considerations and Approaches

The difference between cognitive and exposure interventions is largely arbitrary; both involve some degree of exposure to distressing stimuli (e.g., thinking about the trauma), and both are methods of changing dysfunctional beliefs via exposure to corrective information. Despite these similarities, it is useful to distinguish between cognitive and exposure interventions in order to parse the material covered in this and later chapters. The present chapter will consider the fundamental cognitive restructuring methods used in treating PTSD, including established methods as well as valuable methods that have only recently been applied to this disorder, such as methods for managing worry and rumination. Common problems in effectively implementing cognitive restructuring will also be considered, and some solutions will be offered.

GENERAL PRINCIPLES
OF COGNITIVE RESTRUCTURING FOR PTSD

Overview

When challenging dysfunctional beliefs, the therapist can help the patient understand how the beliefs contribute to PTSD and how the beliefs arose. Specific aims of cognitive restructuring include helping patients view the world as being less dangerous and more predictable, and helping them feel more competent and more in control of their lives. Further goals are to help them regain their appreciation or zest for life, and to shift their self-image from "victim," or "bad" or blameworthy person, to that of a brave person or survivor, who has intrinsic worth as a human being. Cognitive restructuring may involve helping patients come to terms with shattered assumptions by developing revised, adaptive views of themselves and the world. Treatment may also involve helping patients challenge dysfunctional beliefs that have been strengthened by the trauma (e.g., "I was born to suffer") and develop and reinforce more adaptive beliefs (e.g., "I can improve my situation, even though life will continue to have its ups and downs").

As an introduction to cognitive restructuring, the patient can be given Handout 10.1 (pp. 193–194), which lists cognitive distortions commonly associated with PTSD. The distortions arise from dysfunctional beliefs. Patients can be asked to review Handout 10.1 and to identify any errors in their thinking. To avoid the pejorative term "thinking error," the handout refers to these as "unhelpful thinking patterns." Restructuring continues by asking patients to read Handout 10.2 (p. 195), which describes methods for challenging unhelpful beliefs. Patients are also asked to identify their maladaptive thoughts whenever they are distressed and write them down in the "distressing thoughts" column of Handout 10.3 (p. 196–197). In this way, patients learn to label their thoughts (e.g., "This is an example of overestimating danger"). The forms are reviewed during the treatment session, where further cognitive restructuring is conducted.

Tailoring Interventions for Children

Some of the interventions described in this and the following chapter are too sophisticated for use with young children, although with older children (e.g., 8 or 9 years or older), simplified versions of these methods can sometimes be successfully implemented, depending on the child's level of cognitive development. Children 5–9 years old can often be successfully encouraged and trained to use coping statements, combined with simple problem solving (Vernberg & Johnston, 2001). The child is taught to identify negative self-statements and to replace them with more adaptive statements. For example, "I'm to blame that Mommy was beaten" could be replaced with "It was not my fault. I did the best I could." In the same way, self-statements associated with excessive fear, such as "I'm weak—I'm too scared to be alone," can be replaced with "I can be brave."

Style of Questioning

Cognitive restructuring makes use of Socratic dialogue, which consists of guided questioning to help patients identify whether their beliefs are accurate or maladaptive. Socratic dialogue can be used in all stages of treatment, from the initial session onwards. In contrast to the lecture approach, in which the patient is the passive recipient of information presented by the therapist, the Socratic approach encourages patients to do most of the work in questioning their beliefs and in coming up with alternatives. The goal is not to provide patients with all the answers, but instead to help them think for themselves. This method is quite consistent with the treatment engagement methods described in Chapter 8. The following example illustrates the use of Socratic dialogue, in which most of the therapist's dialogue consists of questions and reflections.

THERAPIST: What is the worst thing about the fact that your legs were badly burned in the fire?

PATIENT: The way they look; they're scarred and horrible.

THERAPIST: How does that make you feel?

PATIENT: Really terrible.

THERAPIST: What would life be like for you if you were able to accept your legs the way they are, without feeling terrible?

PATIENT: I haven't thought about that. I suppose life would be better, but I don't know how anyone could feel OK about it.

THERAPIST: OK, I appreciate that it may be difficult to accept what's happened to you. But do you think it would be an important goal? What good things would happen if you didn't feel terrible about your legs?

PATIENT: I guess I wouldn't be thinking about them all the time, and maybe I wouldn't feel like such a freak.

THERAPIST: Those sound like good reasons. What do you think would be a good first step to accepting yourself the way you are?

PATIENT: I really don't know.

THERAPIST: OK. Let's see if we can come up with some ideas. The way a person thinks influences how they feel. Imagine a person with burned and scarred legs who was able to accept themselves. What would they think about their legs?

PATIENT: I suppose they would think they were just legs, that they still worked, and the scarring isn't visible if they wear long pants.

THERAPIST: So, the person would try to look on the bright side, and would remind herself about all the good things about her legs. How is that different from the way you've been thinking about your legs?

PATIENT: I guess I've been focusing on how ugly they look, and I haven't been looking at the big picture.

THERAPIST: That's an important point you've made; it's important to look at the big picture. How do you feel, emotionally, when you look at the big picture? That is, reminding yourself that your legs are in good working order, that you are in no pain, and that the scarring is not visible when you wear pants?

PATIENT: I feel a little bit better about myself.

The following vignette illustrates how this process can even be used with children. In this example, 9-year-old Janie, who was almost abducted by a stranger one afternoon after school, is frightened of returning to school. This example comes from the early stages of therapy, where Janie is understandably shy and reticent.

THERAPIST: I can imagine that you must be pretty scared about going back to school.

PATIENT: I don't want to go back.

THERAPIST: I would feel the same way if I was you. Are you worried about being grabbed by a bad man?

PATIENT: (*Nods, tearfully.*)

THERAPIST: Have you told anyone else that you don't want to go back to school?

PATIENT: Yes, I told my sister, my mom, and my teacher.

THERAPIST: It's good to talk about these things with people you trust. What did they say?

PATIENT: Mom says I have to go back.

THERAPIST: Did she say why?

PATIENT: Because I need to.

THERAPIST: So, you need to go back to school, but at the moment it's too scary for you. Is that right?

PATIENT: (*Nods.*)

THERAPIST: This sounds like a puzzle to be solved. Do you like solving puzzles?

PATIENT: I like the puzzles in the video games we play.

THERAPIST: OK, good. Let's talk some more about the puzzles that you like to play, and then we'll see if we can solve the puzzle of getting back to school. Does that like a good idea?

PATIENT: Yes.

TROUBLESHOOTING

There are several general problems that may be encountered with many of the cognitive interventions described in this chapter. These are considered in this section, and problems in implementing specific interventions are discussed in the relevant sections later in this chapter.

Invalidation

Invalidation occurs when people (including the therapist) appear to deny, dismiss, or trivialize the patient's problems (Linehan, 1993). In PTSD treatment, invalidation can occur if the patient perceives that the therapist does not believe or appreciate the significance of (1) the patient's traumatic experiences, (2) the degree of suffering experienced by the patient, or (3) the patient's beliefs about the trauma, its meaning, and its consequences. Issues (1) and (2) are relatively straightforward to address in therapy, such as by giving patients time to fully describe their experiences and by expressing appropriate empathy. The therapist should wait until the worst of the experiences have been described. Expressing empathy before the patient has finished with his or her narration might lead the patient to perceive the therapist as insincere. The therapist should try to empathize with, and validate, patients' distress about what they have experienced. However, it can be counterproductive to validate their dysfunctional beliefs. It can be challenging to implement cognitive restructuring for these beliefs; on the one hand, you don't want to alienate your patients or trivialize their problems, but on the other hand, it can be important to find some way of challenging their dysfunctional beliefs in order to help them overcome their problems.

One way to prevent invalidation is to avoid telling patients that their thinking is "distorted," "wrong," or "irrational" (Becker & Zayfert, 2001). Dysfunctional or maladaptive beliefs can be framed as "unhelpful" cognitions. If relevant, the therapist could validate the unfairness of the trauma (e.g., "Agreeing to come back to his apartment for a drink in no way justifies what he did to you"). Then the therapist could use psychoeducational methods (Chapter 8) to socialize the patient to the idea that traumatic events can lead to distorted thinking (e.g., "As a result of what you've been through, it's like your brain has been put into self-protection mode, where you distrust anyone who vaguely resembles the abuser"). The goal here is to help the patient understand that everyone has, at some time or other, some form of dysfunctional thinking. Such beliefs can be caused or strengthened by traumatic experiences, and the beliefs can be an extension of the abuse.

"Your ex-husband led you to believe that you were a bad person, and from what you've said you still have that belief about yourself. So, you're still carrying with you a bit of the abuse; the bit that says you're a bad person. To put the abuse in the past, it may be important to deal with that lingering belief. What do you think?"

Reviewing the patient's pretrauma learning experiences can also be useful in helping the patient learn how his or her dysfunctional beliefs arose. To avoid patients blaming themselves for having these beliefs, which would amplify their distress, they can be assured that these beliefs are a common consequence of traumatic experiences.

Unyielding Beliefs

Sometimes the patient's dysfunctional beliefs are held with remarkably strong conviction and are resistant to cognitive restructuring. In such cases the first step is to conduct a thorough assessment of the factors responsible for maintaining belief strength. Are influential friends or significant others reinforcing the patient's beliefs? In such cases it may be difficult to make headway in treatment unless these problems are addressed. If a significant other, for example, appears to be interfering with treatment progress, then this person could be invited, with the patient's permission, to a session with the therapist and patient, in which the significant other's views and concerns are discussed, and any misconceptions can be addressed.

Dysfunctional beliefs also may be strongly held because there is a mismatch between the intervention used by the therapist and the patient's *personal epistemology* (Hofer & Pintrich, 2002), that is, the criteria that the person considers to be valid for gathering knowledge about the world. For some people, advice from an expert, combined with a review of the evidence, meets criteria for valid knowledge. For other people, it is necessary that they go out and do something to prove that the knowledge is valid. For example, a military veteran of the war in Iraq might not be convinced by verbal disputation that it is safe to go to a Middle Eastern restaurant in his Midwestern U.S. hometown. His personal epistemology may require that he actually prove this to himself, by going to such restaurants. In such cases, cognitive restructuring exercises may be of limited value, and exposure exercises may be necessary.

Safety behaviors and safety signals, which were defined in Chapter 3, could also prevent the change of dysfunctional beliefs (e.g., "I'm safe only because potential muggers can tell, by the look in my eyes, that I'm carrying a knife"). Chapter 13 discusses ways that safety behaviors can be gradually dropped and safety signals can be faded out, in order to test the patient's beliefs.

If the patient's trauma-related beliefs are being reinforced by intermittent exposure to genuine danger, then the therapist should reconsider whether these beliefs are truly dysfunctional. If there is a significant risk of danger, then treatment should focus on the patient's safety—via problem solving—instead of helping the patient feel more comfortable about his or her current circumstances.

Beliefs about Recovery

Patients may sometimes be reluctant to complete cognitive restructuring exercises that encourage them to feel good about themselves. Patients might believe that if they feel happy about themselves and the world, they are courting danger by being unable to keep safe or that they will become too happy with themselves and thereby set themselves up for a letdown ("Pride goeth before a fall"). Survivors of traumas in which other people were killed may believe that they are dishonoring the dead by moving on with their lives and may feel guilty at the very thought of feeling good about themselves. Other patients pose the opposite sort of problem; they continually worry about their rate of progress and are concerned that therapy might not work for them ("I'm not getting better as quickly as I should; maybe treatment won't help and I'll be miserable for the rest of my life"). These problems are grist for the cognitive mill. The therapist should identify the relevant beliefs and address them with one or more of the cognitive interventions discussed in this chapter.

Homework Adherence

Homework adherence problems are another set of challenges that may be encountered. Homework in cognitive restructuring consists of monitoring distressing thoughts, using forms such as Handout 10.3, or conducting some other exercises, such as a worry or rumination diary. There are several reasons why patients may not complete these exercises. If the patient has not completed a given homework exercise, then the therapist should check whether the patient understood the rationale for the exercise and how it should be done. Patients will be understandably reluctant to complete an exercise if they don't see why they should do it, or don't understand how it should be done.

Homework adherence problems also could arise because the task is too difficult or distressing. A patient who has difficulty with written expression may be embarrassed by or ashamed of doing any writing (e.g., as in the cognitive restructuring forms) and, as a result, actually feel worse after doing the exercise rather than better. Some patients are worried about doing the exercise "perfectly" because they fear disapproval from the therapist. Other patients avoid cognitive restructuring exercises that cause them to think about distressing thoughts or memories. Logistics problems, such as "not finding the time," can also interfere with homework completion. Trust issues can also get in the way of cognitive restructuring homework. Some patients worry about the confidentiality of the things they write down, especially their private thoughts about experiences that they perceive to be shameful. Each of these issues can be addressed by correcting misunderstandings, or by applying cognitive restructuring to beliefs associated with the problem (e.g., "It's not safe to write down my feelings" or "I have to do my homework perfectly"). The therapist should also check whether the homework assignment is truly relevant to the patient's problems.

EMPIRICAL DISPUTATIONS

Empirical disputations help patients examine the evidence for and against their dysfunctional beliefs. Alternative, adaptive beliefs are generated by the patient and therapist. Evidence to evaluate the beliefs is collected from the patient's own experiences and from other sources. There are several questions that patients can ask themselves to facilitate the process:

- "What evidence do I have for this belief?"
- "Is there any evidence that is inconsistent with the belief?"
- "Is there another explanation or alternative way of looking at things?"

Once the evidence is generated, the patient and therapist decide which belief is best supported. To determine whether this exercise is persuasive, the patient can be asked to rate the strength (0–100) of the dysfunctional and alternative beliefs before and after reviewing the evidence. If the exercise is effective, then it should reduce the strength of the dysfunctional belief and increase the strength of the alternative. The key points from the exercises can be distilled into a pithy statement written on a card, which the patient carries and reviews as needed. Empirical disputations can be conducted with the aid of Handout 10.4 (p. 198), which is used during therapy sessions and as a homework assignment.

During the treatment session, the patient and therapist can generate coping statements, which express the adaptive belief and are reviewed when needed. Consider the belief that "A hurricane could strike at any time." An appropriate coping statement might be "Hurricanes are rare events, and they can be predicted well in advance by meteorologists. So, I can assume I'm safe unless I receive news to the contrary."

TROUBLESHOOTING

Empirical disputations are most effective when they focus on clearly defined beliefs. This permits the therapist and patient to identify evidence that unambiguously supports or refutes the beliefs. Sometimes, however, patients may have difficulty articulating their beliefs because they are embarrassed about them, or because discussing the beliefs makes them feel anxious. Deliberate evasiveness (avoidance) may be suspected when the patient is visibly distressed about discussing the beliefs and attempts to shifts the topic of conversation. The therapist can address this problem by directly but tactfully raising it with the patient and then collaboratively looking for solutions. The therapist should be mindful of the quality of the therapeutic relationship and the way in which the empirical disputations are implemented. Patients will be reluctant to engage in treatment if they feel attacked or criticized for disclosing their beliefs.

Another problem that can arise when conducting empirical disputations concerns the issue of disproving the negative. A patient might say, "How do you know that I won't be on a plane that gets hijacked by terrorists?" These sorts of questions contain an implicit demand for certainty. When they arise in the course of empirical disputations, the therapist can try using a disputation that challenges the demand for certainty (see below).

ADAPTIVE DISPUTATIONS
Highlighting the Cost of Dysfunctional Beliefs

Adaptive disputations involve an analysis of the costs and benefits of holding particular beliefs. To illustrate, Mark was badly beaten and robbed by a gang of youths. In an attempt to prevent this happening again, he tried to avoid leaving his apartment. Although Mark lived in a city with a relatively low crime rate, he believed that "The streets are very dangerous; the best way to stay safe is to remain at home." Mark was asked to consider the adaptiveness of this belief by asking himself the following: "How does this belief impair my quality of life? Is there an alternative, more useful belief I could consider?"

Challenging the Demand for Certainty

Even when the chances of experiencing another traumatic event are very low, patients may still worry about the possibility of it happening. In such cases it can be useful to assess whether the patient has an unrealistic demand for certainty. The latter is reflected in beliefs such as "I can never relax so long as I know that ____ could happen." To challenge demands for certainty, the patient can consider the following questions: Is it useful for me to worry about ____ or are my worries spoiling my life? What sorts of uncertainties *am* I prepared to tolerate? Have I learned to tolerate other uncertainties? How did I do this? The patient and therapist can review the daily low-probability "risks" that the patient already takes, such as breathing smoggy air, freeway driving, or using pedestrian crosswalks. These examples can help patients learn that they already tolerate all kinds of uncertainties, and therefore can learn to accept other low-probability uncertainties.

TROUBLESHOOTING

Sometimes patients readily acknowledge the maladaptiveness of their beliefs but insist that they can't help but worry. In these cases the therapist might shift to an alternative cognitive intervention, such as an empirical disputation to challenge the beliefs or a worry control strategy.

DISTANCING STRATEGIES

Distancing as a Way of Gaining Perspective

Distancing strategies (Leahy, 2003; McMullin, 2000) are methods for helping patients view their beliefs objectively, as assumptions rather than facts. There are several kinds of distancing strategies.

• *Observe, describe, but don't evaluate.* Patients can be asked to record the sequence of events during episodes of distress (in situations in which there is no real danger), objectively observing, as if they were scientists, the sequence of symptoms, thoughts, feelings, and behaviors. The task is simply to observe and describe these events, without evaluating them as good or bad, and without trying to influence them.

• *Shift perspective.* This involves taking another person's perspective. Kasuma, for example, believed that she was a "tainted person" because she had been raped. To challenge this belief she was asked whether she thought that other rape survivors were tainted, and whether other people regard her as tainted. Given that she didn't see other rape survivors as tainted, and there was no evidence that other people think she's tainted, she was able to see that she was not tainted. To consolidate this learning, she decided to join a rape survivors support group, where she gained further evidence that rape survivors come from all walks of life and that there is nothing inherently tainted about them.

- In vivo *labeling of cognitions*. Here, patients are taught to label their beliefs. Whenever Kasuma had the thought "I'm tainted," she responded with the following self-statement: "I'm putting a label on myself, which I don't deserve." This intervention is particularly useful for patients who have too many dysfunctional cognitions to individually challenge. For example, Carl, a combat veteran, had a torrent of thoughts about danger whenever he saw "foreign-looking people." With practice, he became adept at dismissing these thoughts by labeling them as "PTSD thinking."
- *Telescoping*. To put the trauma in perspective, patients are asked to imagine that they are looking back on their life 10 years from now. How would they evaluate their current beliefs in a decade from now? Would they take them seriously or dismiss them?

TROUBLESHOOTING

It requires practice for patients to become adept at distancing themselves from their dysfunctional beliefs. This can be particularly difficult when the beliefs are strongly held. Failure experiences can be discouraging, so it is often best to start practicing with mildly distressing beliefs. With practice, patients can often progress to successfully distancing themselves from more distressing cognitions.

MANAGEMENT OF WORRY AND RUMINATION

Worry consists of a chain of thoughts about threatening events, along with attempts to think of ways of averting or dealing with these events. Rumination consists of persistently thinking over the traumatic event and its aftermath, along with repeatedly asking oneself questions like "Why me?" Patients often report that their worry or rumination is largely involuntary; they might deliberately initiate worry or rumination—to try to solve problems—and then have difficulty discontinuing this pattern of thinking. Alternatively, they may find that worry and rumination are automatically triggered and difficult to terminate.

For patients who believe that prolonged worry and rumination are appropriate things to do, the adaptiveness of these forms of thinking can be explored by considering the costs and benefits. The patient and therapist should try to come up with a realistic estimation of the degree of threat in the patient's life. If worry and rumination are clearly excessive and not justified by the degree of threat in the patient's life, then adaptive disputations could be implemented and behavioral experiments generated, where patients compare their distress levels on days that they did worry versus days they didn't. Borkovec, Wilkinson, Folensbee, and Lerman's (1983) stimulus control exercise is another useful way of reducing worry and rumination, as described in Handout 10.5 (p. 199).

This method can be combined with cognitive restructuring, whereby the material written down in the stimuli control exercises is evaluated by using cognitive disputations. This can be used, for example, to treat ruminative "mental undoing," in which the person repeatedly thinks about what he or she could have done to prevent the trauma. This type of thinking takes the form of "If only . . . " thoughts and usually concerns the person's inaction; "If only I'd cleaned my gun before we went out on patrol, then it wouldn't have jammed and my buddy would still be alive."

To therapeutically address mental undoing, the therapist could empathize that such undoing is a common way of dealing with trauma (Lehman, Wortman, & Williams, 1987), but this sort of thinking doesn't change what happened and doesn't help the person overcome their trauma. In fact, it may perpetuate distress (Davis, Lehman, Wortman, Silver, & Thompson, 1995; Dunmore, Clark, & Ehlers, 1997). Cognitive interventions for guilt-related beliefs (Chapter 11) could also be helpful. It is also worth reviewing whether the patient's "if only" plans would have really worked (Resick & Schnicke, 1993). One can also review whether it would have been reasonable to come up with these plans in the heat of the moment. For example, the therapist could say something like the following.

"You've had 20 years to think about the things you could have done differently. Twenty years to think of all the possible solutions, to reject the bad ones and think about, polish, and refine the good ones. How much time did you have to make a decision that day 20 years ago? You didn't have years; you had to make a split-second decision about an emergency that you'd never encountered before, and you'd never been trained to deal with such an event. Aren't you being unfair to yourself by insisting that you should have done better? Would you criticize one of your buddies if he'd done the same thing that you did?"

For children, stimulus control of worry or rumination can be facilitated by using play therapy techniques, such as the "Worry Can" (Jones, 1997). Here, the therapist produces a can with a plastic lid (such as an empty coffee tin), some colored paper, felt markers, glue, and scissors. The therapist cuts a strip of paper large enough to be completely wrapped around the can and then asks the child to draw the things that he or she finds scary on one side of the paper and color them with the markers. The strip is then glued around the can, and a slot is cut in the lid, large enough for slips of paper to be posted into the can. The child is then asked to write down, on slips of paper, the things that are worrying him or her and to discuss them with the therapist. The purpose of the exercise is essentially the same as the stimulus control exercise used with adults. The child spends some time each day (e.g., a 10-minute worry period) writing down worries and then posts them into the Worry Can. If the worries come to mind at other times in the day, the child defers worry until the worry period (e.g., "I'll think of these things later, during the worry period"). The child is asked to bring the Worry Can to each therapy session, where the child and therapist discuss the worries and try to address them with either problem solving or cognitive restructuring (as appropriate to the developmental level of the child).

TROUBLESHOOTING

A problem with the stimulus control method is encouraging patients to consistently practice the exercise. Patients who "can't find time" to practice could be asked to consider the pros and cons of the procedure and then to schedule a regular time for practice. Patients who believe that worry or rumination is adaptive may be reluctant to use the method. Here, it may first be necessary to implement other interventions (e.g., adaptive disputations) to highlight the maladaptiveness of excessive worry or rumination.

It is not uncommon for patients to report that they try to avoid thinking about the trauma because if they think about it, then they will ruminate for hours. In such cases an adaptive disputation is unlikely to be helpful; these patients know they ruminate too much and they are trying to deal with this through avoidance. An alternative approach is to help them better come to terms with the trauma. This may involve looking at beliefs concerning the meaning and implications of the trauma.

SELECTING AND SEQUENCING COGNITIVE INTERVENTIONS

The choice and timing of interventions depends on many factors, including the treatment plan based on the case formulation and the patient's goals and preferences. If the patient has limited cognitive abilities, or difficulties with the language used in therapy (e.g., English), then cognitive interventions would be greatly simplified, with treatment focusing on other interventions, such as emotion regulation methods and exposure exercises (e.g., imaginal exposure in the patient's native language; see Chapter 12).

If there are problems with the therapeutic relationship, such as difficulty trusting the therapist, then beliefs associated with trust, abuse, and betrayal may need to be addressed early in treatment, along with other interventions to enhance trust (e.g., ensuring that the patient feels the therapist is taking his or her problems seriously, or perhaps offering some appropriate therapist self-disclosure).

Where should you start with patients who have a mélange of dysfunctional beliefs? For example, Anna was in therapy for PTSD arising from an abusive relationship which she had left several years ago. Despite the passage of time, she continued to hold a range of beliefs that appeared to have been formed during the period of abuse, for example, "I'm never safe," "I'm weak and fragile," "He's still a threat—he could be back at any time," "I'm a stupid fool for putting up with his abuse," "I can't control my thinking—I feel like I'm losing my mind," "I'll never have a happy relationship," "You never know who's going to hurt you—people that seem OK on the outside can suddenly turn into weirdos." The risk is that the therapist will feel overwhelmed with this welter of beliefs and try to tackle them all in too short a period of time, or become sidetracked from working on one belief as another belief becomes evident. To deal with this problem, a thorough cognitive assessment (Chapter 6) is important to identify beliefs that are central to the patient's problems. The patient and therapist could then set priorities on which beliefs to tackle first and agree not to get sidetracked on other beliefs unless it is absolutely necessary. Often the most important beliefs are those associated with the greatest distress or functional impairment. In Anna's case, she chose the belief "He's still a threat—he could be back at any time," because this was creating the greatest distress, and her preoccupation with the belief prevented her from effectively doing her job.

The particular types of cognitive factors driving the patient's current level of distress may change over the course of therapy, which can require revisions to the case formulation and treatment plan. This is illustrated in the following case, in which the relative importance of one cognitive factor (a particular dysfunctional belief) was eclipsed by the occurrence of a series of stressors, which fueled another cognitive factor (worry about various life stressors).

For several sessions, Shanice and her therapist were making good progress in helping her feel more comfortable among men, by reviewing the evidence for her belief that "Men will abuse or ridicule me if I express my needs, wants, or preferences." But then treatment was derailed by a series of events. Over a series of weeks, Shanice's mother was diagnosed with lung cancer, Shanice was laid off from her job, and her son was diagnosed with attention-deficit/hyperactivity disorder. As a single, unemployed mother, she felt overwhelmed and was constantly worried about her living circumstances and her mother. Work on her beliefs about men became unimportant to her. Indeed, it appeared that most of her current distress was driven by both realistic and unrealistic (catastrophic) worries about her current difficulties. These factors also appeared to be exacerbating her PTSD symptoms, particularly hyperarousal symptoms. Given this shift in the factors that appeared to be influencing her symptoms, the treatment plan was changed (temporarily, it was hoped) to focus on practical problem-solving and worry management strategies to help Shanice cope with her present difficulties.

SUMMARY

There are several major classes of cognitive intervention, including empirical disputations (i.e., examining the evidence), adaptive disputations (questioning the adaptiveness of a given belief), and methods for controlling thought processes (rumination and worry management). The choice of intervention depends, in part, on the nature of the patient's problems. When implementing cognitive interventions it is important to check the patient's understanding of what was covered in the session, and how the patient experienced the restructuring exercises. This is important to prevent misunderstanding and to identify and address any problems with invalidation.

HANDOUT 10.1. Cognitive Distortions Associated with PTSD

THINKING PATTERNS THAT CREATE DISTRESS

The following are common thinking patterns that create excessive distress in people who have survived a traumatic experience. The trauma can cause or strengthen these thinking patterns. These categories of thinking patterns overlap to some extent, but they are still useful for helping you understand how thinking patterns can influence feelings of trauma-related anxiety, anger, guilt, depression, or shame.

Which of the Following Thinking Patterns Might Contribute to Your Problems?

All-or-nothing thinking. Seeing things in black-and-white categories, ignoring the shades of gray. Examples of all-or-nothing thinking are: "I'm either safe or in danger," "If I'm not a good person then I must be a bad person," "You're either a friend or an enemy." Traumatic experiences can contribute to all-or-nothing thinking, because trauma is often an all-or-nothing situation. For example, a person was either raped or they weren't raped.

Overfocusing on the negatives. Picking out a single negative detail and ignoring the positives. For example, focusing on news reports of murders and ignoring all the evidence that your neighborhood is safe.

Disqualifying the positives. Rejecting positive information. For example, a rape survivor, who wanted to start dating men again, had a nice conversation over coffee with a male friend but said that this positive experience "didn't count" because the man could still have dark, violent secrets that she didn't know about.

Jumping to conclusions. For example, hearing people yelling outside and immediately assuming that someone will be seriously hurt or even killed. Another example is hearing the floorboards creaking at night and jumping to the conclusion that a dangerous burglar has broken into the house.

Catastrophizing. Magnifying in your mind the badness of an event, which then increases how upset you feel. For example, assuming that a flashback means that you're going crazy. Or assuming a fender bender is a terrible disaster.

Overgeneralization. Taking one example as "proof" for a general rule. For example, "Osama bin Laden is from Saudi Arabia; therefore, all Saudis can't be trusted." Another example: "I was mugged by a man who had been drinking; therefore, all men will become violent if they get drunk."

(continued)

Emotional reasoning. Regarding your feelings as facts. For example, "There must be danger because I feel anxious." If emotional reasoning is one of your thinking patterns, then you need to review the evidence in your life to determine whether your emotional reasoning is accurate or inaccurate. For example, how many times have you had the gut feeling or instinct that you are in danger? Of those times, how many times were you wrong and how many times were you right?

Intolerance of uncertainty. Refusing to accept that uncertainty is a part of everyday life and insisting that perfect certainty can and should be obtained. For example, insisting that "I must ensure that I'm completely safe" or "I need to know everything about a person before I'm prepared to trust them."

Superstitious thinking. Assuming that something you do prevents bad things from happening, because the bad events haven't happened so far. For example, "Ever since the assault I've carried a pistol in my bag. I've never been attacked since I've been carrying the pistol, so therefore it must be warding off danger." Notice that carrying a pistol might have had nothing to do with being safe; the person may simply have been staying away from dangerous places. In fact, carrying a pistol could make the person less safe, especially if the person was assaulted again and the assailant got hold of the gun.

HANDOUT 10.2. Methods for Challenging Dysfunctional Beliefs

STOPPING UNHELPFUL THOUGHTS FROM RULING YOUR LIFE

Some types of thoughts are unhelpful and create distress. Those types of thoughts can result from a traumatic event, or they might arise from other life experiences. Examples of unhelpful, upsetting thoughts include the following: "I am never safe," "I can't trust anyone," "I'm incompetent," "I'll be abused if I get close to people," "I have no future," or "My nightmares will never go away." These sorts of thoughts can make a person's life miserable. If you have upsetting thoughts, then it is important to check out whether the thoughts are accurate or helpful, and whether they can be replaced with more useful types of thoughts. For example, the thought "I'll be abused if I get close to people" could be replaced with "I can learn how to spot nonabusive people, so I can get close without being hurt." You can evaluate your thoughts by asking yourself questions such as the following ones:

- Does this thought match one of the unhelpful thinking patterns in Handout 10.1 "Thinking Patterns That Create Distress"?

- Is this a useful thought to have? List all the problems that this thought causes in your life (e.g., unpleasant feelings, excessive avoidance).

- How would your life be different if you didn't have this thought?

- Does this thought contain extreme words, such as "never," "always," and "should"? Are the extremes justified?

- Are you putting labels on yourself or other people (e.g., calling yourself abusive names like "dumb," "incompetent," or "a fool")? Are these labels justified?

- What evidence do you have for and against this thought?

- What advice would you have for a friend who was troubled by this type of thought?

- Is there another way of looking at things? That is, can your upsetting thought be replaced with a more calming thought?

Use one or more of these questions to examine the thoughts you wrote down in the "Thought Recording Form" (Handout 10.3).

HANDOUT 10.3. Cognitive Restructuring Form

THOUGHT RECORDING FORM

Instructions: The purpose of this form is to help you change unhelpful thoughts and behaviors. Please carry this form with you (e.g., in your wallet or purse) and record details of upsetting experiences after they occur, or as soon as possible afterwards. Use extra sheets as needed.

Day and date	Triggers (e.g., an event, person, or bodily sensation)	Thoughts (and strength of belief, 0–100)	Emotion (and intensity of emotion, 0–100)	Behaviors that may be calming in the short term but create problems in the longer term	Rational responses and good coping responses
EXAMPLE	Drove past a car accident.	Dangerous drivers are everywhere. (Believed it 100%)	Anxiety (80%) Anger (50%)	Braked and slowed down as I drove through intersections, even though the lights were green. Other drivers got mad at me because I was driving so slow.	Told myself that I drive past thousands of cars each week and rarely see accidents. Reminded myself that nobody wants to be in an accident, and so most drivers try to be safe. Told myself braking at green lights will cause more harm than good.
EXAMPLE	I had a flashback about my rape; it felt like it was happening all over again.	I'm losing my mind. I'll never get over the trauma. (Both 90%)	Terrified (100%)	Drank some wine to calm down.	Flashbacks are upsetting but they can't hurt me. The rape is in the past. I get over the trauma if I keep working at therapy. I don't need to drink to feel calm; I can go for a walk or take a hot bath instead.

(continued)

Day and date	Triggers (e.g., an event, person, or bodily sensation)	Thoughts (and strength of belief, 0–100)	Emotion (and intensity of emotion, 0–100)	Behaviors that may be calming in the short term but create problems in the longer term	Rational responses and good coping responses

HANDOUT 10.4. Matrix Method for Challenging Dysfunctional Beliefs

	Evidence for the belief	Evidence against the belief
Distressing belief *Example:* "Working as a bank teller is a very dangerous profession."		
Alternative belief *Example:* "People are more likely to die from smoking or overeating than from bank robberies. In other words, working as a bank teller is no more dangerous than the other things I do."		

HANDOUT 10.5. Stimulus Control for Excessive Worry and Ruminative Thinking

CONTROLLING WORRY AND RUMINATIVE THINKING

Worry consists of a chain of thoughts about threatening events, along with attempts to think of ways of averting or dealing with these events. Rumination is a similar pattern of thinking, in which the person persistently thinks about an event. For example, a person who was injured in a boating accident kept going over the accident again and again in his mind, asking himself, "Why me?" A woman who was abused by her former husband kept dwelling on the abuse, and kept thinking, "How can I get even with him for what he's done?" Rumination and excessive worry can ruin your quality of life. If you are troubled by excessive worry or rumination, then try the following:

> **Try stopping.** Are you able to intentionally stop worrying or ruminating? If so, try stopping for a day and see how it feels. If a person thought, for example, that excessive worry kept her safe, then she might try to stop worrying for a day to test whether worry has any effect on safety. If this possibility interests you, then discuss it with your therapist.

If you have difficulty controlling your worry or rumination, then try the following:

1. **Establish a time each day in which you will worry or ruminate.**

   Set aside 30 minutes each day. Try to do all your worrying or ruminating during that period. For example, you might decide that your worry/rumination period will be from 6:00 to 6:30 each night. Don't schedule it too late in the evening; otherwise it might delay you from getting to sleep.

2. **Write out your worries or ruminations**

   Write out all your worries or ruminations during the worry/rumination period. Writing them out can help you view them more objectively. Use the "Thinking patterns that create distress" in Handout 10.1 to see if your worries or ruminations contain any thinking errors. You might also decide to problem-solve some of your concerns, or you might find that some concerns are unnecessary and can be simply dismissed.

3. **Postpone.**

   When you catch yourself worrying or ruminating at other times, try to postpone it until your daily worry or rumination period. You might make a brief note of the worry or rumination in a notebook, and tell yourself, "I'll think about this later."

4. **Practice, practice, practice!**

   The more you practice these exercises the better you will become at controlling your unwanted patterns of thinking.

CHAPTER 11

Cognitive Interventions II
Methods for Specific Types of Beliefs

Among the most exciting developments in cognitive restructuring for PTSD are new methods for targeting specific beliefs that are commonly associated with this disorder, such as beliefs associated with trauma-related guilt, mental defeat, and numbing. These important new methods are covered in the present chapter, along with established methods for addressing other forms of maladaptive, PTSD-related beliefs.

Although patients may hold highly idiosyncratic trauma-related beliefs, most dysfunctional beliefs associated with PTSD can be grouped into a small number of categories, including metaphysical beliefs associated with the meaning of trauma, beliefs about the self (which are often associated with shame and guilt), beliefs about other people and the world, and beliefs about one's symptoms and psychological functioning. Methods for challenging these and other beliefs are discussed in the following sections. These methods are generally more appropriate for adolescents and adults than for children. Simplified versions of the methods could be used with older children (e.g., 8- or 9-year-olds), but for younger children (e.g., 5- to 8-year-olds), simple problem-solving and coping statements are more useful, as described in the previous chapter.

BELIEFS ABOUT THE DANGEROUSNESS OF PEOPLE AND THE WORLD

The challenge in addressing distorted beliefs about the dangerousness of people and the world is that these beliefs contain a grain of truth; people and the world can be unpredictably and uncontrollably dangerous. There is no guarantee that the patient will not experience another traumatic event, such as a disaster or interpersonal violence. To address this issue, cognitive restructuring for beliefs about other people and the world can focus on the person's beliefs about uncertainty, safety, and danger.

The person's tolerance for uncertainty can be explored, as discussed in Chapter 10. The person's beliefs about cues to danger and safety can also be reviewed. Is the person able to identify which situations are likely to be safe or dangerous? It is not uncommon for trauma survivors to over-generalize their conceptions of danger, that is, to assume that all situations are dangerous unless proven otherwise. The adaptiveness of such beliefs can be explored, and available evidence can be reviewed to help the patient develop personally acceptable and empirically justified guidelines for distinguishing safety from danger.

When challenging dysfunctional beliefs about danger, and helping the patient establish reasonable guidelines for distinguishing safety from danger, it is important to consider the *quality* of the evidence. To do this, one needs to distinguish interpretations from facts. Dominique firmly believed that driving downtown was dangerous. His evidence was all the "near misses" and "close calls" he experienced while driving. Further discussion revealed that he used extremely liberal criteria to define these events. An instance of what he considered to be a near miss, for example, consisted of a driver nudging his car out of a side street as Dominique drove past. Dominique and the therapist discussed whether it was helpful for him to label these things as near misses. Such labels led him to be excessively anxious while driving. After some discussion, including a review of how many times these sorts of near misses actually led to accidents, Dominique agreed that it was better to label such events as "things to notice while driving, but no cause for alarm." This, in turn, helped challenge his belief that driving downtown was dangerous. It also helped him distinguish real danger (real near misses) from things that an observant driver would detect (e.g., a car nudging out from a side street) without becoming alarmed.

Another way of addressing danger-related beliefs is to review the evidence that the traumatic event is over, that is, that the danger is in the past. As part of this exercise, the therapist should attend to the language that patients are using; are they using language that gives the trauma an ever-present or unfinished quality? Caterina, for example, was a survivor of spousal abuse. She felt constantly in danger, which was fueled by intermittent, but nonviolent, contacts with her former husband (as part of his child visitation rights). Treatment involved examining the evidence that the abuse was over. There were several pieces of evidence: (1) it had been many years since the last episode of abuse, (2) her ex-husband was no longer using drugs and alcohol, which had fueled past violence, (3) her ex-husband was clearly worried about losing visitation privileges if he acted abusively, and (4) he had completed a court-ordered anger management program and purportedly had very few episodes of anger in all spheres of his life (work, driving, etc.). Although all this evidence did not guarantee that her ex-husband would never again be abusive, after reviewing the evidence Caterina was prepared to accept that the abuse was quite likely over. She was also encouraged to examine the words she used to describe herself and her ex-husband. She regularly called herself "a victim of violence," which had connotations of passivity and powerlessness. She was encouraged to see herself as "a survivor, who has moved on to a better life." She thought of her ex-husband as "my violent husband." The therapist pointed out that this way of thinking about him perpetuated her sense of threat; he was no longer her husband, and he had not been violent for many years. Caterina tried thinking about him as "my formerly violent ex-husband," which she later abbreviated to simply "my ex."

For some patients, one of the most disturbing aspects of the trauma is that their previously held beliefs have been shattered. This could involve the shattering of "just world" assumptions, such as "Bad things don't happen to good people like me" or "My world is fair and just; people only get what they deserve." In such cases, cognitive restructuring can be used to help patients understand the nature of shattered assumptions, and to help them to rebuild their beliefs about the world in a way that avoids the extremes of both cynicism ("Deep down, people are plain bad") and naivety ("The assault was a freak accident; it will never, ever happen again"). This is illustrated in the following vignette, which concerns an 18-year-old university student who was sexually assaulted by an ex-boyfriend. The vignette illustrates an early phase in rebuilding and refining the patient's shattered assumptions about other people.

SUE: I've lost my faith in humanity. Not only was I raped by my ex-boyfriend, but to top it off the first pharmacist I went to refused to fill my prescription for the morning-after pill. I was lucky I didn't get pregnant.

THERAPIST: You've been through some rough times, and I can see how you'd be feeling disillusioned. Can you tell me a bit more about what you mean when you say you've lost faith in humanity?

SUE: I feel cynical, like I can't rely on people. The people who should have been trustworthy have abused me and let me down.

THERAPIST: What was your view of humanity before the rape?

SUE: I suppose I was idealistic. I tended to see the best in people.

THERAPIST: And now your experiences with your ex-boyfriend and the pharmacist have shattered your assumptions about humanity.

SUE: Yes.

THERAPIST: It's easy to become really cynical about other people, especially after the sorts of experiences that you've had, to go from being idealistic to being cynical. How does it feel emotionally to have no faith in all humanity?

SUE: It feels terrible. I feel sad, angry, and hopeless.

THERAPIST: I wonder if there's another way to think about humanity, somewhere in the middle, in between idealism and cynicism. I mean, is there anyone in your life that you have faith in?

SUE: Well, I guess. My family has been really supportive, and so have my friends.

THERAPIST: OK. And did you find a pharmacist who would fill your prescription?

SUE: Yes, she was really nice about it.

THERAPIST: That's good. And what about the campus police? You mentioned earlier that they charged your ex.

SUE: Yes, they were really helpful, especially one of the women police officers.

THERAPIST: OK. So how can we make sense of all this? There are some people who let you down: the pharmacist and your ex. But there also are people who helped you and have stuck by you, like your family, your friends, one of the pharmacists you saw, and the police officers. What does that tell us about humanity?

SUE: It's like, really complicated. There are people I can trust, and people that I should be able to trust who let me down. I'm not sure what I think about humanity.

THERAPIST: So it will take some time to figure out. But that's OK. It's an important start. Maybe you'll emerge from this experience with some hard-won wisdom about the complexity of humanity. That sounds a whole lot better than feeling cynical about everyone.

METAPHYSICAL BELIEFS

Traumatic events often challenge the person's deeply held spiritual beliefs or assumptions about the meaning of life. When addressing such cognitions, the therapist should try to work within the patient's belief system. To illustrate, if the patient was a staunch Roman Catholic, the therapist would ideally want have some familiarity with that religious system in order to conduct optimal cognitive restructuring. In some cases it may be necessary for the patient or therapist to consult a religious or spiritual expert. To illustrate, Angela was tormented with thoughts of why God allowed her young son to drown in a boating accident 2 years ago. She believed that "God has abandoned me. My life now has no purpose." To help make sense of the tragic loss, Angela was encouraged to meet with a local religious leader, to discuss how a just God could permit evil in the world. The therapist first contacted the religious expert to arrange the meeting. Not surprisingly, the religious expert had had this sort of discussion many times, because the question of evil is a commonly discussed theological issue. Angela and her therapist also examined the belief that "My life has no meaning," as illustrated in the following transcript.

THERAPIST: You mentioned that you've been feeling lost and empty because it seems like your life has no meaning, now that Ryan [her son] is gone. What did you see as your meaning or purpose in life before the accident?

ANGELA: Ryan was my world to me. Ever since I split with my husband, it was just Ryan and me. I spent a lot of my time looking after him and making sure he had a good life. I would help him with homework, take him to basketball practice, and everything. Now there's nothing in my life but emptiness.

THERAPIST: Losing a child is a heart-wrenching thing. Do you have any religious or spirit beliefs?

ANGELA: Yes, sort of. I believe in God and Heaven.

THERAPIST: Do you believe that Ryan is in Heaven?

ANGELA: Yes, I'm sure of it. He was such a great boy.

THERAPIST: OK, so Ryan is looking down at you from Heaven. What would *he* want you to do with your life? I mean, would he want you to try to pick up the pieces and move on, to find new purpose in life?

ANGELA: I think he would.

THERAPIST: Then maybe now is the time to start thinking about the sorts of things you would like to do? Maybe we could come up with some ideas.

ANGELA: I would but I feel guilty about moving on, leaving Ryan behind.

THERAPIST: What would he want?

ANGELA: You're right, he would want me to move on.

THERAPIST: Do you think you could move on with your life, while still honoring Ryan's memory?

ANGELA: I think so. I was thinking about getting involved in our town's recreational safety committee.

THERAPIST: That sounds like a really important start.

There are a variety of activities that can help patients gain, or regain, their sense of purpose in life after the trauma has passed. These may include activities that are relevant to preventing similar traumas from befalling others, as in the case of Angela. Other examples include joining a group such as Neighborhood Watch, Mothers Against Drunk Driving, Amnesty International, or a charity organization. Activities need not be trauma related. In fact it is advisable that patients have a range of meaningful activities in their lives, rather than an exclusive focus on trauma-related endeavors. Activities might involve joining a church group, volunteering in a community center (e.g., for a seniors' program), taking up an absorbing avocation, such as pottery, joining a choral society, or taking up a sport such as sailing or jogging.

As illustrated in the case of Angela, for patients who have survived an interpersonal trauma in which someone was killed, it can be very useful to explore their beliefs about what happened to the person after he or she died. Sometimes patients harbor the unexamined assumption that the deceased continues to suffer horribly after death. The plausibility of this belief can be examined in treatment (an example of how this was done in the context of combining cognitive restructuring and imaginal exposure appears in Chapter 12).

MENTAL DEFEAT AND NUMBING

Mental defeat is the perceived loss of all autonomy: a state of giving up in one's mind all efforts to retain one's identity as a human being with a will of one's own (Ehlers et al., 2000). This complex phenomenon, which can arise from interpersonal traumas, is associated with various types of dysfunctional beliefs, for example, "I've been destroyed as a human being," "I'm a hollow person," "I have no control over my life," or "I feel like I'm not part of the human race." These sorts of beliefs are also associated with emotional numbing. Indeed, numbing and mental defeat share many similarities, such as the sense of not feeling fully human and beliefs that one will not be able to achieve important life goals such as having a career or family. Numbing is also associated with beliefs such as "I'll never feel close to people" or "I'll never feel passionate about anything."

For both mental defeat and numbing, the therapist can begin by "unpacking" beliefs like "I'm a hollow person," that is, clarifying what the patient means and identifying any relevant associated beliefs. The following is a therapy transcript with 32-year-old Anne, who was gang-raped as a teenager. During therapy she frequently voiced the belief that she was a hollow person.

> THERAPIST: Anne, to help me understand what things have been like for you, could you tell me what you mean when you say that you're a hollow person?
>
> ANNE: I feel empty inside.
>
> THERAPIST: What is missing?
>
> ANNE: I feel lost, like I have nothing in my life.
>
> THERAPIST: What sorts of things would you like to have?
>
> ANNE: I would like to have friends, and to be in a relationship.
>
> THERAPIST: OK, and is there anything else that would make your life more fulfilling?
>
> ANNE: Um, yes. I have no direction. I would like to go back to school and finish my senior year, but I've lost all confidence.
>
> THERAPIST: OK, so, to summarize, you see yourself as a hollow person because there things missing from your life that you'd like to have, like feeling connected or close to people, having a special person in your life, and feeling like you have a meaningful purpose, like finishing your schooling. And it also sounds like there are some obstacles that prevent you achieving these goals, like feeling unconfident. Does that seem like a reasonably accurate summary?

Notice that the therapist—and perhaps the patient—initially had difficulty pinning down exactly what Anne meant when she called herself a hollow person. Anne associated "hollowness" with things like "something's missing" and "I feel lost." The therapist patiently persisted to help Anne think about what was missing and how she might find direction. Thus, a nebulous self-belief, "I'm a hollow person," was reframed into something more specific, concrete, and therefore attainable: "My life would be more fulfilled if I had friends and a relationship and completed my education." One of the obstacles to achieving these goals was also identified—lack of confidence in her abilities. Thus, therapy began by identifying specific beliefs about concrete things, to be followed by a problem-solving analysis.

Beliefs associated with mental defeat can also be addressed by encouraging patients to engage in planning that involves meaningful aspects of their lives and to increasingly do things that enhance their sense of mastery or control. Examples include assertiveness training, self-defense courses, and other activities that bring a sense of mastery. Numbing can be similarly addressed with mastery and pleasure exercises (see Chapter 9).

To address feelings of alienation or estrangement from others, the therapist can look for relevant beliefs about the reactions of other people (e.g., "My family doesn't want to talk about the accident, so they must blame me for it" or "Everyone can tell by looking at me that I'm a rape victim"). The therapist and patient can explore the evidence and alternative interpretations of the reactions of others. Family members, for example, might avoid discussing the trauma because they do not want to upset the patient. The belief that "people can tell I've been raped" may represent a form of fear-driven reasoning about what other people think, for example, "I'm frightened that other people can tell I've been raped. If they did, they'd think I'm dirty and disgusting. Therefore, I'd better check if people are looking at me. As I'm scanning for disapproval I can see that people are looking at me in a weird manner; they can tell I've been raped!" People may indeed be looking at the patient, but simply because the patient is scanning or staring at them. This possibility can be fruitfully explored in therapy.

Patients can be encouraged to collect information to test beliefs associated with alienation. For example, consider the belief "I can't feel connected to people because nobody could understand what I've been through." This could be addressed by encouraging the patient to join a support group relevant to his or her traumatic experience (e.g., a spousal abuse support group or a veterans group), which typically provides patients with evidence that other people can readily relate to their traumatic experiences.

TRAUMA-RELATED ANGER

Patients with PTSD may have legitimate reasons for feeling angry about what has been done to them. The therapist can empathize with the patient's feelings of anger but also inquire about the costs and benefits of anger. This involves helping the patient to question any beliefs about the positive aspects of excessive anger (e.g., "I can't feel powerful and in charge unless I'm angry"). The evidence for and against the beliefs can also be reviewed. The best way to increase one's chances of being in control in a provocative situation is to focus on one's goals while also trying to remain calm. When reviewing the costs of anger, patients can also be asked to observe its effects on their bodies (e.g., bodily sensations such as a pounding heart, tense muscles, or headache), on their thinking (e.g., anger can cloud one's thinking), on their daily functioning, and on the people they've hurt. Patients can be asked to imagine how life would be different if they were in control of their anger.

Cognitive restructuring for anger also involves teaching patients to take responsibility for their anger instead of attributing it to an external trigger, such as the source of a provocation. The following are examples of responsibility-related coping statements (based on Schiraldi, 2000): "I choose who I let under my skin," "I can choose to talk calmly rather than scream or become violent," "Giving others control of my life—by choosing to let them annoy me—puts me in the victim role and reinforces the feeling of powerlessness," "Violence is not an option; it temporarily relieves tension while destroying inner peace and relationships."

Patients who continually ruminate about past injustices can also be encouraged to replace angry rumination with adaptive coping statements. Here are some famous examples: "Living life well is the greatest revenge" (adapted from the Talmud); "You can't get ahead while you're getting even" (adapted from Sir Francis Bacon); "An eye for an eye would make the whole world blind" (from Mahatma Gandhi); and "When you plan to get even with someone, you are only letting that person continue to hurt you" (from Andy Rooney).

For patients who dwell on fantasies of getting revenge, one method is to ask them to write the fantasy down and share it with the therapist. This is a distancing strategy than can enable the patient to see the futility of such fantasies. For example, June had a fantasy of castrating the man who raped her. She was asked to describe this fantasy in detail, including the aftermath for the castrated man. She realized that acting on such a fantasy would make her an abuser just like him. This led June to consider more effective ways of preventing violence against women, such as getting involved in community programs for rape prevention.

Survivors of interpersonal violence can be asked to consider questions such as the following: What kinds of psychological problems would lead the assailant to do such a thing (e.g., feeling insecure or inferior)? What goals or needs was the assailant trying to fulfill (e.g., a need to feel powerful)? What sorts of childhood or other experiences would have led the assailant to do such things (e.g., abuse from other, more powerful people)? The goal of this exercise is to help the patient understand why the assailant committed the abuse. This helps give meaning to the trauma, and make the patient's world more predictable and controllable. The therapist should emphasize the purpose of this exercise is to help the patient; the goal is not to make excuses for the assailant's unacceptable behavior.

Another useful method consists of guided imagery plus cognitive restructuring. This involves working up a hierarchy of increasingly intense, imaginal anger-provoking situations, combined with the use of coping self-statements, that is, imaginal exercises that simulate exposure to anger-provoking situations and enable the patient to practice coping self-talk (e.g., "I need to focus on my goal of getting the clerk to fill out my disability form; blowing up is not going to help me achieve my goal"). Self-statements are prepared before exposure to the trigger situation (e.g., they can be written on a card). Cognitive restructuring can also be combined with situational exposure exercises, where the patient practices coping statements (and breathing retraining) in increasingly provoking situations. After each exposure exercise the patient should spend some time doing a calming activity (e.g., jogging) rather than engaging in angry rumination. Anger exposure exercises should be especially gradual if the patient has a history of dissociative rage episodes.

Allan developed PTSD and severe road rage after being in a major road traffic collision. He became exceedingly angry whenever another driver cut him off or "provoked" him in some other way. On two occasions Allan angrily ran another car off the road, pulled the other driver from the car, grabbed the driver by the hair, and repeatedly pounded his head onto the hood of the car. Allan had hazy recollections of these episodes; while he was in a state of rage, things seemed unreal and people said that he appeared to be in a daze. When Allan entered treatment, he was asked by his therapist not to drive unless he was absolutely certain that he could avoid provocative situations or leave the situation (e.g., pull over) if his anger started to mount. He was treated with psychoeducation and breathing retraining (Chapter 9), along with cognitive restructuring and very gradual exposure to provocative driving situations. An important goal of therapy was to help Allan control his anger before he slipped into a state of dissociative rage. This was done by helping him identify warning signs. The most effective signs for Allan were jaw tension and the sight of his white knuckles on the steering wheel. When he noticed these signs, he practiced breathing retraining and used coping statements (e.g., "I've got to stay cool or I'll wind up in jail") until his anger had subsided. If these methods did not work, then he switched to "Plan B," which involved pulling over to the side of the road and closing his eyes and relaxing while listening to the radio. Practicing these methods, spurred by Allan's realistic fear that he would end up in prison if his anger was unchecked, led to a substantial reduction in his anger and the elimination of episodes of dissociative rage.

TRAUMA-RELATED SHAME

Cognitive restructuring for shame involves targeting self-related beliefs, especially ones about the person's worth, "badness," or blameworthiness. Here, restructuring may involve disputations about the adaptiveness of imposing labels on oneself (e.g., "Does blaming yourself undo the event or help you deal with the aftermath?"), and disputations concerning over-generalizations (e.g., "How does doing a bad thing make you an entirely bad person? What good things have you done in your life?").

Some patients believe that they need to, or should, feel shame (or guilt) because they believe it motivates them to improve themselves or avoid future trauma or because they believe they deserve punishment (Leahy, 2003). Punishment-related beliefs can be addressed via adaptive disputations, such as reviewing the costs and benefits of self-imposed punishment. Beliefs about the motivational necessity of shame (or guilt) can also be tested by retrospectively reviewing the outcome of days in which patients might not have blamed themselves versus days in which they were highly self-critical. Typically, days associated with low self-criticism are productive and enjoyable, whereas the opposite is true of days of high self-criticism. In fact, it is not uncommon for patients to spend all day in bed, abuse alcohol or drugs, or overeat on high-criticism days. This sort of evidence can be used to challenge the value of self-imposed criticism. This can be followed up with a behavioral experiment in which patients deliberately try, on some days, to suspend self-criticism and compare the outcome of those days with days in which they revert to their pattern of self-criticism.

To facilitate this exercise, patients can use coping statements to help them refrain from self-criticism. These might involve the patient responding to self-critical thoughts with any of the following: (1) Distancing strategies (e.g., "I've just had a self-critical thought; I'm taking a break from those thoughts today, so I don't need to take it seriously. I can simply watch the thought come and go"); (2) response to self-critical thoughts by invoking the advice of an expert (e.g., "Doctor's orders are that today I refuse to listen to self-critical thoughts"); (3) self-soothing or self-acceptance (e.g., "Today I'm going to practice being kind to myself, and accepting me for who I am. That will help me heal"); (4) self-statements that trivialize or make light of self-critical thoughts ("Shame, shame go away, come again another day"). The choice of coping statement would depend on the patient's preferences and what he or she finds helpful. Some patients, for example, find it particularly useful to trivialize their self-critical thoughts, whereas other patients find it more helpful to use self-soothing or self-acceptance.

When challenging trauma-related shame, the therapist can encourage the patient to shift from labeling the self as good or bad to labeling one's actions. This can sometimes be sufficient for reducing shame, especially if patients can forgive themselves for making an error that they can avoid in the future (e.g., "It was a mistake for me to leave my drink unattended. I didn't realize he'd spike it with one of those date-rape drugs. I'll know better next time"). If this is not sufficient, then interventions for trauma-related guilt can be used (see below).

Frequent exposure to shame-related cues or reminders can make it especially difficult to overcome shame. A woman who had a child as a result of a sexual assault, for example, might feel shame at the sight of her child and then might chastise herself for feeling ashamed (Resick & Schnicke, 1993). In such cases, the therapist can help the patient separate the source of shame (the sexual assault) from the outcome of the assault (the birth of the child). Shame-related beliefs concerning the sexual assault can be challenged by reviewing the evidence and by other methods that are used for targeting guilt (described below), for example, "Would you be ashamed of your sister if she was raped?" or "Realistically, how much control did you have to resist the rapist, who was considerably bigger and stronger than you and was threatening you with a knife?" The therapist can also help the patient realize that the child is not simply the "rapist's off spring" (e.g., "Parenting and the environment play an extremely important role in shaping who we are. Your child is a product of your nurturing and the experiences that you have provided. Whatever genetic contribution was made by the rapist is trivial in comparison").

TRAUMA-RELATED GUILT

The most sophisticated, empirically supported interventions for trauma-related guilt have emerged from the work of Kubany and colleagues (e.g., Kubany, 1998; Kubany & Manke, 1995; Kubany & Watson, 2002). The interventions are implemented in a sequential, recursive fashion. The therapist cycles through the sequence of interventions, with each sequence devoted to a single guilt issue. The interventions are: debriefing, hindsight bias analysis, justification analysis, responsibility analysis, and wrongdoing analysis. Each involves psychoeducation and cognitive restructuring.

Debriefing

The patient is asked to give a detailed, nonevaluative account of events prior to and during the trauma. The worst part of the trauma is identified, and associated beliefs and emotions are elicited. Sometimes, simply recounting the trauma in detail is enough to lead the patient to have important insights that correct misconceptions about his or her role in the trauma. "As clients hear themselves describe exactly what happened, they sometimes gain awareness that what they did made more sense than they had previously realized" (Kubany & Manke, 1995, p. 48).

Paula was trapped in an abusive marriage for 15 years until her husband, Jake, was killed in an automobile accident while driving home one night from a bar. She felt guilty about having married Jake (against her parents' wishes), and about having been too frightened to stop Jake during the many times he beat their two young children. During the debriefing the therapist inquired about whether Jake had committed other sorts of violence. Paula recalled that he regularly got into bar fights, which on two occasions led to his being charged with assault. She recalled that on one occasion Jake had savagely beaten a bystander who tried to break up a fight in which Jake was involved. As these details came to light, Paula realized that she too would had been beaten if she had tried to stop him beating their children, and that her attempts to intervene could have worsened the beating the children received. This insight led her to feel somewhat less guilty about been too frightened to stop Jake.

Hindsight Bias Analysis

This intervention involves correcting faulty beliefs about pre-outcome knowledge. The patient is first educated about hindsight bias. This is the "I knew it all along" bias, which involves the tendency to believe, once the outcome is already known, that you would have foreseen it beforehand. It arises because the person's judgments are biased by knowledge acquired after the outcome is known. The therapist determines if the patient falsely believes that he or she knew something prior to the trauma that could have enabled him or her to prevent or avoid it. The therapist then helps the patient realize that it is impossible for knowledge acquired after the event to guide pre-outcome decision making. If the patient insists he or she knew what was going to happen, then the therapist should elicit details of exactly what happened and precisely when the patient knew with certainty what was going to happen (Kubany, 1998).

Paula berated herself for having married Jake. "I should have known better—I should have listened to Mom and Dad." The hindsight bias analysis, however, revealed that prior to the marriage, neither Paula nor her parents had any indication that Jake would become violent. Before marriage, Jake was charming and "a bit wild," but she had no way of knowing that he would become abusive. Her parents' disapproval of Jake had to do with the fact that he did not come from the same religious background as Paula and her parents. Paula realized that even her girlfriends did not expect that Jake would become violent. In fact, many of her friends envied Paula because she was dating such an exciting man. All of this evidence was used to help Paula question her belief that she should have known better.

Justification Analysis

The patient is informed that the best or most justified choice in a given situation is the best choice among the options that were actually considered at the time. Options that would have been ideal but did not exist, and options that came to mind later, should not be included in the analysis of justification. Patients are then asked to describe their reasons for acting as they did and to describe what other courses of action they considered and rejected, along with the reasons for rejection. They are then asked which option, of the options actually considered at the time, was the one most justified, based only on what they knew then.

Two common thinking errors that contribute to distorted beliefs about justification for actions taken are (1) tendencies to overlook positive things associated with actions taken and (2) focusing only on good things that might have happened had alternative courses of action (which were considered at the time) been taken (Kubany & Watson, 2002). When this procedure is used clinically, the option chosen at the time is almost always the best choice of those available at the time.

Paula was asked what made her decide to marry Jake. She recalled several reasons; she was attracted to him, she wanted to escape her controlling, strictly religious parents, and she was also pregnant with her first child. When asked whether she had any other options, Paula said that the only other possibilities were to (1) have an abortion and remain at home, (2) have the child and give it up for adoption, or (3) have the child and try to raise it on her own. Paula recalled that her options were limited, especially because her parents would have told her to leave the family home if she had a child out of wedlock. She realized that marrying Jake was the best option at the time.

Responsibility Analysis

The patient is educated about the distinction between blame and causation; blame involves causation *plus* wrongdoing. The patient is then asked to produce a comprehensive list of people (aside from the patient) and other factors that contributed in some causal way to the trauma. The patient is asked to assign a percentage of importance of each of these causes. The patient is then asked to evaluate his or her own percentage of contribution to the outcome. The total percentages must, of course, add up to 100. Thus, the relative importance of the various causal factors are determined.

Paula felt guilty about Jake's abusive behavior during their marriage: "If I had been a better wife and mother, then maybe Jake wouldn't have turned so nasty." Paula was asked to consider all the factors, apart from herself, that contributed to Jake's violent behavior. She listed several factors: Jake had several upsetting setbacks at work, including being laid off on several occasions; he had fallen in with a group of heavy-drinking guys he met on a construction job; he had rigid beliefs about marital roles (e.g., "The wife should serve the husband"); and he had similarly rigid views about corporal punishment (e.g., "Spare the rod and spoil the child"). The therapist asked Paula whether Jake was in control of his actions. For example, was he able to refrain from beating the children when other people were present, such as his friends or Paula's parents? Paula recognized that, yes indeed, Jake was able to control himself. Paula was then asked whether she would blame her sister if she had been in Paula's position. Paula recognized that, no, she would not hold her sister accountable. This review of the various factors helped Paula realized that she was not responsible for Jake's violent behavior.

Wrongdoing Analysis

Here, the patient is educated that the label of "wrongdoing" is applied when people intentionally cause harm or knowingly violate their moral or ethical code of conduct. The patient is asked whether he or she wanted the trauma to occur and intentionally made it happen. The answer is typically "no," to which the therapist can reply:

> "You didn't want it to happen and did not try to make it happen. In addition, you already concluded that there was no possible way that you could have known better, that what you did was the most justified choice, and that you were minimally responsible for causing what happened. How could what you did be wrong in any way?" (Kubany, 1998, p. 135)

If all the courses of action would have had negative consequences, then the "least bad" choice is the most sound and moral choice. The patient and therapist can also explore whether the patient is discounting or ignoring positive things he or she did to deal with the situation.

Paula felt guilty because she firmly believed it was wrong to use corporal punishment on children, and she failed to prevent the abuse. The therapist and Paula explored whether she was guilty of wrongdoing. Paula had never used corporal punishment and, in fact, had done many things to protect the children from Jake, such as sending them to stay overnight with her parents when she knew Jake would be drinking particularly heavily. She felt guilty about not having called Child Protective Services but then realized that this was an option that she had not considered at the time (hindsight bias), and that involving a government child protection agency could have escalated Jake's rage against her and the children. Paula was able to realize that she did the best she could under very difficult circumstances and that she had done nothing wrong.

For homework, the patient is asked to use a self-monitoring form to keep track of three types of thoughts: (1) Those involving why the trauma occurred and how the patient might have avoided or prevented it (e.g., self-statements containing phrases like "should have," "supposed to," "could

have," "if only," and "why"); (2) self-demeaning thoughts; and (3) "I feel
. . . " self-statements ending in words that are not emotions (e.g., "I feel
like it was all my fault"). The latter types of thoughts are monitored
because merging "I feel" statements with words that are not emotions can
impair patients' ability to objectively appraise themselves and their role in
the trauma (Kubany, 1998). "Why" questions are targeted because they
can perpetuate rumination about the trauma and prevent patients from
moving on with their lives. Self-monitoring is used to enhance the patient's
awareness of when these thoughts arise, which can therefore help them
challenge and reject them.

Paula's self-monitoring contained a lot of "why" questions, such as "Why
didn't I think of calling the police or Child Protective Services?" She was asked
to consider whether this sort of thinking was helpful. Did it, for example, help
or harm her emotional well-being? Did it help or harm her relationship with her
children? Paula recognized that such thoughts led her to feel so guilty that she
would hide away in bed all day, trying to use sleep as a way of avoiding her
painful feelings. This interfered with the quality of her parenting and, importantly, such thinking did not change what had happened. The therapist and
Paula devised a series of coping statements, written on a card that she kept in
her purse, which she consulted whenever she was troubled by these "why"
thoughts. The statements were: "I did the best I could under the circumstances," "Hindsight may be 20/20, but 'why' questions are not helpful," "If I
was perfect I might have been able to do better, but I'm an imperfect person
just like everyone else. I have to accept myself for who I am."

When the Patient Caused the Trauma

In contrast to the examples discussed earlier, in which patients overestimated their degree of responsibility, there are other cases in which it is
fairly clear that the patient played an important role in the trauma. Examples include driving while intoxicated and killing someone in a crash, or
participating in atrocities during wartime. A three-step approach can be
used in these cases. First, analyze the situation, to determine how the
patient became involved in the trauma. This is not to make excuses for the
patient's actions but rather to help them understand how the event
occurred, and how they might prevent a similar thing from happening
again. Second, acknowledge that guilt and shame are expected and normal
reactions, although debilitating shame or guilt does not help anyone; it
doesn't make reparation and doesn't help the patient move on with his or
her life. An important issue here is whether less guilt or shame would make
the patient more likely to commit another crime. If the latter is a likely pos-

sibility, then reducing guilt and shame might not be a target of treatment. Third, explore whether the patient is interested in making reparation or "putting things right" in some fashion. A person who killed a pedestrian while driving intoxicated, for example, might choose to become active in a community road safety program.

Perhaps the most dramatic example of this type of intervention was reported by Kubany (1997), who described the effective treatment of a Vietnam veteran who had PTSD and severe guilt because of the things he had done in combat. Among other things, he had actively participated in atrocities, in which he and other soldiers in his unit mutilated the corpses of the enemy ("overkilling") and cut off the ears of the dead as trophies. Without justifying these actions, the therapist helped the patient understand the social and psychological context in which such things occurred: "The practice of overkilling the enemy and displaying ears as trophies of war was perceived as one way to intimidate the enemy because American troops knew that many Vietnamese believed that a person with a missing body part would be prevented from entering 'whatever heaven was for them' " (p. 237). Overkilling was also intended to warn the enemy to stay away from U.S. troops. The therapist further suggested to the patient that there were two circumstances that might encourage a person to do things that would ordinarily be considered inhumane. First, many U.S. troops were impaired in their capacity to experience compassion, empathy, and guilt because they had become numbed by the trauma of war (along with the social consensus that extreme or brutal behavior was appropriate). Second, research on cue-controlled aggression indicates that tangible and symbolic aggressive cues can trigger impulsive aggression in people who are highly aroused with aversive emotions such as fear or anger. This information enabled the patient to understand how he'd been taught or conditioned to act in particular ways. Other interventions also were used, such as cognitive restructuring for guilt, described earlier in this chapter.

BELIEFS ABOUT SYMPTOMS
AND ABOUT ONE'S PSYCHOLOGICAL FUNCTIONING

There are a range of different beliefs about symptoms and psychological functioning that can contribute to or amplify PTSD symptoms (see Chapter 2). These include beliefs about PTSD symptoms (e.g., "My flashbacks mean I'm going insane"), beliefs about arousal-related symptoms in general (also known as anxiety sensitivity; e.g., "I will have a heart attack if my heart beats too fast"), and beliefs about one's psychological functioning (e.g., "My concentration and memory are bad; my brain must have been damaged by stress"). These beliefs can be addressed with a combination of psychoeducation, cognitive restructuring, and interoceptive exposure exercises (Chapter 12).

PTSD patients often try to suppress their unwanted, intrusive, trauma-related thoughts and images. This can lead to a paradoxical increase in or persistence of intrusive thoughts (Chapter 2). Patients can test the effects of thought suppression by trying to deliberately suppress their thoughts on some days and not suppressing on other days, and keeping track of the frequency of the unwanted thoughts. This exercise can teach them that thought suppression is either ineffective or counterproductive.

Patients can be encouraged to take the same approach to their symptoms in general, that is, practicing *mindfulness* with the symptoms (Kabat-Zinn, 1990): simply observing the symptoms, describing them to oneself without evaluating them, and watching the symptoms naturally come and go without trying to change them. For example, a patient might become startled by a loud noise such as a car backfiring. Startle reactions in PTSD can be quite intense. Patients often become angry or strongly frustrated with themselves, which amplifies the startle-related distress. Patients can be encouraged to use these episodes as opportunities for practicing mindfulness: "Observe the startle response, remind yourself it is a harmless PTSD symptom, and watch it naturally pass, without trying to force it away."

WHICH BELIEFS SHOULD BE TARGETED?

Given the wide range of beliefs that can be associated with PTSD, the challenge is to identify the ones that are most relevant to the patient's problems. These are typically the important targets of cognitive restructuring. It may not be possible, given time constraints, or even necessary to address all of the patient's dysfunctional beliefs. The case formulation, informed by a thorough cognitive assessment (Chapter 6), can help guide the selection of which beliefs to address. Dysfunctional beliefs that are associated with the greatest distress or impairment in social and occupational functioning often play a central role in the case formulation. The patient's goals are also important in selecting beliefs. That is, which beliefs or associated emotional or behavioral problems are most important for the patient to overcome?

In selecting which beliefs are likely to be most important, the therapist should be aware of preconceptions that might bias his or her development of a case formulation and treatment. For example, the presence of prominent trauma-related anger does not necessarily mean that anger-related beliefs play the primary role in the case formulation. There may be other types of beliefs that need to be addressed, as illustrated in the following example.

Anger was one of Joseph's major problems requiring immediate therapeutic attention. The therapist developed a case formulation in which anger-related beliefs played a prominent role. Examples of such beliefs were "People must treat me with dignity" and "My anger protects me." Although Joseph was helped considerably by treatment focusing on anger management and the cognitive restructuring of associated beliefs, he continued to suffer from prominent PTSD symptoms, particularly avoidance and hyperarousal. The case formulation was revisited in order to identify other factors that may have been contributing to his symptoms. The downward arrow method (Chapter 6) was used to assess whether there were any other beliefs associated with his anger-related beliefs. The assessment revealed a series of beliefs about the dangerousness of other people and the world, for example, "People are dangerous; they'll turn on me if they smell fear" and "I'm in constant danger of being attacked." These beliefs were associated with anxiety, not anger. The identification of these beliefs led to a modification of the treatment plan, in which anxiety-related beliefs, in addition to anger beliefs, became important targets of cognitive restructuring.

SUMMARY

The methods described in this chapter focus on the major types of beliefs associated with PTSD, including those summarized in Table 11.1. These are common targets for cognitive restructuring in PTSD. The table also illustrates some of the methods for challenging these beliefs. Cognitive interventions, such as the ones described in this and the previous chapter, are often effective in their own right, and they can be usefully combined with exposure, in ways described in the following chapters.

TABLE 11.1. Major Types of Beliefs Associated with PTSD and Methods for Challenging These Beliefs

Belief domains and examples of beliefs	Examples of interventions
Beliefs about the dangerousness of other people and the world (e.g., "I can never be safe"), often associated with intolerance of uncertainty. Such beliefs may arise from a shattering of previously held assumptions (e.g., "Bad things don't happen to good people") or a strengthening of preexisting beliefs (e.g., "There is more evil than good in the world").	• Review the nature and quality of evidence for the beliefs. • Establish reasonable guidelines for distinguishing danger from safety. • Identify and address black-and-white thinking (e.g., "Is it really true that you're *never* safe?"). • Discuss the adaptiveness of holding particular beliefs (e.g., "Does it help or harm your quality of life to refuse to tolerate any form of uncertainty?").
Metaphysical beliefs, such as particular religious or spiritual beliefs (e.g., "God has forsaken me," "Life no longer has any meaning") and beliefs about the nature of existence after death (e.g., "The soul of my dead sister continues to suffer horribly").	• Work within the patient's belief system to resolve the crisis in religious or spiritual beliefs. This may involve enlisting the assistance of a religious or spiritual expert to provide reassuring information to the patient (e.g., "In our religion, God would not let the soul of your good sister suffer in the afterlife"). • Explore ways of restoring meaning in one's life (e.g., engaging in personally meaningful activities, such as volunteer work to help others). • Review the plausibility of beliefs (e.g., "Just because he was horribly murdered, does that mean he continues to suffer? Could it be that his mutilated body is simply an empty vessel, which his soul has abandoned?")
Beliefs associated with mental defeat and emotional numbing. Examples of beliefs associated with mental defeat include "I've been destroyed as a human being," "I'm a hollow person," and "I have no will or autonomy." Examples of beliefs associated with numbing include "I will never feel close to anyone," "I will never feel passionate about life," and "I will not live long enough to see my children grow to adulthood."	• Unpack the beliefs to identify and clarify the various components (e.g., what is meant by "hollow"?). • Identify what is lacking in the person's life and problem-solve to find ways of making life more fulfilling. This may involve activities that give the person a sense of agency or mastery (e.g., assertiveness training to help patients recognize that they do have a will of their own). • Examine the evidence for beliefs that may contribute to feelings of estrangement from others (e.g., "People think I'm some kind of freak or monster because my face was disfigured by the fire"). • Review the adaptiveness of beliefs such as "I'll never regain my passion for life."

(continued)

TABLE 11.1. *(continued)*

Belief domains and examples of beliefs	Examples of interventions
Beliefs associated with trauma-related . . .	
Anger. This includes beliefs about (1) the culpability of others, (2) the positive or empowering effects of anger, and (c) the responsibility of external sources (e.g., other people) for provoking anger.	• Empathize with the patient about the reasons for being angry (which may be quite legitimate) but also explore the costs of anger. • Examine beliefs about the positive aspects of being angry (e.g., "Anger helps me stand up for my rights") and review whether there are non-angry means of obtaining these benefits (e.g., calm assertiveness). • Review the evidence about the merits of keeping calm in provocative situations (e.g., "When is your thinking clearest, when you are calm or when you're extremely angry?"). • Help the patient generate self-statements to help cope with provocative situations (e.g., "Staying calm and in control, with my breathing exercise, is the best way to deal with tense situations").
Shame. This includes beliefs about one's badness, inferiority, or blameworthiness.	• Adaptive disputation about the costs and benefits of imposing derogatory labels on oneself. Identify and challenge any beliefs about the positive motivating effects of shame or self-blame (e.g., "Do you really need to blame yourself every day in order to stay out of harm's way? Doesn't all this self-blame make you feel so bad that you don't care what happens to you?"). • Identify and challenge overgeneralizations (e.g., "So you made a mistake in deciding to go home with him that night. Does that make you a bad person who deserved to be assaulted?"). As part of this intervention, the patient can be encouraged to label actions as good or bad, but not the self. • Distancing strategies can help the patient gain perspective (e.g., "Would you feel ashamed of your sister if she had been raped? Why not?").
Guilt. This includes beliefs, often exaggerated, about one's role in causing some wrong action (i.e., responsibility and blame: "I should have known better," "If only I'd been a better wife—then he wouldn't have beaten me all the time").	• Kubany's series of cognitive interventions, consisting of debriefing, hindsight analysis, justification analysis, responsibility analysis, and wrongdoing analysis.
Beliefs about symptoms or one's psychological functioning. Examples include "My flashbacks mean I'm going insane," "My memory problems indicate that all the stress has fried my brain," and "I'll have a heart attack if my heart beats too fast."	• Psychoeducation about the nature and realistic consequences of arousal-related sensations in general (e.g., palpitations, concentration problems), and PTSD symptoms in particular (e.g., intrusive recollections or flashbacks). • Cognitive exercises to test beliefs about the effects of trying too hard to control one's thoughts (e.g., suppression vs. nonsuppression, or practicing mindfulness exercises to learn that the unwanted thoughts have no adverse consequences).

CHAPTER 12

Exposure Exercises I

Imaginal and Interoceptive Exposure

Imaginal exposure involves some form of exposure to memories of the trauma, such as by writing a vivid description of the event or narrating it into a tape recorder. Interoceptive exposure, which involves systematic exposure to fear-evoking but harmless bodily sensations, is a new, promising intervention for PTSD. The purpose of interoceptive exposure is to reduce anxiety sensitivity (fear of arousal-related bodily sensations), which plays a role in amplifying anxiety reactions and has been implicated in PTSD (Chapter 2). Although interoceptive exposure is a well-established method for treating panic disorder (Taylor, 2000), it has only recently been found to be useful in treating PTSD, even for patients who do not suffer from panic disorder (Taylor, 2004; Wald & Taylor, 2005a, 2005b). Clinical experience with interoceptive exposure suggests that it often triggers trauma memories, probably because intense, arousal-related bodily sensations occurred at the time of the trauma and so have become part of the patient's recollection of the trauma. Thus, interoceptive exposure involves some degree of imaginal exposure, but it exposes patients to stimuli (bodily sensations) that may not be evoked by conventional imaginal exposure.

GENERAL PRINCIPLES OF EXPOSURE

The following apply to all forms of exposure: imaginal, interoceptive, and situational. Regardless of the form of exposure, a trusting therapeutic relationship is essential for the patient to engage in these exercises.

Precautions and Preparations

Before commencing any form of exposure therapy, the therapist needs to ensure that exposure is safe and suitable for a given patient. The patient needs to have a good understanding of what is involved in treatment. The patient must be physically able to endure some degree of distress associated with imaginal or interoceptive exposure. Also, before conducting interoceptive exposure, the therapist should identify any medical contraindications (see Table 12.1 for examples). When in doubt about using a given exercise, the therapist should either consult with the patient's physician or refrain from using the exercise.

The use of exposure interventions should be avoided, or deferred, if there are indications that the patient may not be able to tolerate the distress associated with exposure. This would be the case if a patient has poor impulse control, a poorly controlled substance use disorder, suicidal ideation or urges, or engages in stress-induced self-injurious behavior. Interventions for dealing with these problems would need to be implemented before using exposure. It is better to wait till the patient is ready for exposure than to engage in an abortive, discouraging attempt.

Marcy had a long history of physical and sexual abuse, including childhood and spousal abuse. Whenever she became distressed in her daily life, such as when she had vivid recollections of previous trauma, she would engage in skin picking on her fingers, face, and sometimes feet. She found this activity to be distracting and soothing. She often dissociated during these episodes, and would "come to" after 30 or 40 minutes to discover that her lips or cuticles were red, raw, and bleeding. Prior to commencing any form of exposure exercise, the therapist and Marcy agreed that it was important to acquire less harmful forms of self-soothing. She learned the emotion coping skills described in Chapter 9 and used methods from a procedure known as habit reversal (Azrin & Nunn, 1973) to reduce the frequency of skin picking: whenever she felt the urge to pick, she engaged in an incompatible, alternative behavior, such as tightly clenching her fists for 1 minute. Gradually, Marcy become skillful at identifying risky periods (i.e., periods when she had a stressful day and was at home alone) and implementing emotion coping skills before her distress escalated. These were combined, as needed, with habit reversal methods. Once her skin picking and dissociation were under control, Marcy and the therapist gradually began a course of exposure exercises.

Exposure Duration and Intensity

Patients should be assured that exposure is always a collaborative venture, and that they always have the option to refrain from or discontinue exposure at any time. Exercises should be challenging (i.e., moderately distress-

TABLE 12.1. Interoceptive Exposure Exercises: Sensations Most Strongly Elicited and Potential Medical Contraindications

Exercise	Sensations most strongly elicited	Potential medical contraindications
Shaking one's head from side to side for 30 seconds	1. Dizziness or faintness 2. Pounding/racing heart 3. Breathlessness/smothering sensations	Cervical pain or disease (e.g., whiplash injury), history of falling due to dizziness or balance disorder[a]
Placing one's head between one's knees for 30 seconds and then lifting the head quickly to the normal position	1. Dizziness or faintness 2. Breathlessness/smothering sensations 3. Numbness/tingling in face or extremities	Postural hypotension, lower-back pain, history of falling due to dizziness or balance disorder[a]
Spinning around (while standing) at a medium pace for 30 seconds	1. Dizziness or faintness 2. Pounding/racing heart 3. Breathlessness/smothering sensations	Pregnancy, history of falling due to dizziness or balance disorder[a]
Hold one's breath for 30 seconds	1. Breathlessness/smothering sensations 2. Pounding/racing heart 3. Dizziness or faintness	Chronic obstructive lung disease
Hyperventilation (i.e., breathing in and out rapidly, as if panting) for 1 minute	1. Breathlessness/smothering sensations 2. Dizziness or faintness 3. Pounding/racing heart	Chronic obstructive lung disease, severe asthma, cardiac conditions, epilepsy, renal disease, pregnancy
Breathing through a narrow straw for 2 minutes, while making sure not to breathe through the nose	1. Breathlessness/smothering sensations 2. Pounding/racing heart 3. Choking	Chronic obstructive lung disease
Staring continuously at a fluorescent light on the ceiling for 1 minute and then trying to read	1. Dizziness or faintness 2. Feeling unreal or as if in a dream (Only two symptoms produced with more than mild intensity)	History of seizures caused by staring at fluorescent or other lights
Staring continuously at oneself in a mirror for 2 minutes	1. Feeling unreal or as if in a dream 2. Dizziness or faintness (Only two symptoms produced with more than mild intensity)	No apparent contraindications

(continued)

TABLE 12.1. (continued)

Exercise	Sensations most strongly elicited	Potential medical contraindications
Staring continuously at a spot on the wall for 3 minutes	1. Feeling unreal or as if in a dream 2. Dizziness or faintness (Only two symptoms produced with more than mild intensity)	No apparent contraindications
Tensing all the muscles of the body for 1 minute	1. Trembling/shaking 2. Breathlessness/smothering sensations 3. Pounding/racing heart	Pain disorders. If pain is localized, patients could tense all but the affected region
Running in place for 1 minute	1. Pounding/racing heart 2. Breathlessness/smothering sensations 3. Chest pain/tightness	Cardiac conditions, severe asthma, lower-back pain, pregnancy
Sitting facing a heater for 2 minutes	1. Breathlessness/smothering sensations 2. Sweating 3. Hot flushes/chills	No apparent contraindications
Placing a tongue depressor at the back of the tongue for 30 seconds	1. Choking 2. Breathlessness/smothering sensations 3. Nausea/abdominal distress	Prominent gag reflex, which may result in vomiting

[a]Some forms of vertigo habituate to these exercises. From Antony, Ledley, Liss, and Swinson (2005), Taylor (2000), and Wald and Taylor (2005b).

ing), without being overwhelming. Exposure-related treatment sessions are typically 60–90 minutes, in which at least half the session is devoted to exposure exercises and the remainder is devoted to other issues, such as reviewing symptoms over the past week, setting up in-session exposure exercises, and planning homework. The duration of exposure should be sufficient to produce at least a 50% reduction in the patient's level of distress (Meadows & Foa, 1998; Turner et al., 2005), as defined on a 0–100 scale, where 0 = no distress, and 100 = maximum distress. Patients should be able to control the degree of distress they are willing to experience, by means of selecting the nature and pace of exposure exercises and by using emotion regulation skills as needed. The therapist also can help titrate the degree of exposure by the altering the amount of detail that the patient is requested to describe. In the first few trials of imaginal exposure, for example, the therapist might ask the patient to imagine the trauma as if it happened to someone else, or as if they were reading about it in a newspaper.

Hierarchic versus Nonhierarchic Approaches

Exposure exercises are often conducted hierarchically, where stimuli are arranged in order of increasing distress. There are two advantages to hierarchical treatment as opposed to starting exposure at the top of the hierarchy (flooding). First, the hierarchical approach is more manageable for patients. Although flooding is quicker, many patients are unable to tolerate the degree of distress evoked by that method and are more likely to successfully complete a hierarchical approach, in which they can control the speed with which they work through the hierarchy. Second, the hierarchal approach teaches patients a skill that they can use on their own once the formal course of treatment ends. This is important because patients often have residual symptoms in need of further, self-directed treatment after a typical course of treatment.

Sometimes it can be difficult to anticipate exposure-related complications, such as severe dissociation or intense emotional reactions such as anxiety, anger, or guilt. Accordingly, during the initial exposure exercises it is generally better to *start low and go slow*. One can begin with short (e.g., 5- to 10-minute) trials of exposure to stimuli that are low in the hierarchy, in order to gauge the patient's responses. Patients themselves generally prefer this approach because most are unsure what to expect from exposure therapy and may be frightened about what might happen. Starting low and going slow is also important even if the patient expresses confidence in his or her ability to tolerate distress. Sometimes patients underestimate their emotional reactions and their ability to cope. These underpredictions can shake the patient's confidence and may strengthen avoidance.

General Procedures for Exposure

Regardless of the type of exposure—interoceptive, imaginal, or situational—the following elements are generally involved:

• The rationale for exposure should be reviewed and emotion regulation skills should be used as needed to deal with anticipatory anxiety. Although patients will have received some information about exposure therapy during the initial psychoeducation at the start of therapy (Chapter 9), it is useful to present more detailed information on exposure (Handout 12.1 [pp. 238–239]) when these exercises are introduced.

• An in-session exposure exercise is planned. For example, the patient might be helped to select a memory to work on via interoceptive exposure.

• The patient's predictions about the effects of exposure can be reviewed. For example, if the patient believed, "If I think about what happened to me, then I could lose control and never stop crying," then the patient and therapist could formulate an alternative prediction, for example, "I'll feel upset and desperate to escape the awful feelings for a while, but soon the feelings will pass and I'll be OK." Note that prediction testing draws on cognitive restructuring methods, as described in previous chapters.

• One or more trials of exposure are conducted, with the number and duration of trials depending on the nature of the exercise (e.g., multiple short interoceptive exercises, or a smaller number of longer, imaginal exposure exercises).

• After each exposure trial, the patient rates the peak degree of distress experienced (on a 0–100 scale). If predictions were made, then the evidence can be reviewed in terms of which prediction was best supported. Then, if there is sufficient session time remaining, the next exposure trial can be implemented.

• Throughout the exposure trials, the therapist periodically offers support and encouragement. This requires only a few supportive words every few minutes during exposure (e.g., "You're doing fine; you're in complete control").

• If exposure exercises evoke very little emotional response, then the therapist can inquire about the avoidance of emotion. One should discourage patients from using relaxation exercises during exposure; they should try to allow themselves to experience their emotions.

• Discourage the patient from talking extensively in between exposure trials. If the patient is highly distressed between trials, a controlled breathing exercise could be briefly used.

• Toward the end of the session, a 5- to 10-minute "wind-down" period is implemented, where the patient is asked to relax. Specific emotion regulation skills can be used, although patients typically calm down quickly without the use of any specific relaxation intervention. During the wind-down period the therapist should review what the exposure session was like for the patient, including what benefits and difficulties were encountered.

• At the end of the session, inquire about any reinterpretations or insights that arose. These may provide useful material for later cognitive restructuring.

• If patients express concern that their distress didn't abate much during exposure, they can be assured that this is not a problem, because there still may be between-session reductions in distress.

• Homework exercises for the coming week are planned. Ways of maximizing the success of the assignments are reviewed, and potential obstacles are reviewed and possible solutions are considered.

• Ensure that patients are physically safe before they leave the session. For example, if they are driving home, make sure that they are not too distressed to drive safely. It may be necessary for them to take some time after the session to do something to further unwind before driving (e.g., by taking a walk or visiting a nearby café for a snack).

Interoceptive Exposure

There are several well-established exercises for inducing arousal-related bodily sensations, as illustrated in Table 12.1, and described in detail elsewhere (Taylor, 2000; Taylor & Asmundson, 2004). Most people with PTSD have elevated anxiety sensitivity, but not all do, so these exercises are not used in all cases. The therapist should review the results of the Anxiety Sensitivity Index (Chapter 6) to determine whether the patient has clinically significant anxiety sensitivity. Then a trial run of each of the interoceptive exercises in the table can be used to gauge the patient's response. For example, a patient might become very anxious when performing only one or two of the exercises, such as hyperventilating and breathing through a narrow straw. These would be the exercises used in subsequent interoceptive exposure exercises.

The exercises are performed in the therapist's office and then as homework assignments. Interoceptive exposure exercises tend to be quite short, requiring at most a few minutes each. The exercises are usually practiced repeatedly in the therapy session and as homework. A patient might perform five trials of each of two exercises in a 60-minute treatment session (10 trials in all), and then practice them for homework. Progress can be monitored by asking patients to record each exercise on a homework rating form (Handout 12.2 [p. 240]).

IMAGINAL EXPOSURE

Format

Imaginal exposure involves systematic, repeated, and prolonged exposure to a traumatic memory, including the aftermath of the trauma, if that was also distressing. This helps reduce the distress associated with traumatic memories and reduces reexperiencing symptoms. Imaginal exposure also teaches patients that the memories of the trauma, and the associated emotions, are not dangerous. Imaginal exposure generally reduces anxiety, anger, and guilt evoked by trauma memories, although exposure alone may not be sufficient for completely reducing these emotions (Stapleton, Taylor, & Asmundson, 2006).

There are several ways to do imaginal exposure. A common approach is to have the patient narrate the traumatic experience into a tape recorder for about 45–60 minutes of the treatment session. The narration can be repeated, if necessary to fill the time period. Patients are asked to listen to the tape each day for homework. Alternatively, the patient can write out the experience as homework. An example showing a fragment of a written imaginal exposure assignment is presented in Figure 12.1.

I'm on my first holiday to another country that I've taken by myself. I just got back to the hotel on the 10th floor watching TV, after a day of visiting some local archaeological ruins. Suddenly, things start shaking and the windows are rattling. There's a construction site next door, so I'm thinking that it's noise from heavy machinery. I get up off the couch to see what's going on, when suddenly the TV goes off, all the power goes out, and the building starts shaking really hard. Then I realize it must be an earthquake. The shaking gets really, really strong. The closet doors are banging open and shut, and things on the dresser are crashing to the floor. I'm starting to panic. I'm running from room to room, not knowing what to do. The cabinet door in the bathroom suddenly swings open, smacking me in the face. My lip feels swollen and numb, and I can taste blood in my mouth. I look down at the bathroom floor. I can see my toothbrush, toothpaste, and pill bottles scattered over the floor.

I feel really trapped, while at the same time I feel like this can't be happening to me. I know I have to get out of there, but I can't think of where I left my shoes and keys. It all feels so unreal, like a movie. The noise is incredible. So loud and deep, and coming from all around me. I'm thrown to the floor because the building is swaying so much. I'm thinking, there's no way the building can withstand this. I'm probably going to die. I try to stand up. I feel really unsteady. My legs feel all rubbery. I'm shaking so hard that I can hardly walk. I'm thinking, "Oh God, please don't let me die!" (Later, this thought surprised me, because I'm not a religious person.)

Then it stops shaking so hard and I'm able to make my way out. In the hallway of my suite I see my bag and keys, and grab them as I leave. I run down the corridor to the fire exit, and start running down the stairs as fast as I can. I'm frightened of falling and hurting myself, and I'm having a hard time controlling my feet as I go. I can see that I'm not wearing any shoes, and my white socks are dirty and they're slipping off my feet. The stairwell smells of dusty concrete.

Finally I get outside and I don't know where to go. There are big cracks in the road and water all over the road. I can see water spouting from one of the cracks. A pipe must have burst. Groups of people are everywhere, standing around. I feel really isolated and I'm standing there, shaking and crying. A police officer comes over and starts yelling at me. I try to tell him that I don't speak the language and can't understand what he's saying. I feel helpless and alone. Women and children are standing around crying.

FIGURE 12.1. Example of imaginal exposure homework: Fragment of a written account of a traumatic event.

An advantage of using a spoken narration is that the intensity of imaginal exposure can be more readily controlled. For example, the therapist can occasionally prompt the patient for details of the trauma (e.g., "Describe what the enemy soldiers looked like"). As the patient's distress from the memories abates over imaginal exposure trials, the vividness of imaginal exposure can be increased. In later exposure trials, for example, the therapist can encourage the patient to speak in the first person, present tense (e.g., "I can smell the alcohol on his breath as he pushes himself on top of me"), and occasionally prompt for details of thoughts, feelings, and bodily sensations that occurred during the trauma.

After the patient finishes each narration, ask him or her to describe which parts of the memory were most distressing (i.e., the "hot spots" of the memory; Richards & Lovell, 1999). Obtain a 0–100 distress rating for the hot spot, and inquire about what emotions were experienced. This rating will be used to chart the patient's progress over the course of the imaginal exposure trials. Patients can be asked to narrate the hot spots numerous times. Sometimes it is useful for patients to imagine that these portions of the trauma are unfolding in slow motion, so as to increase the exposure to these episodes. In other cases, however, patients find the slow motion technique to be distracting.

Throughout imaginal exposure, especially during the most distressing parts of the narration, the therapist should look for cognitive themes or interpretations in the patient's narration. These can provide clues as to the important trauma-related beliefs held by the patient. To elicit more meaning information during imaginal exposure, and thereby enhance the vividness of imaginal exposure, after an exposure trial the therapist can ask, "What does [worst part of trauma] mean to you? Did it influence the way that you see yourself, other people, or the world?" The information gathered can be used in cognitive restructuring.

Methods for Enhancing Imaginal Exposure

There are several methods for increasing the vividness of exposure and for focusing on the most important parts of the traumatic event. Memory aids, such as photographs of the perpetrator or a newspaper report describing the trauma, can be used to enhance vividness. Also, during the narration, the patient can be encouraged to recall incidental details of the trauma, which add to the vividness of the narration. This is illustrated in the following fragment of an imaginal exposure narration, which concerns the aftermath of a terrorist bombing.

"I'm on the ground bleeding and covered glass and debris. . . . As I lay there I notice some people looking at me; a couple of old ladies just standing there staring at me. . . . I start pulling shards of glass out of my arms and hands. I notice that the glass is bluish-green, like the color of a pond or swimming pool."

Imaginal Exposure Homework

Imaginal exposure homework may consist of listening to an audiotape of the traumatic events (e.g., for 60 minutes each day until distress is reduced). Alternatively, the patient might write out or read over a description of the trauma for the same amount of time each day. If written homework is used, patients should be encouraged to write out the trauma without worrying about spelling, grammar, or punctuation. Just as patients might listen to different imaginal exposure tapes derived from their successive exposure sessions, patients using writing as homework should periodically rewrite their narration, adding extra details and insights (e.g., "I realize now that there was no way I could have stopped him"). The therapist can use the added insights as material for cognitive restructuring. (A variant of this is where the patient writes a detailed but unsent letter to the perpetrator, describing the trauma, its effects, and its meaning for the patient.)

Tailoring Interventions for Children

Imaginal exposure for older children (e.g., 8- to 9-year-olds) and adolescents can proceed in much the same manner as for adults. For younger children (e.g., 5–8 years), and sometimes for older children (8–9 years or older), imaginal exposure is more successfully carried out by having them repeatedly draw, in detail, the traumatic experience. For younger children imaginal exposure can also take the form of play, for example, reenacting a road traffic collision with toy cars or sculpting it in clay. However, compared to using toys or clay, there is greater power and flexibility in drawing the trauma. Drawing can better express the idiosyncratic aspects of the trauma, thereby providing exposure to aspects of the trauma that might not be readily available through other means of representation. Graphic and, for many viewers, highly disturbing examples of such drawings were recently published in the *British Journal of Psychiatry* (2004, vol. 184, p. A18; see bjp.rcpsych.org/cgi/reprint/184/5/379-a18). Rwandan orphans were encouraged, as part of therapy, to draw the massacres that they had witnessed, such as women and children being shot, stabbed, or hacked to death with machetes. When they were ready, the children were also encouraged to share their stories with the therapist and with the others in the orphanage, by means of play, drama, or simple storytelling.

For children who are too frightened to draw their traumatic experiences, a gradual, hierarchical method can be used. One approach is the "Party Hats on Monsters" game (Crenshaw, 2001). The therapist first asks children to draw something that makes them feel happy or safe, such as a favorite activity. Once the drawing is completed the therapist engages them in a pleasant conversation about the drawing. The therapist then asks the child to draw something that scares him or her just a little. Next, the therapist asks the child to change the drawing in a way that will make the feared object (e.g., a monster) seem less scary. For example, the child could put a party hat on the monster, or shrink it in size. Then the therapist can say, "It's amazing how many children realize that when they change the picture on paper to make it less scary, they also change the picture in their head so that they are no longer frightened." Over successive sessions the child is encouraged to drawing increasingly more frightening pictures, which are then modified to make them less frightening. In this way the child is eventually able to draw, and thereby gain exposure to, the traumatic event, eventually without the need to modify the drawing to make it less frightening. In some cases, however, it is therapeutic for the child to deliberately modify the drawing of the trauma, particularly if such modifications serve to change maladaptive beliefs. For example, a tsunami survivor might modify the drawing by shrinking the size of the waves and adding people who are happily surfing on them. Such a modification can implicitly challenge beliefs such as "Waves are dangerous."

Drawing methods are also particularly useful for helping children overcome trauma-related nightmares. Here, the child is asked to draw the frightening characters in the nightmare, and to change the elements of the nightmare in a way that makes it less threatening. Nightmares of being carried off by bad men, for example, could be treated by adding to the drawing a superhero, who rounds up the men and hauls them off to prison. Open trials and controlled studies have shown that such nightmare-modification methods are effective in reducing nightmare frequency, for children, adolescents, and adults (e.g., Krakow et al., 2001a, 2001b; Palace & Johnston, 1989). For adolescents and adults it is typically unnecessary to use drawings; imagining the modified nightmare may suffice, either by writing it out or narrating it into a tape recorder. However, in some cases even adolescents and adults may benefit from drawing.

Note that such nightmare reduction strategies are most useful when nightmares are the prominent symptom of the clinical picture. If nightmares are simply one element of an array of reexperiencing symptoms, then imaginal exposure to trauma stimuli typically reduces all reexperiencing symptoms, including nightmares (Taylor, 2004), even when exposure does not specifically target the surreal elements of nightmares.

VARIANTS OF EXPOSURE THERAPY

Adapting Protocols to Special Circumstances

If the patient's first language is not English, one should ask whether it would be more distressing to conduct imaginal exposure in his or her native language or in English, and whether the memory is more vivid when described in one language versus the other. A traumatized refugee from Iran, for example, reported that imaginal exposure was more vivid and emotionally evocative when he described it in his native Farsi. Accordingly, as part of the exposure hierarchy, exposure initially began in English, which had the advantage of providing the English-speaking therapist with information about how the patient was completing the imaginal exposure exercises. The therapist was able to check whether all the sensory modalities were being recalled, and whether the trauma was being described in the present tense. After a few trials of imaginal exposure in English, in which the patient was coached to provide details, there was a sufficient reduction in distress for imaginal exposure to be conducted in Farsi. After each exposure trial, the therapist reviewed the experience with the patient (in English) and checked that exposure was being done optimally.

Imaginal Exposure for Multiply Traumatized Patients

One approach for multiply traumatized patients is to initiate imaginal exposure for the most disturbing memory. By means of generalization, this should reduce, to some extent, the distress associated with memories of other traumatic events. Therapeutic generalization is most likely to occur when the patient has experienced multiple episodes of the same kind of abuse, such as repeated sexual abuse from a single perpetrator. This is because human memory is adapted to store the gist or prototypical elements of repeated experiences (Schacter, 2002). Alternatively, imaginal exposure can be done by focusing on one memory at a time, or by including several memories within each trial of imaginal exposure. The latter approach is used when one memory naturally triggers another, so that it is difficult for the patient to stay focused on a single memory.

A related approach draws on procedures used in *narrative exposure therapy* (Neuner et al., 2004; Schauer et al., 2005). As discussed in Chapter 5, this treatment has been shown to be effective in treating multiply traumatized refugees. The therapist can assist the patient in writing out a detailed, coherent biography of the patient's life, with particular attention to traumatic events, which the patient is asked to narrate in detail. The patient and therapist go over the written document several times, to add details and make other corrections. This helps the patient make sense out of the traumatic events by placing them in the context of his or her life. The patient can also be asked to reread the sections of the biography describing the traumatic events, until distress has been reduced.

Adding Cognitive Restructuring to Imaginal Exposure

The best ways of combining cognitive restructuring and exposure are the focus of ongoing research, and so far there is only clinical experience to serve as a guide. One approach that has proved clinically useful in our treatment studies and those of other clinical investigators (e.g., Gillespie, Duffy, Hackmann, & Clark, 2002; Wald et al., 2004b) is to conduct a trial of imaginal or interoceptive exposure, then implement a short cognitive intervention, followed by another trial of exposure, and so on. In other words, restructuring is incorporated into the debriefing that follows each trial of exposure. The results of cognitive restructuring, such as a new belief or coping statement, are then introduced into subsequent trials of imaginal exposure.

Amanda's imaginal exposure exercises included recalling the many horrendous deaths she attended as a paramedic, including a tragedy in which a young girl was killed and horribly dismembered when she was hit by a truck while bicycling. During the short debriefings that followed each exposure trial, it emerged that Amanda believed that pain and suffering continued after death. As Amanda and her therapist explored this belief, Amanda recognized that she was basing this on the presumption that mutilation is associated with horrible pain. She realized that this would not apply to the deaths she encountered, because these deaths were likely to be instantaneous and virtually painless ("They never knew what hit them"). She was able to successfully replace her belief that "Mutilation, even in a corpse, is associated with horrible pain" with the belief that "Mutilated corpses are 'empty vessels'; they are no longer suffering." After she reinterpreted her experiences in this way, the traumatic memories became much less disturbing.

Another way of integrating cognitive restructuring with imaginal exposure involves written imaginal exposure assignments, in which the patient is asked to write about the trauma from various perspectives (Resick & Schnicke, 1993). Here, the direct goal is cognitive change rather than the extinction of distress, although it is important to remember that exposure and cognitive restructuring both change maladaptive beliefs. There are several ways that these writing assignments can be conducted. The first time patients write about the trauma, for example, they may be simply asked to write a detailed, first-person, present-tense account of the event(s). On subsequent writing exercises, they can be asked to write about the event with particular questions in mind. The questions concern particular issues or problems that need to be addressed. For example, if the therapist and patient agree that issues of trust were shattered by the trauma, then the patient might write about the trauma in terms of his or her beliefs about trust before the trauma, how they were influenced by the trauma, and how the patient currently decides whom to trust. Such exercises involve some degree of imaginal exposure, although the exercise is oriented more toward eliciting material for imaginal exposure. Similarly useful exercises involve writing about the trauma with some other question in mind, such as the following: "What important things did I learn from this experience that can help me be safe and happy in the future?" "Trauma involves a loss of innocence; how can I learn from the trauma without becoming angry and bitter?"

TROUBLESHOOTING

It can be difficult to decide beforehand how best to implement exposure, so even experienced therapists make mistakes. The key is to minimize errors and to ensure that exposure therapy is a self-correcting process, where errors that do occur are detected and remedied. The following are the most common therapist errors in implementing interoceptive and imaginal exposure, along with some solutions.

• Failing to provide the patient with a convincing rationale for exposure, and failing to check the patient's understanding of the rationale. During the early stages of exposure therapy, it is wise to periodically to ask the patient about his or her understanding of the rationale for exposure.
• Failing to establish a sound therapeutic relationship before commencing exposure. Patients need to feel safe and trust their therapist in order for them to be fully engaged in exposure therapy. If a good working relationship has not been established, then the patient may be reluctant to engage in exposure exercises and may be reluctant to share his or her fears or concerns about therapy. To address these problems, the therapist should spend enough therapy time to establish a good working relationship.
• Failing to identify important cognitive factors in the initial assessment, which may be relevant to the case formulation and treatment plan. For example, consider beliefs associated with strong fear of negative evaluation (e.g., "For me to be worthwhile, people need to approve of me," "They won't approve of me if they see that I'm an emotional wreck"). These beliefs can make the patient feel too embarrassed to participate in imaginal or interoceptive exposure exercises during the therapy session. Such beliefs may need to be addressed before conducting exposure.

• Reacting with shock, anxiety, or disgust when hearing the patient's account of the trauma or seeing the patient's emotional response to exposure exercises. Therapists should strive to be unshockable, while still being able to express appropriate empathy and support. If you find yourself become highly distressed by your patient's reactions or experiences, then there are several paths open to you: (1) you may become less disturbed as you gain more experience with PTSD patients and become accustomed to hearing about their experiences and seeing their reactions during treatment; (2) if you are especially disturbed by the degree of emotion expressed by these patients during exposure therapy, then remind yourself that the treatment you are using has a good rationale and established efficacy; (3) seek out supervision or, if necessary, therapy to address your distress; and (4) if working with traumatized patients still continues to be highly disturbing, then perhaps this population is not for you. There are plenty of other types of patients who may benefit from your psychotherapeutic skills.

• Going up the exposure hierarchy too slowly and prematurely aborting exposure trials whenever the patient becomes upset. This reinforces avoidance by conveying the implicit message that distress and harmless trauma-related stimuli are actually dangerous. This problem is compounded when the patient perceives the therapist as lacking confidence and competence in implementing the exposure exercises. It is important to express appropriate confidence that the patient can tolerate exposure to distressing stimuli.

• Going up the hierarchy too fast, or attempting exposure to stimuli that the patient finds to be too distressing or that cause panic or intense bodily reactions (e.g., headache, dizziness, nausea). This too can lead to aborted exposure, and can undermine the patient's confidence in treatment, thereby leading to treatment nonadherence or dropout. An 80% rule can guide the selection of initial exposure exercises (e.g., "We want you to try exercises that are challenging but not overwhelming; I suggest that you only attempt an exercise if you're at least 80% confident of completing it"). In addition, the patient's level of distress should be reduced by at least 50% before moving on to the next item in the exposure hierarchy.

• Abandoning exposure as soon as the patient becomes numb or dissociates. The therapist should bear in mind that numbing and dissociation tend to naturally decline over the course of exposure therapy, even if adjunctive interventions like grounding strategies are not used (Taylor et al., 2003). If the patient becomes numb or dissociates during exposure, then the therapist has two options: (1) if these reactions are not severe, and if the patient is still able to engage in exposure exercises, then the exercises can be continued, while assuring the patient that numbing and dissociation are harmless, temporary reactions that will abate with time; (2) if numbing and dissociation are severe (including the occurrence of flashbacks), then grounding exercises or other emotion coping strategies can be used (Chapter 9), or the patient can simply be given a few minutes to allow numbing or dissociation to dissipate. The causes of numbing and dissociation can then be explored (e.g., were these strategies intentionally used by the patient, because exposure evoked too much distress?). Then the patient and therapist can consider using less distressing types of exposure exercises.

• Talking too much or frequently interrupting the patient during exposure. This is distracting for the patient and dilutes the "dose" of exposure they receive. Anxious therapists sometimes feel the urge to reassure their distressed patients, thereby talking too much to the patient. As therapists become more experienced with exposure therapy, their anxiety should abate.

• Not offering enough support or encouragement during and after exposure trials (e.g., "This is hard, but you're doing excellent work," "That's it, stay with the memory and the feelings"). If patients become highly distressed, the therapist can also gently remind them that they're safe, that the trauma is in the past, and that the memory can't hurt them.

• Avoiding, because of therapist discomfort, the worst of the trauma during imaginal exposure. Graphic details need to be included in the imaginal exposure narration in order for this therapy to be fully effective.

• Failing to identify safety signals and safety behaviors that can interfere with the efficacy of exposure. For example, cognitive avoidance during imaginal exposure (e.g., avoiding details or skipping over the most distressing parts of the trauma) and distraction from feared bodily sensations during interoceptive exposure. Another example of an exposure-interfering safety behavior is when the patient takes anxiolytic medication (e.g., lorazepam) shortly before the exposure exercise. Methods for identifying these problematic behaviors are discussed in Chapter 6. These treatment-interfering factors are also suggested by anomalous reactions to exposure therapy, such as the absence of emotions elicited by exposure or unusually rapid reductions in distress. Poor treatment attendance or consistently arriving late for therapy also raises the question of avoidance. The therapist may need to openly but empathically discuss this with the patient (e.g., "I appreciate that therapy can be unpleasant—just like a visit to the dentist—and so I'm wondering whether you've been feeling the urge to avoid coming to therapy . . . "). Problem solving can be used to address avoidance problems (e.g., proceeding more gradually with exposure and encouraging the patient to let the therapist know if treatment is becoming too difficult). Note also that patients sometimes misuse emotion regulation skills (e.g., relaxation or soothing imagery exercises) for avoidance purposes. Once identified, avoidance, safety signals, and safety behaviors can be omitted or gradually faded out of the exposure exercises, and the therapist can prompt for details of the trauma to help the patient overcome avoidance (e.g., "What did the assailant look like?"). Motivational interviewing methods (Chapter 9) can also be used to address problems with treatment adherence, along with cognitive restructuring to address avoidance-promoting beliefs (e.g., "I'll lose control if I let myself imagine my combat experiences" or "Only crybabies let themselves get emotional").

• Getting sidetracked by other problems that the patient brings up during sessions that are intended to be used for exposure. Sometimes patients bring up minor issues (minor stressors) as a form of avoidance. One way to deal with this is to agree to explore these issues *after* the in-session exposure exercises have been completed. In other cases, the patient may be bringing up important issues that warrant immediate attention. These might include major stressors that have arisen during the course of treatment. Exposure therapy, for example, might be focused on a trauma associated with the patient's PTSD but then become sidetracked because other stressors arise that are in need of clinical attention (e.g., the diagnosis of cancer or the unexpected death of a loved one). Here, getting sidetracked is unavoidable. Nevertheless, the patient can still be encouraged to apply skills learned in therapy to the current crisis (e.g., emotion coping skills), and then the patient and therapist can decide which problem needs to be currently worked on. Sometimes, patients decide to continue on with exposure therapy, focused on the original trauma, while also applying emotion coping skills to handle a more recent stressor.

• Failing to design homework exercises that maximize the chances that they will be completed. This often involves failing to discuss with the patient the details of when, where, and how the exercise will be completed, and failing to identify and overcome likely obstacles to successful homework completion.

SUMMARY

Three forms of exposure—interoceptive, imaginal, and situational exposure—are useful in treating PTSD. Of these, imaginal and situational exposure are well-established interventions, while interoceptive exposure is a promising intervention that remains to be further evaluated. This chapter reviewed the general principles of exposure and provided details on how interoceptive and imaginal exposure can be effectively implemented. Variants on treatment protocols were discussed, and common problems and solutions were considered. Interoceptive and imaginal exposure make it easier for the patient to overcome distress associated with external stimuli, the topic of the next chapter.

HANDOUT 12.1. Description and Rationale for Exposure Exercises

QUESTIONS AND ANSWERS ABOUT EXPOSURE THERAPY

What Is the Purpose of Exposure Therapy?

The goal of exposure therapy is to *desensitize* you to things that are upsetting but objectively harmless. Exposure therapy can reduce distressing emotions associated with the trauma and reduce nightmares and trauma-related fears. This can help you get on with your life without being constantly reminded of awful things that happened in the past. Research has shown that exposure therapy is among the best ways of treating posttraumatic stress disorder (PTSD).

What Exactly Is Involved?

Although your therapist may make suggestions about what exercises are likely to be useful, the choice is completely up to you. There are three sorts of exposure therapy that you may choose to try:

1. Exposure to harmless but often fear-evoking bodily sensations. This called *interoceptive exposure*. For example, many people who suffer from PTSD become very distressed when they experience intense but harmless bodily sensations associated with the trauma, such as thumping heartbeat. If this is a problem for you, then interoceptive exposure can be helpful. It can help you feel less upset when your body becomes physiologically aroused.

2. Exposure to harmless but distressing memories of the trauma. This is called *imaginal exposure*. This involves you recounting the trauma in as much detail as possible, using first person present tense ("I am doing this right now . . . ") and all your senses (e.g., the things you saw, heard, smelled, tasted, and felt), and holding that image until anxiety/distress diminishes. This eventually makes the memory less upsetting and reduces the frequency with which you think about the trauma.

3. Exposure to harmless but distressing real-life reminders of the trauma. This is known as *situational exposure*. This is aimed at helping you become less upset about everyday things that remind you of the trauma. For example, people who have been sexually assaulted usually try to avoid things that remind them of the assault, such as particular people, places, or things. Marion, for example, was sexually assaulted by a man who smoked a cigarette after the rape. From then on, whenever Marion saw someone smoking or smelled tobacco, she felt very upset and panicky. Marion eventually decided to desensitize herself to this unwanted reaction by visiting a cigar bar several times with a trusted friend. If you have problems with being upset by harmless reminders such as these, then situational exposure may be helpful for you. This sort of exposure, like the other forms of exposure therapy, is gradual. We will start with something that you can manage. Then when you are comfortable in that situation we will build up to more uncomfortable situations.

How Does Exposure Therapy Work?

People with PTSD tend to avoid the things that upset them. For example, a person who was in a serious car accident might try to avoid the intersection in which the accident occurred, in

(continued)

order to avoid thinking about the accident. Such avoidance is like a drug such as opium; it provides temporary relief but does not help the person overcome their fears or get over the trauma. Exposure therapy is based on the old saying "If you fall off the horse and are frightened of riding, the way to get over your fears is to get back on the horse." The key is to do this in a way that is gradual and controllable and tolerable for you. That is the goal of exposure therapy. The aim of this treatment is not for you to forget that the trauma ever happened. Rather, you need to work through the event so that you are able to talk about and remember it without great distress or fear.

Is Exposure Therapy Right for Me?

Exposure therapy is helpful for many people who suffer from PTSD, but it is not for everyone. Sometimes, it is necessary to deal with other problems before exposure therapy can be used. For example, if you have a drug or alcohol problem, it may first be necessary to seek help for these problems before receiving exposure therapy. Ask your therapist whether exposure therapy is right for you at the present time.

Is Exposure Therapy an Emotionally Painful Procedure? Will I Be in Control?

Exposure therapy is conducted slowly, so that you do not feel overwhelmed with unpleasant emotions. You will feel some emotional discomfort, but you will be in complete control of how exposure therapy is conducted. Exposure therapy is a bit like a visit to the dentist; there will be some discomfort, but you and your therapist will work to ensure that you don't feel overwhelmed.

Are There Any Side Effects?

There are side effects to every effective treatment, regardless of whether the treatment consists of medication or exposure therapy. The side effects of exposure therapy involve short-term and usually mild increases in symptoms. In the first few weeks of exposure therapy you may experience a slight increase in the frequency of nightmares, or an increase in anxiety or irritability. These are good signs; they indicate that exposure therapy is starting to take effect. You and your therapist can work together to minimize the side effects. This can be done by gradually implementing exposure exercises, starting with exercises that evoke very little distress.

What Are the Long-Term Effects?

Unlike medications, where the effects tend to wear off once the drug is discontinued, evidence suggests that the effects of exposure therapy tend to be long-lasting. This is partly because exposure therapy teaches you practical skills for overcoming your problems in a gradual, step-by-step fashion. In other words, exposure therapy provides you with the skills for overcoming your problems now and in the future.

Further Questions?

Please talk to your therapist, who will be happy to discuss exposure therapy with you in more detail.

HANDOUT 12.2. Exposure Homework Monitoring Form

Date	Homework exercise	Duration	Peak distress (0 = none, 100 = maximum)

Example:

Date	Homework exercise	Duration	Peak distress (0 = none, 100 = maximum)
24/Feb	Listened to tape	50 min	70
25/Feb	Listened to tape	60 min	60
26/Feb	Listened to tape	60 min	45

CHAPTER 13

Exposure Exercises II

Situational Exposure

Situational exposure involves exposure to safe, harmless external stimuli that resemble or remind the patient of the trauma. The choice of stimuli is determined largely by the patient's goals regarding the stimuli for which they want to overcome their distress. Stimuli used in situational exposure exercises include places (e.g., the scene of a bank robbery), situations (e.g., having conversations with authority figures), things associated with the trauma (e.g., a piece of clothing worn when the patient was raped), and symbolic reminders (e.g., particular movies, photographs, or pieces of music associated with the trauma). Situational exposure tends to be most effective when the stimuli evoke fear or anxiety, rather than anger, shame, or guilt. Cognitive restructuring is more useful for the latter three emotions, although trauma-related anger and guilt have been shown to be reduced by situational exposure exercises (Stapleton et al., 2006). Situational exposure, like other forms of exposure therapy, can be fruitfully combined with cognitive restructuring. Situational exposure is also typically combined with other forms of exposure. For example, treatment could consist of a series of sessions on interoceptive and imaginal exposure, followed by situational exposure sessions involving therapist-assisted (in session) exposure and exposure homework assignments.

GENERAL PRINCIPLES OF SITUATIONAL EXPOSURE

Precautions and Preparations

The precautions and preparations, and homework monitoring forms, for situational exposure are much the same as those for imaginal and interoceptive exposure, although there are some exceptions. The therapist em-

phasizes the importance of *safe* situational exposure exercises that can be
practiced regularly. Patients can be advised that situational exposure exercises will not make them become reckless or foolhardy.

Safety and Risk Tolerance

Sometimes it can be challenging to help patients distinguish safe from dangerous exposure situations. In planning exposure assignments, useful questions that the patient can consider are "Did this seem dangerous to me
before the trauma?" and "Do other people see this situation as dangerous?" (Meadows & Foa, 1998). If the patient lives in an objectively dangerous neighborhood or has a hazardous occupation, exposure exercises
should not involve additional exposure to risk; instead, the patient should
be encouraged to find ways of minimizing risk, such as moving to a safer
neighborhood or occupation or taking precautions to ensure safety, such as
walking with trusted others in a dangerous area or carrying a whistle at
night (Meadows & Foa, 1998).

In other cases, patients may be overestimating danger or insisting on
complete certainty that they will be safe. For many exposure situations—as
in life in general for all of us—there is no 100% guarantee that a given situation is safe. A drive on the freeway, a visit to the bank, a flight on a plane,
or a social outing with friends—each carries some degree of risk, even if the
risk is small. The patient, like everyone else, needs to decide on what is a
personally acceptable degree of risk, balancing safety and quality of life. If
patients tend to overestimate danger or have an intolerance of uncertainty,
then cognitive restructuring can be used to address these issues.

Elements of Exposure Exercises

Situational exposure is typically conducted in a hierarchical fashion, starting with the least distressing stimulus (see Handout 13.1 on p. 258). The
hierarchy could consist of, say, the dozen most relevant stimuli for a given
trauma, including those that best represent the main aspects of the trauma
as well as the stimuli that the patient most wants to become comfortable
with. However, exposure tends to be most beneficial when it is conducted
in multiple contexts, including exposure to different variations of the exposure stimulus, and at different times of day (Bouton, 2002). For patients
who have been exposed to multiple traumas, it may be necessary to work
through more than one exposure hierarchy, beginning with the currently
most distressing trauma, or the trauma associated with stimuli that are
causing the greatest interference in the patient's daily life.

The patient works through the hierarchy at his or her own pace, and
the therapist encourages the patient to tackle challenging but not overwhelming exposure exercises. Toward the end of exposure therapy, the in-

session situational exposure exercises are gradually faded out (spaced further apart in time) in order to wean the patient off therapist-assisted exposure, while at the same time the patient continues to practice self-directed exposure in the form of homework assignments.

Exposure trials need to be long enough, and to be repeated enough, for enduring distress reduction to occur. A commonly used clinical guideline is that exposure continue until there is at least a 50% reduction in distress. Alternatively, one can plan for 45 minutes of in-session exposure and 60 minutes of homework exposure trials. If distress reduction does not occur by the end of a therapy session, then the patient can be given a few minutes to unwind, or an emotion regulation exercise can be used. Patients can be advised that even if their distress has not abated during a session (within-session extinction), they still may show between-session distress reduction (e.g., Taylor et al., 2003).

Before each exposure trial, the patient can use an emotion regulation skill (e.g., breathing retraining) to deal with anticipatory anxiety. During exposure, however, it is important that the patient allow him- or herself to feel the full range of emotions elicited by the stimulus. After an exposure trial, the patient could use an emotion regulation skill to calm down. However, this is often unnecessary. Patients typically calm down naturally without the need for specific exercises. In fact, if the therapist insists on using relaxation exercises or other calming methods at the end of each exposure trial, that could give the patient the misleading impression that emotion arousal is dangerous and something that needs to be quickly contained.

Reducing Reliance on Safety Signals and Safety Behaviors

Over the course of exposure exercises, patients are encouraged to discontinue relying on unnecessary safety signals and safety behaviors. Safety signals are stimuli that the person associates with the absence of danger (e.g., carrying pepper spray around the office). Safety behaviors are things that the person does to needlessly avert danger, such as avoidance, checking, and escape, as well as vigilance and scanning of the environment, and tensing one's muscles in preparation for action.

Jim, who developed PTSD after being rear-ended by another driver, developed a range of maladaptive safety behaviors, including braking at green lights, traveling well under the speed limit on freeways, and trying to make eye contact with the driver behind him through his rearview mirror when he was about to stop at a traffic light. These behaviors actually increased Jim's odds of being in another road collision, so it was important that his situational exposure exercises be designed specifically to involve the intentional discontinuation of such behaviors.

A further example is the combat veteran who, as a civilian living in a safe neighborhood, resorted to several safety behaviors that perpetuated his sense of danger. For example, he always kept his blinds drawn at home and frequently checked the windows for strangers walking past his house, he repeatedly checked the locks each night before retiring, when on the street he often turned to check people who passed him to make sure that they continued on their way, and, when he went out to a restaurant, he always insisted on a seat that enabled him to have his back to the wall, so nobody would sneak up behind him. Performing these behaviors served as a recurrent reminder of "possible" threats. Exposure therapy involved gradually dropping these needless behaviors, which eventually helped him feel more comfortable in his daily life.

Fading out such needless sources of safety can help patients test their maladaptive beliefs (e.g., "If I don't remain vigilant then I'll be harmed"). These exercises are usefully combined with cognitive restructuring that focuses on the advantages and disadvantages of relying on such perceived sources of safety. Of course, patients are encouraged to continue using adaptive forms of safety, such as being escorted by security personnel to one's car in a dimly lit parking garage late at night.

DEVELOPING SITUATIONAL EXPOSURE EXERCISES: ILLUSTRATIVE EXAMPLES

One of the challenges in conducting situational exposure is to come up with safe, feasible exercises, which can be conducted during therapy sessions and as homework assignments. The therapist may need to be creative in coming up with suitable exposure exercises. The Internet can be a useful source of exposure stimuli (e.g., images of combat or natural disasters). Several examples will be included here in order to help therapists with the important but challenging task of developing exposure exercises.

Generic and Idiosyncratic Stimuli

Patients can rent commercially available movies to use as a form of exposure to trauma-related stimuli. Table 13.1 provides some examples for various types of trauma. Before recommending a movie as an exposure assignment, the therapist should first view the film to ensure that it is relevant for a given patient. Some films are likely to be more disturbing than others. For patients with PTSD associated with domestic violence, for example, the film *Once Were Warriors* may be more distressing than *Sleeping with the Enemy*. The therapist should use clinical judgment in selecting appropriate films. The list in Table 13.1 is illustrative rather than exhaustive. Patients

TABLE 13.1. Examples of Films That Can Be Used as Exposure Stimuli

Trauma category	Title	
Childhood abuse (physical and/or sexual)	• The Boys of St. Vincent • A Thousand Acres • Bastard Out of Carolina • Mommie Dearest • The Prince of Tides	• Radio Flyer • Sleepers • The 400 Blows • The Celebration • This Boy's Life
Combat	• Apocalypse Now • Black Hawk Down • Full Metal Jacket • Hamburger Hill • Saving Private Ryan	• The Killing Fields • Pearl Harbor • Platoon • Jarhead • War Photographer
Disasters	• Airport (1970, 1975, 1977, or 1979 versions) • The Poseidon Adventure • Dante's Peak • Fearless	• The Perfect Storm • Alive • The Towering Inferno • Twister
Domestic violence	• The Stalker (2002 version) • Once Were Warriors • Sleeping with the Enemy • The Burning Bed	• The Color Purple • The Shining • Enough
Physical assault (adult)	• A Clockwork Orange (physical and sexual assault) • Psycho (1960 or 1998 versions) • The Passion of the Christ • Fight Club • Henry: Portrait of a Serial Killer	• Panic Room • The Godfather • Cape Fear • The Professional • American Psycho
Road traffic collisions	• Duel • Gone in 60 Seconds • Open Your Eyes	• Vanilla Sky • Speed
Sexual assault (adult)	• I Spit on Your Grave • The Strength to Resist • Rape and Marriage • Rape Is . . .	• Rape of Love • The Accused • Monster (2003)
Terrorism	• Collateral Damage • Executive Decision • The Great New Wonderful • Hijacking Catastrophe 9/11	• September 11 • Fahrenheit 9/11 • The Terrorist
Torture and genocide	• Auschwitz: Inside the Nazi State • Death and the Maiden • Shake Hands with the Devil • Nobody Listened	• Schindler's List • Hotel Rwanda • The Pawnbroker

Note. Thanks to Gordon Asmundson, Nick Carleton, Amy Janeck, Jennifer Stapleton, Andrew Urquhart, and Jaye Wald for their contributions in preparing this table.

themselves may be aware of other films that they have been deliberately avoiding because they serve as reminders of the trauma.

Initially, the patient might choose to watch the movie with a supportive person present, and then watch the film alone. Movie-related exposure typically proceeds by having the patient view the entire film two or three times, and then, on subsequent exposure trials, watch the most disturbing scenes over and over again. The films should be viewed in a nondistracting setting. The patient should also be discouraged from watching the movie from the perspective of a film critic. Attention to the technical details (e.g., the accuracy of Vietnam combat details), acting ability, and realism can serve as a distraction, thereby undermining the effects of the exposure exercise. Patients should be encouraged to immerse themselves in the film, while suspending judgment on its quality. However, if patients find that they are becoming too upset by the film, then they can remind themselves that it's only a movie.

Regarding other commonly used stimuli, the site of the trauma (providing it is safe) is a commonly used stimulus for exposure exercises. This could include the site of a road traffic collision, the house or school in which one was abused, the factory in which one was injured, the restaurant or nightclub in which an assault occurred, places where an earthquake destroyed one's former dwelling, or the bank in which a holdup took place. Trigger stimuli that evoke reexperiencing symptoms or avoidance are also potential candidates for exposure stimuli. These would be identified during the initial assessment. Other examples of safe and readily available stimuli for exposure exercises for various classes of trauma are presented in Table 13.2.

Generic stimuli are a good starting place for formulating ideas about situational exposure exercises to suit the goals and needs of a given patient. To be optimally effective, stimuli that are specific to the patient's trauma experiences need to be included in the exposure exercises. These can be variations on the stimuli described in Table 13.2, or they may be idiosyncratic stimuli for a given patient. To illustrate the latter, some assault survivors feel highly anxious if they can't be vigilant for sounds of intruders in their house. So, showering with the door closed, running the vacuum cleaner, watching the TV with the volume turned up, or listening to loud music through headphones at home all would be potential exposure exercises. Some survivors of sexual assault become anxious if they dress in ways that accentuates their appearance, such as wearing makeup or attractive clothes. These can be the source of safe, appropriate exposure exercises.

For some trauma survivors, exposure to particular odors may be used as stimuli because they evoke memories of the trauma. Such stimuli might include the cologne the assailant was wearing, the smell of diesel or gasoline reminiscent of a vehicular or aircraft crash, the smell of disinfectant

TABLE 13.2. Examples of Potential Stimuli for Situational Exposure Exercises

Trauma category	Stimulus
Childhood abuse (physical and/ or sexual)	• Childhood memorabilia or photographs, such as photographs of parents or perpetrators, or of the patient as a child. • Watching, from a discreet distance, parents interacting with children in a park or playground. • Objects that resemble those used to punish the patient as a child (e.g., a cane or paddle). • Visiting churches and talking with clergymen (if the patient was assaulted by someone affiliated with a church group).
Domestic violence	• Photographs or other reminders of the perpetrator, such as particular pieces of music or colognes preferred by the perpetrator. • Practicing being assertive (e.g., voicing one's opinion to men). • Writing out, and reading out loud, abusive words or phrases used by the perpetrator. • Going to places where men are gesticulating and yelling, such as sporting events.
Physical assault (adult)	• The sight of weapons, such as knives or guns. These can be viewed in gun stores, army surplus stores, museums, and in hunting or camping stores, or they can be kitchen knives from department stores. • Standing in line at the bank without scanning the surroundings. • Attending a boxing or martial arts match. • Going to a hockey match.
Sexual assault (adult)	• Gymnasiums or sporting facilities that involve the use of locker rooms (for survivors of same-sex assault). • Patient looking at his or her naked body in the mirror. • Scheduled medical examinations (e.g., mammogram or cervical exam) • Going out for coffee, alone or with a friend, in coffee shops in which men are seated.
Road traffic collisions	• Car travel, either as a driver or passenger. • Taking driving lessons or an advanced driving course. • Performing driving maneuvers that are reminiscent of the collision (e.g., making left-hand turns or watching others make such turns, or driving on freeways or through busy intersections). • Attending a car race, such as a demolition derby.
Terrorism	• Books, documentaries, or newspaper articles on terrorism. • Being in crowded public places such as a market or railway station (if the patient experienced a terror attack in such a situation). • Photographs of people killed by terrorist. • Photographs of the terror suspects.

(continued)

TABLE 13.2. (continued)

Trauma category	Stimulus
Combat	• Gravesites, photographs, or memorials to fallen soldiers. • Museum displays about warfare or about wars relevant to the patient's experiences. • Taking a public tour of a military school or base. • Visiting places where there are people in uniforms (e.g., visiting shopping malls in which there are uniformed security guards).
Torture or genocide	• Museum exhibitions (e.g., the Holocaust Museum). • Books or documentaries about specific genocides. • Photos of people who "disappeared" as a result of torture or genocide. • Viewing objects that were used as instruments of restraint and torture (e.g., electrical cables in hardware stores, toy handcuffs in novelty stores).
Disasters	• Riding in a glass elevator to the top of a tall building (for survivors of earthquake trauma). • Riding in planes, boats, or trains (as relevant) for survivors of crashes involving those modes of transportation. • Visiting dams or large, swollen rivers (for flood survivors). • Walking on the beach or in a park on a windy, rainy day (for hurricane survivors).

Note. The patient and therapist should ensure that situations are reasonably safe before planning to use them in exposure exercises.

associated with childhood abuse in an orphanage, or the smell of alcohol associated with the breath of a sexual abuser.

For other trauma survivors, particular sounds may be especially evocative of the trauma. Particular pieces of music, for example, may have been playing in the background of a trauma such as an assault, and therefore serve as fear-evoking stimuli. The sounds of crying babies or children may be trauma stimuli for a formerly battered woman who was abused by her husband whenever their young children cried "too much." Many survivors of domestic violence become anxious when they hear raised voices or arguing. Here, graded exposure to raucous TV programs or loud but safe community activities (e.g., football games) may be included as part of their exposure exercises.

Foods can also be exposure stimuli. One male patient, who was repeatedly orally raped in childhood while attending a residential school, became distressed whenever people encouraged him to eat salty snacks (e.g., peanuts or pretzels) because the taste triggered memories of his sexual abuse experiences. He was even anxious about entering places in which such foods were sold, such as convenience stores. These places and stimuli were included in his exposure exercises. Similarly, exposure exercises for a U.N. peacekeeper involved trips to local butcher shops, supermarkets, and open markets in which butchered livestock was sold. Meat-related stimuli reminded him of exposure to bodies he had seen.

The Exposure Hierarchy

Figure 13.1 illustrates part of a situational exposure hierarchy for a woman who was sexually assaulted while jogging through a park one evening. She was dragged off the jogging path and raped. The exposure hierarchy entails two main themes, which were simultaneously addressed in treatment: proximity to the scene of the assault and proximity to unknown males.

Exposure situation (e.g., place, object, person, or activity)	Anticipated peak level of distress while completing the task (0 = none, 100 = maximum)
Walking through the open, public areas of the park in which I was assaulted (in broad daylight, by myself).	90
Working out in a local fitness center during the day, where there are lots of guys exercising (by myself).	80
Walking through the open, public areas of the park in which I was assaulted (in broad daylight, with a friend).	75
Swimming in the local pool in which there are men in bathing suits (by myself).	70
Working out in a local fitness center during the day, where there are lots of guys exercising (with a friend).	65
Swimming in the local pool in which there are men in bathing suits (with a friend).	50
Reading and rereading the police report of the assault.	45
Listening to music containing explicit sexual lyrics.	40
Having morning coffee at a café in which male strangers are seated nearby (by myself).	30
Having morning coffee at a café in which male strangers are seated nearby (with a friend).	15
Wearing the jogging clothes that I wore when I was assaulted.	10

FIGURE 13.1. Exposure hierarchy for a patient who was assaulted while jogging through a park one evening.

One of the challenges in developing an exposure hierarchy is that the latter is based on the patient's anticipated level of distress in each of the exposure situations. Patients may over- or underestimate the actual level of distress they experience. Underestimations are more of a problem than overestimations, because unexpectedly severe distress can undermine the patient's confidence in completing exposure assignments and thereby strengthen the patient's avoidance tendencies (Taylor & Rachman, 1994). Accordingly, the patient and therapist should not be too ambitious in the types of exercises chosen as the first exposure exercises. It is generally better to start with an easily tolerated, low-distress exercise that the patient is likely to successfully complete.

A further challenge is that there is often some degree of uncertainty or unpredictability in exposure exercises, especially exercises that involve other people. For example, some of the exercises in Table 13.2 involve entering public places (e.g., going to a fitness center). It is possible (although unlikely) that such a situation would be unexpectedly highly distressing (e.g., if a fight broke out between two of the men working out). Or a trip to the bank for a survivor of a bank robbery could result in the patient being exposed to another holdup. There is no way of avoiding such rare but possible outcomes. When the therapist and patient are discussing the safety of exposure exercises (along with a discussion of the patient's risk tolerance in general), these low-probability aversive outcomes could be discussed, and patients can be advised that a goal of exposure exercises is to help them become comfortable in situations in which the realistic risk of harm is low, but that in these situations, like in the rest of their lives, there is no way of absolutely eliminating the risk of harm. Nevertheless, the patient and therapist should discuss the cues or warning signs that indicate that the patient should leave, or not enter, a situation that is likely to turn hazardous.

Virtual Reality Exposure Therapy

There is encouraging preliminary evidence that effective situational exposure exercises can be carried out in the form of virtual reality simulations (e.g., Difede & Hoffman, 2002; Rothbaum, Ruef, Litz, Han, & Hodges, 2004). The company Virtually Better is the leading source of virtual reality software for exposure purposes (www.virtuallybetter.com), including software for virtual exposure to heights, aircraft travel, and combat-related stimuli. Advantages to virtual reality exposure include the fact that exposure exercises can be readily conducted for situations that can be difficult to arrange in real life (e.g., plane travel or exposure to combat scenes), and the patient and therapist have complete control over these stimuli. Disadvantages include the limited range of exposure simulations that are currently available, and the unrealistic, cartoon-like quality of the simulations. The usefulness of virtual reality exposure therapy should improve once these issues have been addressed.

Application to Children

Situational exposure for adults, adolescents, and children proceeds in much the same way. The exception is that for children (and sometimes adolescents), it may be useful for the therapist to first demonstrate (model) the exposure exercise. To illustrate, an 11-year-old boy was treated for PTSD that arose after he witnessed the violent death of his female cousin, who was immolated by her angry boyfriend (Abrahams & Udwin, 2000). Thereafter, the boy was extremely frightened of anything related to fire. Situational exposure included exercises in which the boy's mother would model (in a nonthreatening manner) the safe lighting of the kitchen gas stove.

As this example shows, when treating children, it can be very useful to involve a parent as a coach or guide during exposure-related homework assignment. Here, the role of the parent is similar to the role of significant others (e.g., spouses) in assisting in the exposure exercises of adults. The therapist trains the caregiver or significant other in how they can provide support and encouragement for exposure exercises, while at the same time not forcing the patient to engage in any unwanted exposure activities. The therapist routinely reviews the results of these assisted exposure assignments, in order to offer support and constructive feedback.

INTEGRATING SITUATIONAL EXPOSURE WITH COGNITIVE RESTRUCTURING

Cognitive restructuring can be implemented before, during, and after situational exposure. Before exposure, cognitive restructuring can be used to set up a behavioral experiment or to prepare a coping statement for use before and during exposure. After exposure, cognitive restructuring can be used to evaluate the exposure exercise, for example, which predictions were supported or refuted? Postexposure cognitive restructuring is also important for correcting any distorted appraisals of the exposure experience (e.g., misinterpreting a partially completed exercise as a "complete failure").

Coping Statements

Coping statements can be used to help the patient deal with anticipatory anxiety prior to exposure (e.g., "The worst of it is the anticipatory period;

all I need to do is stay with my feelings and I'll be fine") and during expo-sure (e.g., "I'm safe walking into the bank; the chance of another armed holdup is slim"). If coping statements are used during exposure, the patient and therapist should ensure that they are not being misused as a form of distraction or as safety behaviors (e.g., "I have to calm myself down or I'll lose control"). After the exposure exercise the patient and therapist can review the effects of the coping statements. Were the statements helpful? If not, then how might they be revised? Were the statements a distraction from the exposure experience? If so, then they might be dropped in subse-quent exposures.

Behavioral Experiments

A useful way of integrating situational exposure and cognitive restructuring is to use situational exposure exercises as behavioral experiments. Behav-ioral experiments are forms of situational exposure in which explicit pre-dictions of the outcome are made beforehand, derived from the patient's maladaptive (e.g., danger-related) beliefs and an alternative, adaptive belief statement that the patient and therapist have formulated during the course of cognitive restructuring.

Melik narrowly escaped being crushed to death in an earthquake while visiting relatives in Turkey. When he returned to his home in Vancouver he had an intense fear and avoidance of entering "old looking" buildings, for fear that an earthquake could strike and the building would collapse. His belief ran counter to the fact that building-destroying earthquakes in Vancouver were extremely rare events. Melik and his therapist agreed on a behavioral experiment to help make him feel more comfortable in buildings. The experiment involved going into old-looking buildings. The prediction based on his maladaptive belief was "Old buildings are dangerous; if I go into one I'll be courting fate. An earth-quake will strike, and it will collapse." The adaptive alternative was "Old build-ings in this city are just as safe as new buildings. They might remind me of the earthquake, but that's where the similarity ends." The behavioral experiment involved Melik entering a number of old-looking public buildings and sitting in the lobby and traveling the elevator of each until he felt comfortable that the building would not collapse.

Behavioral experiments are efficacious interventions, although there is no empirical evidence that situational exposure is enhanced when this form of exposure is used in the form of behavioral experiments. Even so, the therapist has the option of deciding, on a case-by-case basis, whether tradi-tional situational exposure or behavioral experiments will be more useful for a given patient. Regardless of which method is used, it is important that situational exposure be properly implemented.

In principle, behavioral experiments can be much shorter than traditional forms of situational exposure. All that is needed for behavioral experiments is sufficient exposure to test the maladaptive and adaptive beliefs. This could be a matter of minutes or less. Traditional situational exposure requires the person to be exposed to the trauma-related stimulus until his or her level of distress has sufficiently abated. Although behavioral experiments can be conducted much more quickly than traditional exposure, in clinical practice it is a good idea to employ behavioral experiments for the same amount of time that one would use traditional situational exposure, that is, until the patient's distress level has been reduced by at least 50%. This is for two reasons. First, some patients attempt to abort behavioral experiments early by settling for weak test of their beliefs (e.g., "Thirty seconds in the old building was all I needed to see that it wouldn't collapse if an earthquake suddenly struck. . . . What? You want me to go in there for a longer period of time. No way! It could, um, collapse . . . "). Thus, the patient's understandable desire to avoid distressing stimuli could compromise his or her ability to properly conduct behavioral experiments. The second, related, reason for tying the duration of behavioral experiments to the degree of distress reduction (50% or more) is based on the idea that the patient's level of distress (e.g., assessed on a 0–100 scale) is an index or marker of the success of the behavioral experiment. If the exposure assignment truly refutes the patient's maladaptive beliefs (e.g., the belief that "Old buildings are dangerous") and supports the adaptive alternative (e.g., "Earthquakes are highly rare where I live, so I don't need to avoid old buildings"), then the behavioral experiment should reduce the patient's level of distress. If the patient is exposed to the trauma-related stimulus (e.g., an old building) and still feels highly distressed, then clearly the patient still strongly adheres to the maladaptive (danger-related) belief.

Postexposure Processing

After each situational exposure exercise, the patient and therapist can review the similarities and differences between the exposure experience and the actual trauma. This can help the patient establish a time perspective and help in discriminating the harmless stimuli that happened to coincide with the trauma from the dangerous stimuli encountered during the traumatic event (Ehlers & Clark, 2000). Patients can also be asked to review what they learned from the exposure exercise. This can help underscore the safety of the exposure experience or, in some cases, can reveal information about the following:

- Trauma-related triggers that the patient might not have previously recognized. For example, a discussion of his exposure experience led John to realize why driving under sunny conditions was always distressing for him; his car accident occurred during a particularly sunny day, which was made all the more salient because it came after weeks of overcast, rainy weather.

- The use of safety signals or safety behaviors (e.g., "I was fine, but I felt safe only because you were with me when I went into the bank").

- Distorted appraisals of the exposure experience, particularly "near miss" or "close call" appraisals. That is, the person regards the exposure exercise as involving a "lucky escape" rather than providing evidence that the situation was safe. Often, such appraisals can be identified during the assessment interview, when the therapist assesses the patient's posttrauma experiences with stimuli that resemble or remind the patient of the trauma. In other cases, especially with highly avoidant patients, the therapist might not identify these types of appraisals until the situational exposure exercises are under way.

Tom developed PTSD after he was involved in an aircraft accident in which several other passengers were seriously injured and one was killed. Tom was making steady progress with his situational exposure assignments, which involved going on sightseeing flights and taking flights on small commercial aircraft. Despite his steady progress, he arrived visibly shaken at a session one day. Tom said he had been on a flight that "nearly crashed." A review of the incident revealed that the flight was turbulent and the landing bumpy. The therapist and Tom reviewed the evidence about whether the flight nearly crashed or whether it was simply a rough flight. Tom was asked to collect further evidence on this issue by talking with a flight instructor, who advised him that rough flights are quite common and it is very rare for such a flight to be hazardous. He realized that he had overestimated the seriousness of the rough flight. This information, along with other information gleaned from the flight instructor (e.g., information about the safety features of aircraft and safety training of pilots), reduced his anxiety about flying, which in turn made it much easier for him to continue with the air travel exposure exercises.

TROUBLESHOOTING

Extreme Distress, Pain, or Dissociation Evoked by Exposure

It can be difficult for the patient and therapist to accurately predict the degree of distress evoked by situational exposure exercises. Accordingly, intense emotional reactions can occur. Intense distress or panic attacks occurring during exposure exercises are not necessarily a problem, unless they make the exposure situation dangerous (e.g., panicking while flying a plane), or if they prompt the patient to flee the situation or resort to some form of maladaptive coping behavior (e.g., abuse of sedating drugs or alcohol). If patients can safety tolerate intense emotions then exposure exercises can be continued if the patient so desires. In our clinic we have treated a number of patients who are so determined to overcome their PTSD that they are willing to persist even with highly distressing exposure exercises. Other patients, however, are understandably unwilling to endure high levels of exposure-induced distress or panic. In such cases, an easier exposure exercise can be tried. Either way, after an intense exposure exercise the patient can be given a few minutes to unwind and discuss the experience with the therapist. The therapist can empathize with the patient's distress and provide praise for his or her courage in enduring emotional distress, and then the therapist and patient can plan what to do next. If the patient experiences intense exposure-related pain (e.g., headaches or muscle spasms), then plans should be made for less distressing, more gradual exposure exercises in the future, combined with relaxation training or other pain management strategies.

If the patient experiences intense dissociation during an exposure exercise, then a grounding exercise could be used (Chapter 9) and, once the patient has sufficiently recovered, a less distressing exposure exercise could be planned. As mentioned in the previous chapter, mild levels of exposure-induced dissociation are usually not a problem because these reactions typically diminish over the course of exposure. Intense dissociation can be hazardous if it occurs in a situation in which the person is operating vehicles or machinery. Exposure exercises need to be tailored to reduce the risk of harm.

When Exposure Seems to Fail

If the patient doesn't seem to be benefiting from situational exposure exercises, then the therapist should consider (1) patient goals and related issues concerning adherence to the exercises, (2) the presence of safety signals or safety behaviors, and (3) the types of emotions elicited by exposure (e.g., intense anger, guilt, or shame, which may require cognitive restructuring).

A patient may refuse to complete exposure exercises if they do not match his or her goals. This can occur even if the case formulation suggests that these exercises are an important part of the treatment plan. In such cases it may be necessary to revise the treatment plan to better match the patient's goals, or explore whether the patient is willing to consider a change of goals (e.g., "If you were better able to manage your anxiety, would that have any impact on the goals that you might choose about resuming driving on busy streets?").

In terms of adherence, patients may be unwilling to properly complete exposure exercises if the exercises are too difficult for them, if they don't understand the rationale, or if there are incentives for them not to complete exposure exercises (e.g., the loss of disability payments if they recover). Accordingly, the therapist should assess for these possibilities and also look for possible safety signals or safety behaviors that might interfere with exposure exercises. Some patients, for example, consume benzodiazepines (e.g., lorazepam) or alcohol before attempting situational exposure homework. Or patients may use distraction or soothing imagery so that they can imagine that they are not actually in the exposure situation. The patient might not disclose using these strategies unless the therapist explicitly inquires.

Exposure-Related Perceptual Distortions

Some patients experience perceptual distortions when they are exposed to trauma-related stimuli. For example, for PTSD associated with motor vehicle accidents it is not uncommon for patients to report the illusion that cars are looming toward them or veering into the wrong lane, or that the traffic around them is driving extremely fast or is very close to one's vehicle. These distortions can happen during naturally occurring exposures and during situational exposure exercises.

These distortions appear to be characteristic of the "looming vulnerability" commonly observed in anxious people, in which they have mental representations of dynamically intensifying danger and rapidly escalating risk (Riskind & Williams, 2006). In other words, the perceptual distortions commonly involve qualities such as exaggerated velocity or acceleration of threat.

Some patients fear that the illusions are dangerous because they might place themselves in jeopardy by acting on them, for example, crashing into a telephone pole as a result of swerving away from a car that is perceived to be crossing the center lane. Some patients may be at risk for such hazardous actions, but clinically, such risks are rare. In most cases, distortions are distressing but not dangerous and usually disappear over the course of exposure therapy. Even so, the therapist and patient should evaluate the evidence for and against the idea that the illusions place the patient at risk. Such disputations can similarly be used if the patient strongly believes the illusion (especially when it is occurring), and sees him- or herself as the direct target of threat (e.g., "Cars are deliberately swerving toward *me*").

Distancing strategies can be used to help patients cope with trauma-related perceptual distortions. This is done by (1) providing an explanation of the distortion (i.e., it's a fear-related illusion, perhaps arising from cognitive simulations of feared threats to the self); (2) informing the patient that distortion typically abates when fear abates over the course of the exposure exercises; (3) informing the patient that he or she can cope with the distortion by not taking it seriously (e.g., "Remind yourself that it's just a harmless illusion that will eventually disappear"); and (4) ensuring that exposure exercises are conducted in such a way that the distortions do not create a hazard.

It is also helpful to conduct imaginal exposure for looming-related stimuli. A graded approach can be used, starting with imagining non-looming (nonthreatening) stimuli, such as imagining cars passing without swerving into one's lane or imagining traffic moving slowly. This can also serve as a distancing strategy (i.e., by reinforcing the message that the patient is experiencing a harmless illusion). After the patient's level of distress has abated due to these modified images, then he or she can receive imaginal exposure to increasingly distorted images, such as imagining increasing fast-moving traffic, including traffic that is moving much more rapidly than it does in reality. When distress evoked by these images is reduced, then the real-life distortions and distress also tend to abate (Riskind & Williams, 2006).

SUMMARY

Situational exposure is an integral part of the cognitive-behavioral treatment of PTSD. It builds on, and is integrated with, other interventions such as imaginal exposure and cognitive restructuring. The choice of situational exposure exercises depends on the patient's goals concerning the types of stimuli that he or she would like to feel comfortable with. Situational exposure can be more challenging to implement than other sorts of exposure, because there are more uncontrolled variables in situational exposure, and it can be challenging to find exposure activities that the patient can readily, frequently, and safely practice. Further development of virtual reality programs, such as more realistic programs for a wider range of trauma situations, may offer a partial solution to this problem. However, such programs are no substitute for real-life exposure.

HANDOUT 13.1. Situational Exposure Hierarchy Form

This form is designed to help you identify **harmless, but distressing** real-life situations. These should be situations related to your traumatic event(s), situations that you find upsetting or tend to avoid. Please try to come up with 10 situations. In therapy you and your therapist will use this form to help desensitize you to these situations. After you list each situation, please rate how distressed or upset you would be in this situation. Do this by choosing a number between 0 and 100, where 0 = none, and 100 = extremely. Try to choose situations that cover the full range of the scales, e.g., some that are mild (0–30 on the scale), some moderate (e.g., 30–60), and some severe (higher than 60).

Example: Here is an example to help you complete this form. Consider a woman who was tied up with a belt and sexually assaulted by a man in a public park. The following might appear on her hierarchy:

Situation (e.g., place, object, person, or activity)	How upset would you be in this situation? (0–100)
Walking through the park in which I was assaulted (in broad daylight, by myself)	90
Working out at the local fitness during the day (where there are a lot of sweaty guys)	80
Walking through the park in which I was assaulted (in broad daylight, with a friend)	75
Looking at belts in the men's wear section of a department store	60
Listening to rock music that contains sexual lyrics	45
Having morning coffee at a coffee house with one of my male friends	30

Your hierarchy:

Situation (e.g., place, object, person, or activity)	How upset would you be in this situation? (0–100)

CHAPTER 14

Adjunctive Methods and Relapse Prevention

The case formulation and treatment plan provide guidelines about the types of interventions likely to be helpful in treating a given patient's problems. Usually, treatment involves some combination of interventions discussed in the preceding chapters. Relapse prevention, as described in this chapter, is also an important component of treatment. Adjunct interventions—such as interpersonal skills training and couple and family interventions—are useful in some cases, which are described in this chapter. The chapter concludes with some suggestions about what can be done to treat "treatment failures," that is, to help a small but important subgroup of patients who have derived little or no benefit from a course of CBT.

INTERPERSONAL SKILLS TRAINING

Overview

Trauma survivors may experience interpersonal problems for a variety of reasons. In some cases the person has failed to acquire skills, or has learned maladaptive patterns of interaction, as a result of long-standing abuse, such as childhood abuse. In other cases, the PTSD symptoms themselves lead to interpersonal problems. For example, after being mugged several times as an adult, Jane became anxious and unassertive around men in general because she feared another assault. After he was nearly killed in a mudslide, Andy was horrified to find that his neighbors wouldn't help him search the debris for his missing family members; they were too busy trying to salvage their possessions. As a result of this experience, Andy has trouble trusting people and has become suspicious, guarded, and sometimes hostile in his personal and professional relationships.

Cognitive-behavioral interventions focusing on PTSD symptoms, such as those described in previous chapters, can often have beneficial effects on interpersonal problems. However, for some patients the interpersonal problems persist even after the PTSD symptoms have been treated. Such patients may benefit from interpersonal skills training. This type of training not only improves skills, it also serves as a form of *in vivo* exposure. Interpersonal skills training also is a potent vehicle for eliciting maladaptive beliefs about interactions with others (Levitt & Cloitre, 2005), which can be targeted with cognitive restructuring. Finally, skills training can reduce the risk of subsequent trauma exposure, for example, by reducing the risk of retraumatization.

Reducing the Risk of Retraumatization

Reasons for Retraumatization

Even patients successfully treated for PTSD tend to be at increased risk for future trauma exposure and PTSD, compared to people who have never been traumatized or developed PTSD (see Chapter 1). Patients can be informed of this risk toward the end of treatment, in a frank but nonalarmist manner. You might tell your patient something like the following:

> "People who have been exposed to trauma and develop PTSD tend to be, on average, at somewhat greater risk for future trauma and PTSD. This doesn't mean this will necessarily happen to you, and even if it did, that would simply mean another course of treatment for PTSD. But to be on the safe side, it would be useful for us to consider whether there is anything in your living situation that could put you at risk for future trauma."

There is a small but growing empirical literature on the possible causes, although much more work is required. Several explanations have been offered, and different factors may be relevant to different patients. Accordingly, the patient's risk for retraumatization needs to be examined on a case-by-case basis. Clearly, PTSD patients who live in dangerous neighborhood or who have dangerous occupations should be encouraged to change their jobs or living circumstances to reduce their risks of future trauma exposure and PTSD. Other reasons for retraumatization, and possible solutions, include the following.

Risk Perception

There is some evidence that increased risk of retraumatization is correlated with an increased latency in detecting cues to interpersonal danger
(Messman-Moore & Long, 2003). These findings need to be interpreted
with caution, especially if they are shared with patients, because they could
be misinterpreted as blaming the victim. The fact remains that rape or other
interpersonal violence is morally wrong, regardless of the reaction time of
the victim. Toward the end of PTSD treatment, however, it can be useful to
review ways that the patient can reduce the risk of subsequent trauma. This
may involve reviewing the warning signals of the patient's previous trauma
(e.g., a rape, mugging, or some other assault) and devising guidelines for
identifying threat. Susan, for example, was raped after agreeing to leave her
friends at the bar and go off with some strangers to a party. At the party
her drink was spiked with a hypnotic drug (likely flunitrazepam; i.e.,
Rohypnol) and then she was sexually assaulted. Working with her therapist, she came up with a list of warning signs that would serve her in the
future (avoiding going off with complete strangers, not leaving her drink
unattended, etc.).

As a further example, Kubany and Watson (2002) offered several useful suggestions about how formerly battered women can identify potential
abusers and avoid revictimization. Such signs, evident early in a dating relationship, include the following.

> Possessiveness, jealously (often perceived early on as flattery), wanting to rush
> into a serious relationship, unreliability (e.g., lateness), always checking on or
> wanting to know his girlfriend's whereabouts (e.g., calling her several times a
> day), overcontrolling about how, where, and with whom his girlfriend spends
> her time, disliking his girlfriend's friends or relatives, lying or secrecy (about
> activities, whereabouts, or previous relationships), subtle put-downs, trying to
> impose his opinion and worldviews on his girlfriend, known to have been
> physically aggressive or otherwise abusive with someone else, a bad temper
> (even if he is "happy-go-lucky" most of the time), and a history of heavy use of
> alcohol or drugs. (p. 122)

Personality or Behavioral Patterns

Impulsive, antisocial, or excitement-seeking personality traits or behaviors
can increase the risk of retraumatization (Jang et al., 2003; see also Chapter
1). Some people are drawn to exciting, risky occupations or recreational
pursuits. That is, they have high scores on personality measures of sensation seeking or related measures. Such people are at risk for PTSD if they
also have high scores on personality measures of negative emotionality

(neuroticism). In other words, they are liable to put themselves, sometimes inadvertently, in dangerous situations, and then liable to react with intense negative emotions, such as fear or horror. In such cases it can be helpful to share this formulation with the patient and then work to find more adaptive, nonhazardous ways of seeking excitement. Sometimes, intense sensation seeking may be acquired in the traumatic situation, rather than being a long-standing personality trait. But even here, the principle of treatment remains the same: to redirect the tendency to seek excitement into more adaptive channels.

Gene, a war veteran developed PTSD from his combat experiences but also regarded his war experiences as the most exciting, meaningful experiences of his life. When he returned to civilian life, he generally felt emotionally numb and detached from others and suffered from other PTSD symptoms. But he also periodically engaged in highly risky behaviors, such as deliberately venturing into dangerous parts of the town, frequenting seedy bars, and walking down dark alleyways. He carried a combat knife with him for protection. Although he never had to use the knife, he got into frequent fistfights. Gene wasn't able to clearly articulate his reasons for placing himself in these risky situations. On the one hand he felt terrified by the things he did. But on the other hand he felt masterful, in control, and "more alive" than he felt during his routine, emotionally numb everyday life. Clearly, Gene's activities were putting him at risk for further trauma, but they also served an important psychological need for him. Gene and his therapist explored this dilemma in an effort to find a more adaptive compromise. The therapist asked Gene to describe the activities that he formerly found to be exciting, including those that predated his war experiences. It turned out that he had formerly enjoyed amateur boxing. Gene and the therapist discussed whether a return to boxing would be a satisfactory, safe alternative to his hazardous nocturnal activities. Gene agreed that this seemed to be a good alternative and agreed to leave his knife at home when he went out to work out at the training gym.

Trauma survivors may also acquire other behavioral patterns that can put them at risk for subsequent traumatization. For example, some survivors of childhood abuse are taught that their needs don't matter, and that they should put the needs of others ahead of their own. This can lead the person to get into relationships in which they assume the role of the overused or even abused caretaker. For example, Jasminder was raised in an emotionally and sometimes physically abusive household, in which she was repeatedly told by her father that she shouldn't be so selfish as to think of herself, and that she should look after her ailing mother and her handicapped younger brother. Jasminder was later raped as a teenager, blamed for the rape by her parents, and subsequently had an abortion. Although she made good progress in treatment for her PTSD, her therapist noted that Jasminder had a pattern of getting into abusive relationships. Specifically, Jasminder, now as an adult, tended to be drawn to needy men who were "down on their luck." Thus, she got into several relationships with men she tried to "save," including men with gambling or substance abuse problems. In addition to her desire to help people she also voiced the opinion that "Fucked-up relationships is all I can get." The result was often physical or financial abuse. Although Jasminder had successfully dealt with her PTSD, her current pattern of relationships was a risk factor for further trauma. This became an important topic of therapy.

Assertiveness Training

Assertiveness problems are also associated with the risk for retraumatization. Assertiveness involves standing up for one's rights or preferences, without trampling on the rights of others (Paterson, 2000). Assertiveness also involves being able to express one's feelings to others, whether they be tender feelings (e.g., telling a spouse that you love him or her) or negative feelings (e.g., discussing a problem you have with a coworker). Assertiveness problems—such as unassertive or aggressive behaviors—merit treatment in their own right, and are all the more important to address when they contribute to PTSD. Unassertiveness, for example, can worsen avoidance symptoms, and aggressive behaviors can fuel hyperarousal There are many good assertiveness training guides available, among the best being Paterson's (2000) short but highly informative and practical workbook.

The first step involves assessing assertiveness difficulties and helping the patient identify and understand where he or she is interpersonally skillful, and where problems tend to arise. This can be done as part of a more general assessment, where interpersonal problems are identified, and the patient's goals are identified. As discussed earlier in this volume, an important goal of treatment is to ensure patient safety. Accordingly, assertiveness exercises (e.g., homework assignments in which patients practice standing up for their rights) should be planned only for those situations in which the patient will be safe. In some situations it can be dangerous to practice assertiveness (e.g., a patient might be beaten if she asserted herself to her former husband during child visitation). Under such circumstances, other interventions would be more appropriate (e.g., having a witness or protective person present during the visits).

If assertiveness training seems appropriate, then the patient and therapist can discuss ways of dealing with each situation, and role plays with feedback can be conducted in session. Homework assignments then can be planned, such as practicing particular skills in particular situations (e.g., saying "No" using the Broken Record technique, where the patient simply repeatedly declines an unwanted request, without apologizing or needing to provide explanations or excuses). Role plays and homework exercises can be hierarchically arranged, beginning with the easiest (in which the patient is most likely to succeed) and then working up to more difficult ones. After each exercise the patient and therapist conduct a "postmortem" to analyze what happened, identify successful behaviors, and develop strategies for overcoming any problems that arose. Throughout assertiveness training, the patient and therapist should try to identify relevant maladaptive beliefs, such as beliefs contributing to unassertiveness or aggressiveness (e.g., "I have to work myself up and get mad in order for people to take me seriously"). Cognitive restructuring can be used to address these beliefs.

Ellen had been in a long-standing abusive marriage with an alcoholic man who eventually committed suicide. After several months of therapy her PTSD symptoms had abated, and she was no longer tormented by the web of tangled feelings she had for her former husband, such as fear and anger, and guilt about wishing him dead and then discovering that he killed himself. Despite her many gains in therapy, she still had problems, primarily concerning her teenage son. She had difficulty asserting herself to him, especially making requests for him to do his share of the chores. When she tried to assert herself, he bristled with indignation, which reminded Ellen of how her former husband behaved before beating her. Although her son has never been aggressive toward her or anyone else, Ellen believed that "If I ask him to do something, he may fly into a rage and attack me." She tried coping with her fears by doing the chores herself, and by avoiding her son. She felt guilty about avoiding him, because she loved him and believed that he loved her. During therapy, Ellen and her therapist reviewed the evidence that her son would become violent, and reviewed evidence that he would actually do the chores. Ellen tentatively concluded that he was likely to comply, but the real test would be to ask him. Accordingly, the therapist and Ellen planned a series of assertiveness exercises, starting with one involving a minor request (i.e., asking him to pick up some milk on the way home from soccer practice). This request was role-played during the session, and then Ellen tried it as homework. This was successful, which encouraged her to continue practicing assertiveness. Although her son grumbled at some of the requests, there was no violence. Ellen was not always successful in her requests but learned that there was nothing dangerous about or wrong with negotiating with her son, and she no longer felt the urge to avoid him.

The therapist should take care in the way that feedback in assertiveness training is expressed. People who have experienced interpersonal violence, especially long-standing violence (e.g., childhood abuse or involvement in an abusive marriage) may be highly sensitive to perceived criticism. They may become angry and defensive, or ashamed and withdrawn if they believe they are being told that they're "doing it all wrong" (Levitt &

Cloitre, 2005). They also may engage in excessive self-criticism and therefore may fail to identify any positive aspects of their performance during an assertiveness exercise. Sensitivity to criticism and self-criticism can both undermine the skills- and confidence-building goals of assertiveness training.

There are several ways of providing effective feedback. The following is one method. Before conducting any role plays or assertiveness homework, the therapist can inform the patient that there are all kinds of ways of being assertive or dealing with interpersonal problems. There rarely is any single "correct" approach. The patient can also be encouraged to take a nonjudgmental, problem-solving approach to assertiveness: to experiment via trial and error with different ways of relating to others, while trying to suspend any self-criticism. The focus is on behavior, not on labeling the self. Then, after each assertiveness exercise, the patient can be asked to first summarize the strengths of his or her performance. Self-criticism should be discouraged, and patients should be encouraged to find something positive about their performance. If necessary, the therapist can prompt the patient to elicit positive comments. Next, the patient can be asked whether there was anything about the way he or she handled the assertiveness situation that could be improved, or anything that might have been done differently. The therapist can reinforce (praise) the patient's efforts at coming up with solutions. Then the therapist can provide his or her feedback, beginning with the positives (including those that might not have been identified by the patient). Then, building on what the patient has identified as things that could be improved, the therapist could offer some suggestions. These are presented simply as alternatives, the efficacy of which can only be ascertained by trying them out.

Other Skills Training

Self-Defense

Important goals of skills training involve reducing the objective risk of harm and reducing exaggerated expectations of danger. For survivors of interpersonal violence, both goals can be achieved by encouraging the patient to take a self-defense course. Consistent with this, a recent literature review concluded that the most effective avenue for preventing sexual assault is self-defense training (Söchting et al., 2004). This could involve a women-only self-defense course aimed at reducing the risk for rape (e.g., the *Dr. Ruthless* program) or it could involve joining a martial arts club. The therapist could periodically review the patient's experiences in such training to ensure that the acquired skills were not being misused. An optimal outcome of such training would be to strengthen beliefs such as "I can avoid objectively dangerous places and I can protect myself in other situations." Other sorts of beliefs may be less adaptive, such as "Now that I know kung fu, I never have to worry about my safety" or "I'm safe against men so long as I vigorously practice my karate training." In such cases the therapist would do well to encourage the patient to review whether such beliefs are useful or realistic. Also, if the patient takes a self-defense program that encourages the use of a deterrent, such as a handgun or Mace, then the deterrent may become a safety signal, associated with beliefs such as "I'm safe outdoors only as long as I have my hand on my pepper spray." Such safety signals and beliefs can perpetuate a sense of current danger and therefore can perpetuate PTSD. Accordingly, the beliefs and behaviors may need to be addressed via cognitive restructuring.

Driving

For patients who have developed PTSD after being involved in a serious road traffic collision, it can be useful to take a defensive driving course or even driving lessons. The goal of defensive driving is to teach people how to proactively avoid dangerous situations. Such courses are useful for a variety of reasons; they can serve as *in vivo* exposure, and they encourage patients to improve their driving skills and drop any maladaptive safety behaviors. And, perhaps most importantly, they can help the patient develop and strengthen important *interpersonal* skills—that is, skills about how to anticipate and respond to the actions of other drivers. Many people with PTSD associated with motor vehicle accidents are frightened about the actions of other drivers (Koch & Taylor, 1995). Such actions may be perceived as unpredictable, uncontrollable, and potentially lethal. A defensive driving course or driving lessons can teach patients how to anticipate the actions of other drivers, and how to effectively deal with emergency situations. This can improve the patient's driving confidence and reduce unrealistic beliefs about the dangerousness of driving.

Applications to Children

Many of the skills training exercises, such as assertiveness or self-defense training, can be used with children in much the same way as they are used with adults or adolescents. Skills training can also be used for children who engage in developmentally inappropriate sexual behaviors (e.g., imitating intercourse or inserting one's tongue into the mouth of another person), which is more commonly displayed by sexually abused than nonabused children (Deblinger & Heflin, 1996). The nonoffending parent plays an important role in shaping the child's behaviors. For example, he or she may reward appropriate behaviors (i.e., catching the child being good). Inappropriate behaviors can be dealt with via verbal admonishment, "time-out," or other strategies. A detailed discussion is provided in Deblinger and Heflin's (1996) treatment manual.

Training to help children identify and avoid risky situations can be provided by school-based educational programs, such as the "Good Touch/ Bad Touch" program for reducing the risk of sexual abuse. Such programs educate children about the difference between being touched in appropriate versus inappropriate ways by other people. There is some evidence that these programs can reduce the risk of sexual assault (Gibson & Leitenberg, 2000), although concerns have also been raised about such programs, including whether young children can make appropriate distinctions between "good" and "bad" touches (DeYoung, 1988; Hebert & Tourigny, 2004).

Another form of risk reduction is to reduce the exposure of children and adolescents to inappropriate sexual material on the Internet. At this stage, the only effective methods are parentally administered filtering or blocking software. This is associated with only a modest reduction in exposure, which suggests that it is helpful but far from foolproof (Mitchell, Finkelhor, & Wolak, 2003a). A related problem involves protecting the child and adolescent from sexual solicitation or harassment on the Internet. Research is currently under way to find effective ways of addressing this problem, such as educating and encouraging youth to report these unwanted contacts (Mitchell, Finkelhor, & Wolak, 2001, 2003b).

COUPLE AND FAMILY INTERVENTIONS

Symptoms of PTSD—particularly fears, preoccupation with the trauma, emotional numbing (e.g., lack of affection), avoidance, and irritability— play themselves out in the patient's interpersonal world. Relationships may become strained, disrupted, or even disintegrate. Cognitive-behavioral interventions, such as those covered in previous chapters, can reduce PTSD and thereby improve relationship functioning. However, this does not invariably happen, so couple or family interventions may be warranted once the course of PTSD-focused treatment has been completed. In other circumstances the case formulation may suggest that PTSD and relationship problems mutually exacerbate one another. Irritability and avoidance, for example, could alienate and antagonize the spouse, who responds to the patient in ways that increase the patient's hyperarousal. As we saw in Chapter 5, poor outcome for PTSD treatment tends to occur when patients live with angry or critical significant others (i.e., live in environments with high expressed emotion). Family members may blame the patient for the trauma (e.g., blame them for a sexual assault or for enlisting in the military) and may blame the patient for being "too weak" to get over the PTSD. In such situations, and in other circumstances where interpersonal problems and PTSD appear to mutually maintain one another, the optimal treatment may involve the simultaneous implementation of PTSD treatments described in previous chapters and couple or family interventions.

It can be useful to implement exercises from *behavioral couple or family therapies*, combined with psychoeducation for the significant others about PTSD. Based on social learning principles, these treatments involve a collection of strategies emphasizing communication training and interpersonal problem solving. Interventions include constructive expression of emotions, empathic listening, training in conflict resolution and anger management, negotiation training, and methods for increasing the exchange of positive interactions and decreasing aversive ones. An important goal is to reduce mutual blaming and to encourage a problem-solving approach to interpersonal difficulties. Detailed descriptions of behavioral couple and family treatments are available elsewhere (e.g., Baucom et al., 2002; Jacobson & Margolin, 1979).

The following vignette illustrates how some relatively simple couple or family interventions can be usefully integrated into individual PTSD treatment. The example also illustrates how problems in treatment can lead to a revision in the case formulation and treatment plan in order to overcome the difficulties.

Six sessions of individual CBT with Ron had been largely ineffective. The therapist believed that she had developed a sound formulation of his problems and a good treatment plan. Ron readily agreed with the formulation and the plan. But treatment failed to reduce his PTSD symptoms. Part of the problem was that Ron often seemed to forget to complete his homework assignments or said that he couldn't find the time. Given these problems, the therapist and Ron decided to revisit the case formulation and to attempt to identify the source of the difficulties. Incidental comments from Ron in previous sessions suggested that there may have been important but overlooked interpersonal factors that were relevant to the case formulation at treatment plan. It turned out that Ron's girlfriend and his parents were critical of his decision to enter therapy, and they often criticized or subtly mocked him whenever he tried to go out on situational exposure assignments or to practice other therapeutic exercises, such as diaphragmatic breathing or cognitive restructuring worksheets. His girlfriend and mother told Ron that he should stop complaining about his symptoms and get over them. Both parents also implied to Ron that it was shameful that he was a "mental patient." The identification of these interpersonal factors suggested that the high expressed emotion in Ron's social environment may have been exacerbating his symptoms and undermining his attempts at completing homework assignments. Compounding matters, Ron seemed to be overly dependent on his girlfriend and parents. Given these revisions to the case formulation, the treatment plan was revised. The first step was to try to reduce the level of criticism from his girlfriend and parents. The therapist, with Ron's permission, decided to invite his girlfriend to meet with them in order to help her better understand his problems. Two informational sessions with Ron's girlfriend proved successful in enhancing her understanding and curbing her criticism. A subsequent family intervention was planned in which Ron, his girlfriend, and the therapist would meet with his parents to try to help them better understand the nature of his problems, and to help them understand that it was wise and courageous for Ron to seek therapy, rather than a source of shame. This was sufficient to enable Ron to resume his homework exercises to work on his PTSD symptoms. The therapist and Ron agreed that once these symptoms had abated sufficiently, they would reassess his interpersonal relations to determine whether his dependency on his girlfriend and parents was still a problem. It was predicted that once Ron gained more confidence about overcoming his fears and other PTSD symptoms, he might feel less reliant on his girlfriend and parents.

INTERVENTIONS FOR THE FINAL STAGES OF TREATMENT

Treatment Tapering

Most therapy protocols developed and evaluated in treatment research typically consist of 8 to 16 sessions. In general clinical practice, however, the duration of treatment is determined by many factors, including logistic constraints such as the number of sessions provided by an insurance company as well as the patient's degree of treatment response. If you are able to provide, say, 12 sessions of treatment, the planning for treatment tapering may begin in session 8. If there are no constraints on the number of sessions, you may wish to treat the patient until either he or she has made a good response to therapy (e.g., at least a 50% reduction in symptoms), or has drawn as much benefit as he or she is likely to gain from cognitive-behavioral treatment. The greatest degree of treatment response typically occurs in the first several sessions (Taylor, 2004). Regardless of the duration of treatment, it is useful to allow for at least 4 sessions of treatment tapering and 1 or 2 sessions for relapse prevention.

As the formal course of PTSD treatment draws to a close, the treatment sessions should be spaced increasingly further apart, so as to fade out reliance on the therapist and encourage the patient to take an increasingly active role in extending and maintaining treatment gains. The final 4 treatment sessions might be successively spaced 2, 4, 8, and 12 weeks apart. During the tapering period, patients should be encouraged to continue working, on their own, on any remaining clinical problems, using whatever cognitive-behavioral methods they have found useful. Progress can be monitored during the tapering sessions, and problem solving can be used to address any difficulties that are encountered.

Maintaining and Extending Treatment Gains

In the final one or two sessions the patient and therapist should review the progress made over the course of therapy and determine the extent to which the patient's goals were attained. Scores on PTSD symptom scales (Chapter 6) can also be used to assess progress.

As part of the treatment review, the patient should be asked to identify the interventions that were most helpful, and to plan how he or she could continue to use these methods to work on any remaining problems. As part of this exercise, patients can be encouraged to identify what *they* did to reduce their symptoms, instead of attributing all the gains to the skill of the therapist. This is important for building self-confidence in patients and for increasing the odds that they will continue to practice the interventions on their own. To this end, patients could be asked to write a description of what they found to be the most useful methods for working on their PTSD. This would involve generating a list of specific interventions, the steps involved in their implementation, and the rationale for each intervention. Interventions should be described in specific, concrete terms. This is done in a collaborative fashion, with the therapist using careful questioning to have the patient come up with most of the information.

The general elements of a plan for maintaining and extending gains (and preventing relapse) are presented in Table 14.1. The patient and therapist should also develop a set of written plans for maintaining and extending treatment gains. Problems that remain to be addressed can be ranked in order of importance. Plans, based on the skills learned in CBT, can then be developed for each problem. The patient can be encouraged to work through each problem, beginning with the most pressing concern. Of course, if these problems are severe, then the patient and therapist may decide to extend the course of therapy.

Dealing with Lapses and Relapses

In the last session or two, written guidelines are also developed, specific to a given patient's needs, for identifying "high-risk" situations (i.e., situations that may cause a reemergence of PTSD). Preparation for relapse prevention obviously should be done in a manner that does not alarm patients or make them believe they are fated to encounter future trauma. In order to successfully maintain treatment gains, it is important that a setback or lapse—

TABLE 14.1. General Elements of a Program for Maintaining and Extending Gains and Preventing Relapse

Review treatment progress.
- What problems have diminished during treatment?
- What problems remain to be addressed?
- What interventions were most useful?

Establish appropriate expectations for posttreatment functioning.
- Some ongoing practice of some treatment exercises may be required to address outstanding problems.
- Setbacks may occur, especially if major stressors are encountered in the future.
- Coping strategies can overcome setbacks.

Develop a written maintenance plan.
- Write a list of ongoing coping strategies and therapeutic exercises.
- Remind patient to keep and periodically review the therapy handouts.

Develop a plan for relapse prevention.
- Distinguish between setback and relapse.
- Identify high-risk situations and times (e.g., the anniversary of the trauma).
- Develop plans for coping with setbacks, using hypothetical scenarios.
- Ensure the patient understands that although future trauma exposure and PTSD is a possibility, it is not inevitable.

Arrange for periodic check-in with therapist.
- Booster sessions, if needed.
- Telephone or e-mail consultations.

defined as a moderate increase in symptoms—does not progress into a full-blown relapse of PTSD. The maintenance program should provide patients with relapse prevention strategies. These should be written down so patients can consult them in the future, if necessary. The points to convey are described below and can be supplemented by a written handout or worksheet such as Handout 14.1 (pp. 276–278). Important points include the following:

- Life is full of ups and downs. There will be times when the patient feels anxious and distressed in response to stressors. These reactions are no cause for alarm; it is normal to feel anxious at times.
- A lapse (setback) is not a relapse. A future occurrence of PTSD symptoms does not mean that the patient has lost all the gains that he or she made during treatment. It simply means that it's time to practice the exercises learned in therapy.
- Lapses can be framed as *opportunities* for continuing to practice the skills learned in therapy. Patients can be asked to write out a plan of what methods they would use if they encountered another severe stressor and they developed PTSD symptoms. As part of this exercise, patients can write

out and challenge any dysfunctional beliefs they have about the recurrence of their problems (e.g., "If my problems return then that means I'm doomed to despair"). It is important that patients realize that, as a result of therapy, they have acquired effective skills for dealing with setbacks.

• If a setback does occur, then the patient should attempt to analyze the situation to identify any dysfunctional beliefs or other factors that may have been involved. Once they are identified, the patient can use cognitive and exposure strategies learned in therapy to evaluate these beliefs. Patients are encouraged to restrict the lapse before it gets worse, using the approach described in Handout 14.1.

• Encourage the patient to put the lapse in perspective: if you're overcome the effects of past trauma, then you can deal with future stressors. If a lapse occurs, patients could ask themselves how they would view it in 5 or 10 years. Would this be seen as another short-lived hassle in life's bumpy ride?

• If the patient is unable to manage the setback, then the therapist should be contacted for one or more telephone contacts or face-to-face booster sessions. Consultation should focus on the cause of the setback and should thereby lead to a plan for correcting the problem.

As part of the maintenance plan, arrangements can be made for the patient to periodically check in with the CBT practitioner in order to review progress and discuss any ongoing problems. This can be done by brief telephone, e-mail, or face-to-face booster sessions. Check-in sessions can be arranged, say, 3, 6, and 12 months after the end of a formal course of, say, 12 CBT sessions. Such contacts are used to assess the maintenance of treatment gains, to reinforce the patient's efforts, to provide assistance in helping the patient deal with any new or enduring problems, and to develop plans for ongoing exposure or other therapeutic exercises. Patients should write down what they learned from these contacts so the information is not forgotten.

Jason was a bank teller who had experienced multiple armed robberies, including one in which the assailant thrust the barrel of a sawed-off shotgun into his mouth, breaking Jason's upper front teeth. Jason resigned from that job and joined an accounting firm. He responded well to treatment for the PTSD associated with these experiences but had a partial relapse when he witnessed an armed robbery in a jewelry store in a local shopping mall. The lapse was associated with thoughts like "Danger follows me around." After two weeks of becoming increasingly anxious and avoidant, he consulted the relapse prevention plan he developed in therapy. Using that plan he devised a series of exposure exercises, which involved returning to the mall, the jewelry store, and other stores selling jewelry until his fears had abated. He responded well to the booster session, and even realized that he had overlooked the 2-year anniversary of the day he quit working at the bank, which was the day of the robbery. Jason e-mailed his therapist about these developments and was greatly encouraged by the therapist's praise for handling the situation so well.

TREATING TREATMENT FAILURES

The interventions described in this volume have proven useful, in clinical practice and in controlled clinical trials, for most PTSD patients. But that does not mean that they are effective for all patients. Some patients partially respond to treatment, while a small proportion fails to benefit at all. What can be done to help these partial responders and nonresponders? Fortunately, many options are available. The first step is to develop a formulation of the factors that could lead the patient to have little or no response to treatment. Developing such a formulation may require further clinical assessment. There are all sorts of reasons for an unsatisfactory treatment response. Such reasons, and their possible solutions, are as follows:

Treatment may not have been delivered properly by the therapist. For example, inappropriate interventions may be used (e.g., targeting beliefs that are not central to the patient's problems) or the timing and pacing of interventions may be inappropriate. The therapist could reevaluate the case formulation and treatment plan to determine if this is the source of the problem. It also may be useful to consult with a colleague experienced in cognitive-behavioral treatment of PTSD. Sometimes a fresh perspective can help find ways of improving the case formulation and treatment plan.

Treatment may fail because of a mismatch between patient and therapist, in a way that significantly interferes with the therapeutic relationship and with treatment progress. For example, Sharon reluctantly agreed to see a male therapist for PTSD stemming from childhood sexual abuse by an uncle. She reasoned to herself that she had worked with other male therapists in the past (for other problems), so she should be able to work with this one. The therapist reviewed Sharon's problems and openly, and respectfully, asked whether she was comfortable working with a male therapist. Sharon said she was, but as therapy progressed she became increasingly uncomfortable about working with the therapist. Her attendance at therapy sessions became erratic and she frequently refused to work on in-session exposure exercises, such as imaginal exposure. The problem was that his physical appearance, hair style, and even his cologne reminded Sharon of her uncle. She was too embarrassed to discuss this with the therapist. As treatment continued to stall, the therapist referred the patient for a second opinion. Sharon was able raise the problem with the consultant, even though the consultant was also male (but, fortunately, bore no resemblance to Sharon's uncle). Sharon was encouraged by the consultant to openly discuss this issue with her therapist, so they could decide whether to work on this issue or to arrange for a referral to another therapist. The consultant offered to facilitate the process. In the end, Sharon decided that it was in her own interests to stick with her current therapist, and to discuss—rather than avoid—his unsettling resemblance to her uncle.

Stressors arising during the course of treatment can exacerbate the patient's PTSD symptoms and derail treatment. The treatment plan may need to be modified, either to focus mainly on crisis management or, preferably, to focus on helping the patient develop skills for anticipating, avoiding, and coping with life stressors. In some circumstances optimal treatment may be focused largely on generic stress management.

Family members or other environmental factors could be interfering with treatment progress. For example, one PTSD patient, who had been in sustained abstinence from alcohol dependence for many years, regularly attended Alcoholics Anonymous (AA). As PTSD treatment progressed, he became less adherent with homework assignments, more likely to miss treatment sessions, and more skeptical of the treatment rationale. An assessment revealed that the source of the problem lay with the patient's AA sponsor, who was actively criticizing the patient's decision enter cognitive-behavioral therapy. The solution was to invite the sponsor to meet with the therapist to dispel any misconceptions (e.g., the patient had been in stable remission for many years and there was no evidence that PTSD treatment was putting the patient at risk for relapse).

In rare cases the failure to respond to treatment may be due to frank malingering or symptom exaggeration, motivated by incentives such as compensation payments. PTSD treatment is not the treatment of choice in such cases; it is more important to identify the problem and discuss it with the patient in a frank but nonaccusatory manner (for further discussion of the detection and management of malingering in treatment-seeking patients, see Taylor, Frueh, & Asmundson, in press).

In some cases the therapist will have fully explored these possibilities, reassessed the patient and revisited the case formulation and treatment plan, worked diligently on enhancing patient motivation for treatment, ensured that the duration of treatment has been adequate (e.g., 6 months of weekly sessions), and consulted with colleagues—but still the patient does not benefit from treatment. What then? There are several options: (1) Treatment may be more appropriate at a later date than at the present time; (2) treatment may be more effective if the patient is referred to another cognitive-behavioral therapist (i.e., another perspective on the case, and another therapist's style may be better suited in a given case); or (3) refer the patient for a different form of empirically supported therapy altogether. This could be an alternative or adjunctive treatment, such as pharmacotherapy as the sole intervention or pharmacotherapy combined with ongoing cognitive-behavioral treatment.

SUMMARY

Adjunctive interventions such as those described in this chapter can be valuable in treating aspects of PTSD that may have not been adequately addressed by interventions described in previous chapters. Adjunctive interventions are typically insufficient by themselves but can powerfully augment the effects of other interventions. Relapse prevention is another important component in the treatment of PTSD. It can be used in all cases, except, of course, with that minority of patients who fail to make any gains in treatment. In those cases there are no relapses to prevent. This chapter offered a number of guidelines for helping such patients overcome their problems. Thus, even for "treatment failures" there is reason to be hopeful about an eventually positive clinical outcome. Clinicians and patients are in the fortunate position of having many treatment options at their disposal, which increases the chances that there will be at least some interventions that may be effective for even the most recalcitrant forms of PTSD.

HANDOUT 14.1. Relapse Prevention Exercises

PTSD RELAPSE PREVENTION

Everyone feels stressed out at some time or other. It is important to cope with these episodes when they arise. This is important for preventing a minor *setback* or lapse (i.e., some return of your PTSD symptoms) from turning into a major *relapse* (the full return of PTSD). This handout is intended to help you design a relapse prevention program for your particular problems so that you can cope with setbacks in the future. Let us begin by considering some examples of how two people coped poorly with their setbacks:

Examples of Poor Coping

Jim developed PTSD after surviving a traumatic train derailment. He had successfully overcome most of his problems over the course of therapy. But one day while driving to work he was involved in a freeway pile-up, in which seven cars were wrecked. He started having nightmares about the pile-up and anxiety about driving and tried to avoid freeway driving whenever he could. Jim thought, "Therapy hasn't helped me! This time, I'm losing it; I'm back at square 1." As a result of these thoughts, Jim didn't use the coping skills he learned in therapy, and so his driving anxiety continued to worsen.

Janice had successfully overcome her rape-related PTSD, and was no longer anxious about dating. But one evening, while walking home from work, she was grabbed by a masked man and dragged into an alleyway, where she was punched and robbed. Janice was understandably distraught. She took time off work and avoided all of her friends. She even stopped answering the phone. Janice thought, "I'm doomed to be abused; nothing can help me." She neglected all the things she had learned in therapy and felt helpless to deal with the return of fears of men.

Good Coping

Write down 3 things that Jim could have done to better cope with his anxieties.
(Hint: How might Jim's thoughts influence his anxiety? Does his lapse really mean that he's back at "square 1"? What sorts of things could Jim do to deal with his driving anxiety?)

1. _____
2. _____
3. _____

Now write down 3 things that Janice could have done to better cope with her fears.
(Hint: What sorts of things could she do in a step-by-step fashion to tackle her fears? Would it help if Janice figured out how to avoid potentially dangerous situations? Does avoidance help her overcome her fear of men?)

1. _____
2. _____
3. _____

(continued)

DEVELOPING YOUR PERSONALIZED RELAPSE PREVENTION PROGRAM

Preparing to Cope with Setbacks

Preventing relapse consists of several steps. The first step comes *before* you have experienced any setbacks.

1. Write down all the things you have learned about the *causes* of your PTSD. Use additional pages if necessary.

   _____

   _____

2. Write down the things that might help you in the short term but make your symptoms *worse* in the longer term. (Hint: Think about excessive avoidance.)

   _____

   _____

3. What sorts of things have you learned to help you cope with, or even overcome, your problems?
   (Hint: These might involve the way you think about things or the way you do things, or they might involve practicing particular exercises.)

   _____

   _____

Administering Emotional First Aid In the Event of a Setback

Now let us develop some strategies for coping with setbacks when they occur. If you begin to experience PTSD symptoms (e.g., nightmares, anxieties, excessive avoidance), then complete the following:

1. *Is the setback a catastrophe?* Write out your reasons.
   (Hint: Have you had a full relapse or was it just a temporary failure to cope? If you have had a full relapse, is it a catastrophe? Why or why not?)

   _____

   _____

2. *Analyze the situation.* Try to learn why the setback occurred. Write out the frightening thoughts you had during the stressor or period of anxiety, including thoughts of what you feared might happen.

   _____

   _____

3. Now *review the evidence* for and against your frightening thoughts.

   _____

   _____

(continued)

4. *Practice other exercises you learned in therapy,* such as (a) exposure exercises (imaginal exposure or live exposure to harmless but distressing situations), or (b) stress management exercises (the relaxation or breathing exercises). Write down the exercises you used. What was the outcome?

_____

_____

5. *Restrict the setback:* Refrain from doing things that make anxiety worse, such as excessive avoidance of fear-evoking things. Please list the things that you are trying to refrain from doing.

_____

_____

6. *Return to any harmless situations that you are starting to avoid.* Do this as soon as possible. Develop a step-by-step plan for returning to these situations. If an avoided situation is too anxiety-provoking to enter, then try an easier, similar situation and then gradually work up to more difficult situations. Example: Janice overcame her fear of men by no longer avoiding the males working in her office. She also reminded herself that although particular situations could be hazardous (e.g., walking down dark streets at night), almost all of her encounters with men were completely safe.

_____

_____

Write down the situations that you are avoiding because of excessive fear. Then list the steps for gradually exposing yourself to these situations, in order to overcome the fear.

_____

_____

7. If these methods haven't helped you, then *contact your therapist* to discuss the problem or to arrange for further therapy sessions.

Therapist's name: _____

Therapist's telephone number or e-mail address: _____

References

Abrahams, S., & Udwin, O. (2000). Treatment of post-traumatic stress disorder in an eleven-year-old boy using imaginal and in vivo exposure. *Clinical Child Psychology and Psychiatry, 5,* 387–401.

Alarcón, R. D., Libb, J. W., & Boll, T. J. (1994). Neuropsychological testing in obsessive-compulsive disorder: A clinical review. *Journal of Neuropsychiatry and Clinical Neurosciences, 6,* 217–228.

Ali, T., Dunmore, E., Clark, D., & Ehlers, A. (2002). The role of negative beliefs in posttraumatic stress disorder: A comparison of assault victims and non victims. *Behavioural and Cognitive Psychotherapy, 30,* 249–257.

Allen, J. G., Huntoon, J., & Evans, R. B. (1999). Complexities in complex posttraumatic stress disorder in inpatient women: Evidence from cluster analysis of MCMI-III personality disorder scales. *Journal of Personality Assessment, 73,* 449–471.

Alonzo, A. A. (1999). Acute myocardial infarction and posttraumatic stress disorder: The consequences of cumulative adversity. *Journal of Cardiovascular Nursing, 13,* 33–45.

American Academy of Child and Adolescent Psychiatry. (1998). Practice parameters for the assessment and treatment of children and adolescents with posttraumatic stress disorder. *Journal of the American Academy of Child and Adolescent Psychiatry, 37*(Suppl. 10), 4–26.

American Psychiatric Association. (1980). *Diagnostic and statistical manual of mental disorders* (3rd ed.). Washington, DC: Author.

American Psychiatric Association. (1994). *Diagnostic and statistical manual of mental disorders* (4th ed.). Washington, DC: Author.

American Psychiatric Association. (2000). *Diagnostic and statistical manual of mental disorders* (4th ed., text rev.). Washington, DC: Author.

Amir, N., Stafford, J., Freshman, M. S., & Foa, E. B. (1998). Relationship between trauma narratives and trauma pathology. *Journal of Traumatic Stress, 11,* 385–392.

Anderson, M. C., Ochsner, K. N., Kuhl, B., Cooper, J., Robertson, E., Gabrieli, S.

W., et al. (2004). Neural systems underlying the suppression of unwanted memories. *Science, 303,* 232–235.

Antony, M. M., Ledley, D. R., Liss, A., & Swinson, R. P. (2005). Responses to symptom induction exercises in panic disorder. *Behaviour Research and Therapy, 44,* 85–98.

Asmundson, G. J. G., Coons, M. J., Taylor, S., & Katz, J. (2002). PTSD and the experience of pain: Research and clinical implications of shared vulnerability and mutual maintenance models. *Canadian Journal of Psychiatry, 47,* 930–937.

Asmundson, G. J. G., Stapleton, J. A., & Taylor, S. (2004). Are avoidance and numbing distinct PTSD symptom clusters? *Journal of Traumatic Stress, 17,* 467–475.

Avenell, A., Brown, T. J., McGee, M. A., Campbell, M. K., Grant, A. M., Broom, J., et al. (2004). What interventions should we add to weight reducing diets in adults with obesity? A systematic review of randomized controlled trials of adding drug therapy, exercise, behaviour therapy or combinations of these interventions. *Journal of Human Nutrition and Dietetics, 17,* 293–316.

Avina, C., & O'Donohue, W. (2002). Sexual harassment and PTSD: Is sexual harassment diagnosable trauma? *Journal of Traumatic Stress, 15,* 69–75.

Azrin, N. H., & Nunn, R. G. (1973). Habit-reversal: A method of eliminating nervous habits and tics. *Behaviour Research and Therapy, 11,* 619–628.

Baker, D. G., West, S. A., Orth, D. N., Hill, K. K., Nicholson, W. E., Ekhator, N. N., et al. (1997). Cerebrospinal fluid and plasma beta endorphin in combat veterans with post traumatic stress disorder. *Psychoneuroendocrinology, 22,* 517–529.

Ballenger, J. C., Davidson, J. R. T., Lecrubier, Y., Nutt, D. J., Foa, E. B., Kessler, R. C., et al. (2000). Consensus statement on posttraumatic stress disorder from the International Consensus Group on Depression and Anxiety. *Journal of Clinical Psychiatry, 61*(Suppl. 5), 60–66.

Başoğlu, M., Ekblad, S., Baarnhielm, S., & Livanou, M. (2004). Cognitive-behavioral treatment of tortured asylum seekers: A case study. *Journal of Anxiety Disorders, 18,* 357–369.

Başoğlu, M., Livanou, M., Şalcioğlu, E., & Kalender, D. (2003). A brief behavioural treatment of chronic post-traumatic stress disorder in earthquake survivors: Results from an open clinical trial. *Psychological Medicine, 33,* 647–654.

Baucom, D. H., Epstein, N., & LaTaillade, J. J. (2002). Cognitive-behavioral couple therapy. In A. S. Gurman & N. S. Jacobson (Eds.), *Clinical handbook of couple therapy* (3rd ed., pp. 26–58). New York: Guilford Press.

Baxter, L. R., Schwartz, J. M., Bergman, K. S., Szuba, M. P., Guze, B. H., Mazziotta, J. C., et al. (1992). Caudate glucose metabolic rate changes with both drug and behavior therapy for obsessive-compulsive disorder. *Archives of General Psychiatry, 49,* 681–689.

Beck, A. T., & Emery, G. (1985). *Anxiety disorders and phobias: A cognitive perspective.* New York: Basic Books.

Beck, A. T., Freeman, A., Davis, D. D., & Associates. (2003). *Cognitive therapy of personality disorders* (2nd ed.). New York: Guilford Press.

Beck, A. T., Rush, A. J., Shaw, B. F., & Emery, G. (1979). *Cognitive therapy of depression.* New York: Guilford Press.

Beck, A. T., Steer, R. A., & Brown, G. K. (1996). *Manual for the Beck Depression Inventory-II.* San Antonio, TX: Psychological Corporation.

Becker, C. B., & Zayfert, C. (2001). Integrating DBT-based techniques and concepts to facilitate exposure treatment for PTSD. *Cognitive and Behavioral Practice, 8,* 107–122.

Beckham, J. C., Crawford, A. L., & Feldman, M. E. (1998). Trail Making Test performance in Vietnam combat veterans with and without posttraumatic stress disorder. *Journal of Traumatic Stress, 11,* 811–819.

Bendel, O., Bueters, T., von Euler, M., Ögren, S. O., Sandin, J., & von Euler, G. (2005). Reappearance of hippocampal CA1 neurons after ischemia is associated with recovery of learning and memory. *Journal of Cerebral Blood Flow and Metabolism, 25,* 1586–1595.

Ben-Ezra, M. (2002). Trauma 4,000 years ago? *American Journal of Psychiatry, 159,* 1437.

Ben-Ezra, M. (2003). Flashbacks and PTSD. *British Journal of Psychiatry, 183,* 75.

Benham, E. (1995). Coping strategies: A psychoeducational approach to posttraumatic symptomatology. *American Journal of Psychosocial Nursing, 33,* 30–35.

Bernstein, E. M., & Putnam, F. W. (1986). Development, reliability, and validity of a dissociation scale. *Journal of Nervous and Mental Disease, 174,* 727–734.

Berntsen, D., Willert, M., & Rubin, D. C. (2003). Splintered memories or vivid landmarks? Qualities and organization of traumatic memories with and without PTSD. *Applied Cognitive Psychology, 17,* 675–693.

Birmes, P., Hatton, L., Bruner, A., & Schmitt, L. (2003). Early historical literature for post-traumatic symptomatology. *Stress and Health, 19,* 17–26.

Bisson, J. I. (2003). Single-session early psychological interventions following traumatic events. *Clinical Psychology Review, 23,* 481–499.

Bisson, J. I., Shepherd, J. P., Joy, D., Probert, R., & Newcombe, R. G. (2004). Early cognitive-behavioural therapy for post-traumatic stress symptoms after physical injury: Randomised controlled trial. *British Journal of Psychiatry, 184,* 63–69.

Blake, D. D., Weathers, F. W., Nagy, L. M., Kaloupek, D. G., Gusman, F. D., Charney, D. S., et al. (1995). The development of a clinician-administered PTSD scale. *Journal of Traumatic Stress, 8,* 75–90.

Blanchard, E. B., Buckley, T. C., Hickling, E. J., & Taylor, A. E. (1998). Posttraumatic stress disorder and comorbid major depression: Is the correlation an illusion? *Journal of Anxiety Disorders, 12,* 21–37.

Blanchard, E. B., & Hickling, E. J. (2004). *After the crash: Psychological assessment and treatment of survivors of motor vehicle accidents* (2nd ed.). Washington, DC: American Psychological Association.

Blanchard, E. B., Hickling, E. J., Devineni, T., Veazey, C. H., Galovski, T. E., Mundy, E., et al. (2003). A controlled evaluation of cognitive behavioral therapy for posttraumatic stress disorder in motor vehicle accident survivors. *Behaviour Research and Therapy, 41,* 79–96.

Bleich, A., & Moskowits, L. (2000). Post traumatic stress disorder with psychotic features. *Croatian Medical Journal, 41*, 442–445.

Borkovec, T. D., Wilkinson, L., Folensbee, R., & Lerman, C. (1983). Stimulus control applications to the treatment of worry. *Behaviour Research and Therapy, 21*, 247–251.

Bouton, M. E. (2002). Context, ambiguity, and unlearning: Sources of relapse after behavioral extinction. *Biological Psychiatry, 52*, 976–986.

Bozzuto, J. C. (1975). Cinematic neurosis following "The exorcist": Report of four cases. *Journal of Nervous and Mental Disease, 161*, 43–48.

Bracha, H. S., Ralston, T. C., Matsukawa, J. M., Williams, A. E., & Bracha, A. S. (2004). Does "fight or flight" need updating? *Psychosomatics, 45*, 448–449.

Brecht, M.-L., von Mayrhauser, C., & Anglin, M. D. (2000). Predictors of relapse after treatment for methamphetamine use. *Journal of Psychoactive Drugs, 32*, 211–220.

Brehm, J. W. (1962). *A theory of psychological reactance.* New York: Academic Press.

Bremner, J. D. (2001). Hypotheses and controversies related to effects of stress on the hippocampus: An argument for stress-induced damage to the hippocampus in patients with posttraumatic stress disorder. *Hippocampus, 11*, 75–81.

Bremner, J. D., Vermetten, E., Afzal, N., & Vythilingam, M. (2004). Deficits in verbal declarative memory function in women with childhood sexual abuse-related posttraumatic stress disorder. *Journal of Nervous and Mental Disease, 192*, 643–649.

Breslau, N. (2002). Epidemiologic studies of trauma, posttraumatic stress disorder, and other psychiatric disorders. *Canadian Journal of Psychiatry, 47*, 923–929.

Breslau, N., & Davis, G. C. (1992). Posttraumatic stress disorder in an urban population of young adults: Risk factors for chronicity. *American Journal of Psychiatry, 149*, 671–675.

Breslau, N., Davis, G. C., Andreski, P., & Peterson, E. (1991). Traumatic events and posttraumatic stress disorder in an urban population of young adults. *Archives of General Psychiatry, 48*, 216–222.

Brewin, C. R. (2001). A cognitive neuroscience account of post-traumatic stress disorder. *Behaviour Research and Therapy, 39*, 373–393.

Brewin, C. R. (2003). *Posttraumatic stress disorder: Malady or myth?* New Haven, CT: Yale University Press.

Brewin, C. R., Andrews, B., & Valentine, J. D. (2000). Meta-analysis of risk factors for posttraumatic stress disorder in trauma-exposed adults. *Journal of Consulting and Clinical Psychology, 68*, 748–766.

Brewin, C. R., & Beaton, A. (2002). Thought suppression, intelligence, and working memory capacity. *Behaviour Research and Therapy, 40*, 923–930.

Brewin, C. R., Dalgleish, T., & Joseph, S. (1996). A dual representation theory of posttraumatic stress disorder. *Psychological Review, 103*, 670–686.

Brewin, C. R., & Holmes, E. A. (2003). Psychological theories of posttraumatic stress disorder. *Clinical Psychology Review, 23*, 339–376.

Brewin, C. R., McNally, R. J., & Taylor, S. (2004). Point/counterpoint: Two views on traumatic memories and posttraumatic stress disorder. *Journal of Cognitive Psychotherapy, 18*, 99–114.

Brewin, C. R., & Smart, L. (2005). Working memory capacity and suppression of obsessional thoughts. *Journal of Behavior Therapy and Experimental Psychiatry, 36*, 61–68.

Briere, J. (1995). *Trauma Symptom Inventory professional manual.* Odessa, FL: Psychological Assessment Resources.

Briere, J. (2004). *Psychological assessment of adult posttraumatic states* (2nd ed.). Washington, DC: American Psychological Association.

Brittlebank, A. D., Scott, J., Williams, J. M. G., & Ferrier, I. N. (1993). Autobiographical memory in depression: State or trait marker? *British Journal of Psychiatry, 162*, 118–121.

Brooks, N., & McKinlay, W. (1992). Mental health consequences of the Lockerbie disaster. *Journal of Traumatic Stress, 5*, 527–543.

Brown, D., Scheflin, A. W., & Hammond, D. C. (1998). *Memory, trauma treatment, and the law.* New York: Norton.

Brown, M. C. J., & Guest, J. F. (1999). Economic impact of feeding a phenylalanine-restricted diet to adults with previously untreated phenylketonuria. *Journal of Intellectual Disability Research, 43*, 30–37.

Bryant, R. A., & Guthrie, R. M. (2005). Maladaptive appraisals as a risk factor for posttraumatic stress: A study of trainee firefighters. *Psychological Science, 16*, 749–752.

Bryant, R. A., & Harvey, A. G. (1997). Attentional bias in posttraumatic stress disorder. *Journal of Traumatic Stress, 10*, 635–644.

Bryant, R. A., & Harvey, A. G. (2002). Delayed-onset posttraumatic stress disorder: A prospective evaluation. *Australian and New Zealand Journal of Psychiatry, 36*, 205–209.

Bryant, R. A., Moulds, M. L., Guthrie, R. M., Dang, S. T., & Nixon, R. D. V. (2003). Imaginal exposure alone and imaginal exposure with cognitive restructuring in treatment of posttraumatic stress disorder. *Journal of Consulting and Clinical Psychology, 71*, 706–712.

Bryant, R. A., Sackville, T., Dang, S. T., Moulds, M., & Guthrie, R. (1999). Treating acute stress disorder: An evaluation of cognitive behavior therapy and supportive counseling techniques. *American Journal of Psychiatry, 156*, 1780–1786.

Buckley, T. C., & Kaloupek, D. G. (2001). A meta-analytic examination of basal cardiovascular activity in posttraumatic stress disorder. *Psychosomatic Medicine, 63*, 585–594.

Bulik, C. M., Sullivan, P. F., & Kendler, K. S. (2003). Genetic and environmental contributions to obesity and binge eating. *International Journal of Eating Disorders, 33*, 293–298.

Burgess, A. W., & Holmstrom, L. L. (1976). Coping behavior of the rape victim. *American Journal of Psychiatry, 133*, 413–417.

Burns, D. D. (1980). *Feeling good: The new mood therapy.* New York: Morrow.

Bury, A. S., & Bagby, R. M. (2002). The detection of feigned uncoached and coached posttraumatic stress disorder with the MMPI-2 in a sample of workplace accident victims. *Psychological Assessment, 14*, 472–484.

Bustamante, V., Mellman, T. A., David, D., & Fins, A. I. (2001). Cognitive functioning and the early development of PTSD. *Journal of Traumatic Stress, 14*, 791–797.

Butcher, J. N. (2005). *MMPI-2: A practitioner's guide*. Washington, DC: American Psychological Association.

Butcher, J. N., Dahlstrom, W. G., Graham, J. R., Tellegen, A., & Kaemmer, B. (1989). *MMPI-2: Minnesota Multiphasic Personality Inventory–2*. Minneapolis: University of Minnesota Press.

Cabe, N. (2001). Relaxation training: Bubble breaths. In H. G. Kaduson & C. E. Schaefer (Eds.), *101 more favorite play therapy techniques* (pp. 346–349). Northvale, NJ: Jason Aronson.

Caffo, E., & Belaise, C. (2003). Psychological aspects of traumatic injury in children and adolescents. *Child and Adolescent Clinics of North America, 12,* 493–535.

Cahill, L., & McGaugh, J. L. (1998). Mechanisms of emotional arousal and lasting declarative memory. *Trends in Neurosciences, 21,* 294–299.

Cahill, S. P., Rauch, S. A. M., Hembree, E. A., & Foa, E. B. (2003). Effect of cognitive-behavioral treatments for PTSD on anger. *Journal of Cognitive Psychotherapy, 17,* 113–131.

Cassiday, K. L., McNally, R. J., & Zeitlin, S. B. (1992). Cognitive processing of trauma cues in rape victims with post-traumatic stress disorder. *Cognitive Therapy and Research, 16,* 283–295.

Chan, A. O., & Silove, D. (2000). Nosological implications of psychotic symptoms with established posttraumatic stress disorder. *Australian and New Zealand Journal of Psychiatry, 34,* 522–525.

Chard, K. M. (2005). An evaluation of cognitive processing therapy for the treatment of posttraumatic stress disorder related to childhood sexual abuse. *Journal of Consulting and Clinical Psychology, 73,* 965–971.

Charney, D. S. (2004). Psychobiological mechanisms of resilience and vulnerability: Implications for successful adaptation to extreme stress. *American Journal of Psychiatry, 161,* 195–216.

Chemtob, C., Novaco, R. W., Hamada, R. S., & Gross, D. M. (1997). Cognitive-behavioral treatment for severe anger in posttraumatic stress disorder. *Journal of Consulting and Clinical Psychology, 65,* 184–189.

Chemtob, C., Roitblat, H. L., Hamada, R. S., Carlson, J. G., & Twentyman, C. T. (1988). A cognitive action theory of post-traumatic stress disorder. *Journal of Anxiety Disorders, 2,* 253–275.

Cheung, E., Alvaro, R., & Colotla, V. A. (2003). Psychological distress in workers with traumatic upper or lower limb amputations following industrial injuries. *Rehabilitation Psychology, 48,* 109–112.

Chu, J. A. (1998). *Rebuilding shattered lives*. New York: Wiley.

Clifft, M. A. (1986). Writing about psychiatric patients: Guidelines for disguising case material. *Bulletin of the Menninger Clinic, 50,* 511–524.

Cloitre, M., Koenen, K., Cohen, L. R., & Han, H. (2002). Skills training in affective and interpersonal regulation followed by exposure: A phase-based treatment for PTSD related to childhood abuse. *Journal of Consulting and Clinical Psychology, 70,* 1067–1074.

Coffey, S. F., Saladin, M. E., Drobes, D. J., Brady, K. T., Dansky, B. S., & Kilpatrick, D. G. (2002). Trauma and substance cue reactivity in individuals with comorbid posttraumatic stress disorder and cocaine or alcohol dependence. *Drug and Alcohol Dependence, 65,* 115–127.

Cohen, J. A. (2003). Treating acute posttraumatic reactions in children and adolescents. *Biological Psychiatry, 53,* 827–833.

Conway, M. A., Singer, J. A., & Tagini, A. (2004). The self and autobiographical memory: Correspondence and coherence. *Social Cognition, 22,* 491–529.

Cooke, A. L., & Shear, M. K. (2001). Treatment of a 50-year-old African woman whose chronic posttraumatic stress disorder went undiagnosed for over 20 years. *American Journal of Psychiatry, 158,* 866–870.

Corcoran, K., & Fischer, J. (2000). *Measures for clinical practice: A sourcebook* (2 vols., 3rd ed.). New York: Free Press.

Cox, B. J., & Taylor, S. (1999). Anxiety disorders: Panic and phobias. In T. Millon, P. Blaney, & R. Davis (Eds.), *Oxford textbook of psychopathology* (pp. 81–113). New York: Oxford University Press.

Creamer, M., Burgess, P., & Pattison, P. (1992). Reaction to trauma: A cognitive processing model. *Journal of Abnormal Psychology, 101,* 452–459.

Creamer, M., & Forbes, D. (2004). Military populations. In S. Taylor (Ed.), *Advances in the treatment of posttraumatic stress disorder: Cognitive-behavioral perspectives* (pp. 153–173). New York: Springer.

Crenshaw, D.A. (2001). Party hats on monsters. In H. G. Kaduson & C. E. Schaefer (Eds.), *101 more favorite play therapy techniques* (pp. 124–127). Northvale, NJ: Jason Aronson.

Dalgleish, T. (2004). Cognitive approaches to posttraumatic stress disorder: The evolution of multirepresentational theorizing. *Psychological Bulletin, 130,* 228–260.

Daly, R. J. (1983). Samuel Pepys and posttraumatic stress disorder. *British Journal of Psychiatry, 143,* 64–68.

Davey, G. C. L. (1992). Classical conditioning and the acquisition of human fears and phobias: A review and synthesis of the literature. *Advances in Behaviour Research and Therapy, 14,* 29–66.

Davidson, J. R. T. (1996). *Davidson Trauma Scale.* Toronto: Multi-Health Systems.

Davies, M. I., & Clark, D. M. (1998). Thought suppression produces a rebound effect with analogue post-traumatic intrusions. *Behaviour Research and Therapy, 36,* 571–582.

Davis, C. G., Lehman, D. R., Wortman, C. B., Silver, R. C., & Thompson, S. C. (1995). The undoing of traumatic life events. *Personality and Social Psychology Bulletin, 21,* 109–124.

Davis, M., Myers, K. M., Ressler, K. J., & Rothbaum, B. O. (2005). Facilitation of extinction of conditioned fear by D-clycloserine: Implications for psychotherapy. *Current Directions in Psychological Science, 14,* 214–219.

Davis, M., & Whalen, P. J. (2001). The amygdala: Vigilance and emotion. *Molecular Psychiatry, 6,* 13–34.

Davis, W. B., Mooney, D., Racusin, R., Ford, J. D., Fleischer, A., & McHugo, G. J. (2000). Predicting posttraumatic stress after hospitalization for pediatric injury. *Journal of the American Academy of Child and Adolescent Psychiatry, 39,* 576–583.

Deahl, M. P., Gillham, A. B., Thomas, J., Searle, M. M., & Srinivasan, M. (1994). Psychological sequelae following the Gulf War: Factors associated with subsequent morbidity and the effectiveness of psychological debriefing. *British Journal of Psychiatry, 165,* 60–65.

Dean, E. T. (1997). *Shook over hell: Post-traumatic stress, Vietnam, and the Civil War.* Cambridge, MA: Harvard University Press.

Deblinger, E., & Heflin, A. H. (1996). *Treating sexually abused children and their nonoffending parents: A cognitive behavioral approach.* Thousand Oaks, CA: Sage.

Deblinger, E., McLeer, S. V., & Henry, D. (1990). Cognitive behavioral treatment for sexually abused children suffering post-traumatic stress: Preliminary findings. *Journal of the American Academy of Child and Adolescent Psychiatry, 29,* 747–752.

De Jong, J. T. V. M., Komproe, I. H., van Ommeran, M., El Masri, M., Araya, M., Khaled, N., et al. (2001). Life events and posttraumatic stress disorder in 4 postconflict settings. *Journal of the American Medical Association, 286,* 555–562.

Delahanty, D. L., Raimonde, A. J., & Spoonster, E. (2000). Initial posttraumatic urinary cortisol levels predict subsequent PTSD symptoms in motor vehicle accidents. *Biological Psychiatry, 48,* 940–947.

Devilly, G. J., & Foa, E. B. (2001). Comments on Tarrier et al.'s study and the investigation of exposure and cognitive therapy. *Journal of Consulting and Clinical Psychology, 69,* 114–116.

DeYoung, M. (1988). The good touch/bad touch dilemma. *Child Welfare, 67,* 60–68.

Dickinson, J. J., Poole, D. A., & Bruck, M. (2005). Back to the future: A comment on the use of anatomical dolls in forensic interviews. *Journal of Forensic Psychology Practice, 5,* 63–74.

Dienstbier, R. A. (1989). Arousal and physiological toughness: Implications for mental and physical health. *Psychological Review, 96,* 84–100.

Difede, J., & Hoffman, H. G. (2002). Virtual reality exposure therapy for World Trade Center post-traumatic stress disorder: A case report. *CyberPsychology and Behavior, 5,* 529–535.

DiNardo, P., Brown, T. A., & Barlow, D. H. (1994). *Anxiety disorders interview schedule for DSM-IV.* New York: Graywind.

Dunmore, E., Clark, D. M., & Ehlers, A. (1997). Cognitive factors in persistent versus recovered post-traumatic stress disorder after physical or sexual assault: A pilot study. *Behavioural and Cognitive Psychotherapy, 25,* 147–159.

Dunmore, E., Clark, D. M., & Ehlers, A. (1999). Cognitive factors involved in the onset and maintenance of posttraumatic stress disorder (PTSD) after physical or sexual assault. *Behaviour Research and Therapy, 37,* 809–829.

Dunmore, E., Clark, D. M., & Ehlers, A. (2001). A prospective study of the role of cognitive factors in persistent posttraumatic stress disorder (PTSD) after physical or sexual assault. *Behaviour Research and Therapy, 39,* 1063–1084.

Easterbrook, J. A. (1959). The effect of emotion on cue utilization and the organization of behavior. *Psychological Review, 66,* 183–201.

Ehlers, A., & Clark, D. M. (2000). A cognitive model of posttraumatic stress disorder. *Behaviour Research and Therapy, 38,* 319–345.

Ehlers, A., Clark, D. M., Dunmore, E., Jaycox, L., Meadows, E., & Foa, E. B. (1998a). Predicting response to exposure treatment in PTSD: The role of mental defeat and alienation. *Journal of Traumatic Stress, 11,* 457–471.

Ehlers, A., Clark, D. M., Hackmann, A., McManus, F., Fennell, M., Herbert, C., et al. (2003). A randomized controlled trial of cognitive therapy, a self-help booklet, and repeated assessments as early interventions for posttraumatic stress disorder. *Archives of General Psychiatry, 60,* 1024–1032.

Ehlers, A., Hackmann, A., Steil, R., Clohessy, S., Wenninger, K., & Winter, H. (2002). The nature of intrusive memories after trauma: The warning signal hypothesis. *Behaviour Research and Therapy, 40,* 995–1002.

Ehlers, A., Maercker, A., & Boos, A. (2000). Posttraumatic stress disorder following political imprisonment: The role of mental defeat, alienation, and perceived permanent change. *Journal of Abnormal Psychology, 109,* 45–55.

Ehlers, A., Mayou, R. A., & Bryant, B. (1998b). Psychological predictors of chronic posttraumatic stress disorder after motor vehicle accidents. *Journal of Abnormal Psychology, 107,* 508–519.

Ehlers, A., & Steil, R. (1995). Maintenance of intrusive memories in posttraumatic stress disorder: A cognitive approach. *Behavioural and Cognitive Psychotherapy, 23,* 217–249.

Elbert, T., & Schauer, M. (2002). Burnt into memory. *Nature, 419,* 883.

Elhai, J. D., Gray, M. J., Naifeh, J. A., Butcher, J. J., Davis, J. L., Falsetti, S. A., et al. (2005). Utility of the Trauma Symptom Inventory's atypical response scale in detecting malingered posttraumatic stress disorder. *Assessment, 12,* 210–219.

Elhai, J. D., Ruggiero, K. J., Frueh, B. C., Beckham, J. C., & Gold, P. B. (2002). The infrequency-posttraumatic stress disorder scale (Fptsd) for the MMPI-2: Development and initial validation with veterans presenting with combat-related PTSD. *Journal of Personality Assessment, 79,* 531–549.

Emmons, K. M., & Rollnick, S. (2001). Motivational interviewing in health care settings: Opportunities and limitations. *American Journal of Preventive Medicine, 20,* 68–74.

Engelhard, I. M., Macklin, M. L., McNally, R. J., van den Hout, M. A., & Arntz, A. (2001). Emotion- and intrusion-based reasoning in Vietnam veterans with and without chronic posttraumatic stress disorder. *Behaviour Research and Therapy, 39,* 1339–1348.

Engelhard, I. M., van den Hout, M., Arntz, A., & McNally, R. J. (2002). A longitudinal study of "intrusion-based reasoning" and posttraumatic stress disorder after exposure to a train disaster. *Behaviour Research and Therapy, 40,* 1415–1424.

Fairbank, J. A., DeGood, D. E., & Jenkins, C. W. (1981). Behavioral treatment of a persistent post-traumatic startle response. *Journal of Behavior Therapy and Experimental Psychiatry, 12,* 321–324.

Farrell, S. P., Hains, A. A., & Davies, W. H. (1998). Cognitive behavioral interventions for sexually abused children exhibiting PTSD symptomatology. *Behavior Therapy, 29,* 241–255.

Fedoroff, I. C., Taylor, S., Asmundson, G. J. G., & Koch, W. J. (2000). Cognitive factors in traumatic stress reactions: Predicting PTSD symptoms from anxiety sensitivity and beliefs about harmful events. *Behavioural and Cognitive Psychotherapy, 28,* 5–15.

Feeny, N. C., Hembree, E. A., & Zoellner, L. A. (2003). Myths regarding exposure therapy for PTSD. *Cognitive and Behavioral Practice, 10,* 85–90.

Fellous, J.-M., Armony, J. L., & LeDoux, J. E. (2002). Emotional circuits and computational neuroscience. In M. A. Arbib (Ed.), *Handbook of brain theory and neural networks* (2nd ed., pp. 1–6). Cambridge, MA: MIT Press.

Feske, U. (2001). Treating low-income and African-American women with posttraumatic stress disorder: A case series. *Behavior Therapy, 32,* 585–601.

First, M. B., Spitzer, R. L., Gibbon, M., & Williams, J. B. W. (1996). *Structured Clinical Interview for DSM-IV.* New York: New York State Psychiatric Institute.

First, M. B., Spitzer, R. L., Gibbon, M., Williams, J. B. W., & Lorna, B. (1994). *Structured Clinical Interview for DSM-IV Axis II Personality Disorders (SCID-II) (Version 2.0).* New York: New York State Psychiatric Institute.

Flannery, R. B. (2002). Addressing psychological trauma in dementia sufferers. *American Journal of Alzheimer's Disease and Other Dementias, 17,* 281–285.

Fletcher, K. E. (1996). Childhood posttraumatic stress disorder. In E. Mash & R. Barkley (Eds.), *Child psychopathology* (pp. 242–276). New York: Guilford Press.

Flynn, B. W., & Norwood, A. E. (2004). Defining normal psychological reactions to disaster. *Psychiatric Annals, 34,* 597–603.

Foa, E. B. (1995). *The Posttraumatic Diagnostic Scale (PDS) manual.* Minneapolis, MN: National Computer Systems.

Foa, E. B. (2000). Psychosocial treatment of posttraumatic stress disorder. *Journal of Clinical Psychiatry, 61*(Suppl. 5), 43–48.

Foa, E. B., Dancu, C. V., Hembree, E. A., Jaycox, L. H., Meadows, E. A., & Street, G. P. (1999a). A comparison of exposure therapy, stress inoculation training, and their combination for reducing posttraumatic stress disorder in female assault victims. *Journal of Consulting and Clinical Psychology, 67,* 194–200.

Foa, E. B., Davidson, J. R. T., & Frances, A. (1999b). Treatment of PTSD: The NIH expert consensus guideline series. *Journal of Clinical Psychiatry, 60*(Suppl. 16), 4–76.

Foa, E. B., Ehlers, A., Clark, D. M., Tolin, D. F., & Orsillo, S. M. (1999c). The posttraumatic cognitions inventory (PTCI): Development and validation. *Psychological Assessment, 11,* 303–314.

Foa, E. B., & Hearst-Ikeda, D. (1996). Emotional dissociation in response to trauma: An information-processing approach. In L. K. Michelson & W. J. Ray (Eds.), *Handbook of dissociation: Theoretical and clinical perspectives* (pp. 207–222). New York: Plenum Press.

Foa, E. B., Hearst-Ikeda, D., & Perry, K. J. (1995a). Evaluation of a brief cognitive-behavior program for the prevention of chronic PTSD in recent assault victims. *Journal of Consulting and Clinical Psychology, 63,* 948–955.

Foa, E. B., Hembree, E. A., Cahill, S. P., Rauch, S. A. M., Riggs, D. S., Feeny, N. C., et al. (2005). Randomized trial of prolonged exposure for posttraumatic stress disorder with and without cognitive restructuring: Outcome at academic and community clinics. *Journal of Consulting and Clinical Psychology, 73,* 953–964.

Foa, E. B., & Kozak, M. J. (1986). Emotional processing of fear: Exposure to corrective information. *Psychological Bulletin, 99,* 20–35.

Foa, E. B., Molnar, C., & Cashman, L. (1995b). Change in rape narratives during exposure therapy for posttraumatic stress disorder. *Journal of Traumatic Stress, 8,* 675–690.

Foa, E. B., & Rauch, S. A. M. (2004). Cognitive changes during prolonged exposure alone versus prolonged exposure and cognitive restructuring in female assault survivors with PTSD. *Journal of Consulting and Clinical Psychology, 72,* 879–884.

Foa, E. B., & Riggs, D. S. (1993). Posttraumatic stress disorder in rape victims. In J. Oldham, M. B. Riba, & A. Tasman (Eds.), *American Psychiatric Press review of psychiatry* (Vol. 12, pp. 273–303). Washington, DC: American Psychiatric Press.

Foa, E. B., Riggs, D. S., Massie, E. D., & Yarczower, M. (1995c). The impact of fear activation and anger on the efficacy of exposure treatment for posttraumatic stress disorder. *Behavior Therapy, 26,* 487–499.

Foa, E. B., & Rothbaum, B. O. (1998). *Treating the trauma of rape.* New York: Guilford Press.

Foa, E. B., Rothbaum, R. O., Riggs, D. S., & Murdock, T. B. (1991). Treatment of posttraumatic stress disorder in rape victims: A comparison between cognitive-behavioral procedures and counseling. *Journal of Consulting and Clinical Psychology, 59,* 715–723.

Foa, E. B., Steketee, G., & Rothbaum, B. O. (1989). Behavioral/cognitive conceptualizations of post-traumatic stress disorder. *Behavior Therapy, 20,* 155–176.

Foa, E. B., Zinbarg, R., & Rothbaum, B. O. (1992). Uncontrollability and unpredictability in post-traumatic stress disorder: An animal model. *Psychological Bulletin, 112,* 218–238.

Foa, E. B., Zoellner, L. A., Feeny, N. C., Hembree, E. A., & Alvarez-Conrad, J. (2002). Does imaginal exposure exacerbate PTSD symptoms? *Journal of Consulting and Clinical Psychology, 70,* 1022–1028.

Fontana, A., Litz, B., & Rosenheck, R. (2000). Impact of combat and sexual harassment on the severity of posttraumatic stress disorder among men and women peacekeepers in Somalia. *Journal of Nervous and Mental Disease, 188,* 163–169.

Forbes, D., Creamer, M., Hawthorne, G., Allen, N., & McHugh, T. (2003). Comorbidity as a predictor of symptom change after treatment in combat-related posttraumatic stress disorder. *Journal of Nervous and Mental Disease, 191,* 93–99.

Frueh, B. C., Elhai, J. D., Gold, P. B., Monnier, J., Magruder, K. M., Keane, T. M., et al. (2003). Disability compensation seeking among veterans evaluated for posttraumatic stress disorder. *Psychiatric Services, 54,* 84–91.

Frueh, B. C., Elhai, J. D., Grubaugh, A. L., Monnier, J., Kashdan, T. B., Sauvageot,

J. A., et al. (2005). Documented combat exposure of US veterans seeking treatment for combat-related post-traumatic stress disorder. *British Journal of Psychiatry, 186*, 467–472.

Fullerton, C. S., Ursano, R. J., & Wang, L. (2004). Acute stress disorder, posttraumatic stress disorder, and depression in disaster or rescue workers. *American Journal of Psychiatry, 161*, 1370–1376.

Furmark, T., Tillfors, M., Marteinsdottir, I., Fischer, H., Pissiota, A., Langstrom, B., et al. (2002). Common changes in cerebral blood flow in patients with social phobia treated with citalopram or cognitive-behavioral therapy. *Archives of General Psychiatry, 59*, 425–433.

Galliano, G., Noble, L. M., Travis, L. A., & Puechl, C. (1993). Victim reactions during rape/sexual assault. *Journal of Interpersonal Violence, 8*, 109–114.

Gallup, G. G., & Rager, D. R. (1996). Tonic immobility as a model of extreme stress of behavioral inhibition: Issues of methodology and measurement. In M. Kavaliers (Ed.), *Motor activity and movement disorders* (pp. 57–80). Totowa, NJ: Humana Press.

Garland, E. J. (2004). Facing the evidence: Antidepressant treatment in children and adolescents. *Canadian Medical Association Journal, 170*, 490–491.

Geracoti, T. D., Baker, D. G., Ekhator, N. N., West, S. A., Hill, K. K., Bruce, A. B., et al. (2001). CSF norepinephrine concentrations in posttraumatic stress disorder. *American Journal of Psychiatry, 158*, 1227–1230.

Gewirtz, J. C., McNish, K. A., & Davis, M. (2000). Is the hippocampus necessary for contextual fear conditioning? *Behavioural Brain Research, 110*, 83–95.

Gibson, L. E., & Leitenberg, H. (2000). Child sexual abuse prevention programs: Do they decrease the occurrence of child sexual abuse? *Child Abuse and Neglect, 24*, 1115–1125.

Gilbertson, M. W., Shenton, M. E., Ciszewski, A., Kasai, K., Lasko, N. B., Orr, S. P., et al. (2002). Smaller hippocampal volume predicts pathologic vulnerability to psychological trauma. *Nature Neuroscience, 5*, 1242–1247.

Gillespie, K., Duffy, M., Hackmann, A., & Clark, D. M. (2002). Community based cognitive therapy in the treatment of posttraumatic stress disorder following the Omagh bomb. *Behaviour Research and Therapy, 40*, 345–357.

Ginsberg, D. L. (2004). Women and anxiety disorders: Implications for diagnosis and treatment. *CNS Spectrums, 9*, 1–16.

Glover, H. (1984). Survival guilt and the Vietnam veteran. *Journal of Nervous and Mental Disease, 172*, 393–397.

Goldapple, K., Segal, Z., Garson, C., Lau, M., Bieling, P., Kennedy, S., et al. (2004). Modulation of cortical-limbic pathways in major depression. *Archives of General Psychiatry, 61*, 34–41.

Golier, J., & Yehuda, R. (2002). Neuropsychological processes in post-traumatic stress disorder. *Psychiatric Clinics of North America, 25*, 295–315.

Grace, M. C., Green, B. L., Lindy, J. D., & Leonard, A. C. (1993). The Buffalo Creek disaster: A 14-year follow-up. In J. P. Wilson & B. Raphael (Eds.), *International handbook of traumatic stress syndromes* (pp. 441–449). New York: Plenum Press.

Graham, J. R. (1999). *MMPI-2: Assessing personality and psychopathology.* New York: Oxford University Press.

Gramzow, R., & Tangey, J. P. (1992). Proneness to shame and the narcissistic personality. *Personality and Social Psychology Bulletin, 18,* 369–376.

Gray, J. A. (1988). *The psychology of fear and stress* (2nd ed.). Cambridge: Cambridge University Press.

Gray, M., Bolton, E. E., & Litz, B. T. (2004). A longitudinal analysis of PTSD symptom course: Delayed-onset PTSD in Somalia peacekeepers. *Journal of Consulting and Clinical Psychology, 72,* 909–913.

Green, B. L., Lindy, J. D., Grace, M. C., Gleser, G. C., Leonard, A. C., Korol, M., et al. (1990). Buffalo Creek survivors in the second decade: Stability of stress symptoms. *American Journal of Orthopsychiatry, 60,* 43–54.

Grillon, C., & Morgan, C. A. (1999). Fear-potentiated startle conditioning to explicit and contextual cues in Gulf War veterans with posttraumatic stress disorder. *Journal of Abnormal Psychology, 108,* 134–142.

Grossman, R., Buchsbaum, M. S., & Yehuda, R. (2002). Neuroimaging studies in post-traumatic stress disorder. *Psychiatric Clinics of North America, 25,* 317–340.

Grunert, B. K., Devine, C. A., Matloub, H. S., Sanger, J. R., Yousef, N. J., Anderson, R. C., et al. (1990). Psychological adjustment following work-related hand injury: 18-month follow-up. *Annals of Plastic Surgery, 29,* 537–542.

Gurvits, T. V., Gilbertson, M. W., Lasko, N. B., Tarhan, A. S., Simeon, D., Macklin, M. L., et al. (2000). Neurologic soft signs in chronic posttraumatic stress disorder. *Archives of General Psychiatry, 57,* 181–186.

Halligan, S. L., Clark, D. M., & Ehlers, A. (2002). Cognitive processing, memory, and the development of PTSD symptoms: Two experimental analogue studies. *Journal of Behavior Therapy and Experimental Psychiatry, 33,* 73–89.

Halligan, S. L., Michael, T., Clark, D. M., & Ehlers, A. (2003). Posttraumatic stress disorder following assault: The role of cognitive processing, trauma memory, and appraisals. *Journal of Consulting and Clinical Psychology, 71,* 419–431.

Harvey, A. G., & Bryant, R. A. (2002). Acute stress disorder: A synthesis and critique. *Psychological Bulletin, 128,* 886–902.

Harvey, A. G., Bryant, R. A., & Dang, S. T. (1998). Autobiographical memory in acute stress disorder. *Journal of Consulting and Clinical Psychology, 66,* 500–506.

Hebert, M., & Tourigny, M. (2004). Child sexual abuse prevention: A review of evaluative studies and recommendations for program development. In S. P. Shohov (Ed.), *Advances in psychology research* (Vol. 29, pp. 123–155). Hauppauge, NY: Nova.

Heidt, J. M., Marx, B. P., & Forsyth, J. P. (2005). Tonic immobility and childhood sexual abuse: A preliminary report evaluating the sequela of rape-induced paralysis. *Behaviour Research and Therapy, 43,* 1157–1171.

Hellawell, S. J., & Brewin, C. R. (2004). A comparison of flashbacks and ordinary autobiographical memories of trauma: Content and language. *Behaviour Research and Therapy, 42,* 1–12.

Hembree, E. A., Foa, E. B., Dorfan, N. M., Street, G. P., Tu, X., & Kowalski, J. (2003). Do patients drop out prematurely from exposure therapy for PTSD? *Journal of Traumatic Stress, 16,* 555–562.

Henderson, D., Hargreaves, I., Gregory, S., & Williams, J. M. G. (2002). Autobiographical memory and emotion in a non-clinical sample of women with and without a reported history of childhood sexual abuse. *British Journal of Clinical Psychology, 41,* 129–141.

Heresco-Levy, U., Kremer, I., Javitt, D. C., Goichman, R., Reshef, A., Blanaru, M., et al. (2002). Pilot-controlled trial of D-cycloserine for the treatment of posttraumatic stress disorder. *International Journal of Neuropsychopharmacology, 5,* 301–307.

Herman, J. L. (1997). *Trauma and recovery* (rev. ed.). New York: Basic Books.

Hinton, D. E., Chhean, D., Pich, V., Safren, S. A., Hofmann, S. G., & Pollack, M. H. (2005). A randomized controlled trial of CBT for Cambodian refugees with treatment-resistant PTSD and panic attacks: A cross-over design. *Journal of Traumatic Stress, 18,* 617–629.

Hinton, D. E., Pham, T., Tran, M., Safren, S. A., Otto, M. W., & Pollack, M. H. (2004). CBT for Vietnamese refugees with treatment-resistant PTSD and panic attacks. *Journal of Traumatic Stress, 17,* 429–433.

Hofer, B. K., & Pintrich, P. R. (2002). *Personal epistemology: The psychology of beliefs about knowledge and knowing.* Mahwah, NJ: Erlbaum.

Horowitz, M. J. (1975). Intrusive and repetitive thought after experimental stress. *Archives of General Psychiatry, 32,* 1457–1463.

Horowitz, M. J. (2001). *Stress response syndromes* (4th ed.). Northvale, NJ: Jason Aronson.

Hungerford, A. (2005). The use of anatomically detailed dolls in forensic investigations: Developmental considerations. *Journal of Forensic Psychology Practice, 5,* 75–87.

Hyer, L., & Sohnle, S. J. (2001). *Trauma among older people: Issues and treatment.* New York: Brunner-Routledge.

Hyer, L., Summers, M. N., Braswell, L., & Boyd, S. (1995). Posttraumatic stress disorder: Silent problem among older combat veterans. *Psychotherapy, 32,* 348–364.

Hyler, S. E. (1994). *Personality Diagnostic Questionnaire–4.* New York: New York State Psychiatric Institute.

Hyman, S. M., Gold, S. N., & Cott, M. A. (2003). Forms of social support that moderate PTSD in childhood sexual abuse survivors. *Journal of Family Violence, 18,* 295–300.

Jacobsen, L. K., Southwick, S. M., & Kosten, T. R. (2001). Substance use disorders in patients with posttraumatic stress disorder: A review of the literature. *American Journal of Psychiatry, 158,* 1184–1190.

Jacobson, N. S., & Margolin, G. (1979). *Marital therapy.* New York: Brunner/Mazel.

Jang, K. L., Stein, M. B., Taylor, S., Livesley, W. J., & Asmundson, G. J. G. (2003). Exposure to traumatic events and experiences: Aetiological relationships with personality function. *Psychiatry Research, 120,* 61–69.

Janoff-Bulman, R. (1989). Assumptive worlds and the stress of traumatic events: Applications of the schema construct. *Social Cognition, 7,* 113–136.

Janoff-Bulman, R. (1992). *Shattered assumptions.* New York: Free Press.

Jaycox, L. H., & Foa, E. B. (1996). Obstacles in implementing exposure therapy for PTSD: Case discussions and practical solutions. *Clinical Psychology and Psychotherapy, 3,* 176–184.

Johnston, D. (2000). A series of cases of dementia presenting with PTSD symptoms in World War II combat veterans. *Journal of the American Geriatric Society, 48,* 70–72.

Jones, B. P., Duncan, V. V., Brouwers, P., & Mirsky, A. F. (1991). Cognition in eating disorders. *Journal of Clinical and Experimental Neuropsychology, 13,* 711–728.

Jones, C., Griffiths, R. D., & Humphris, G. (2000). Disturbed memory and amnesia related to intensive care. *Memory, 8,* 79–94.

Jones, D. S. (1997). Worry can. In H. G. Kaduson & C. E. Schaefer (Eds.), *101 favorite play therapy techniques* (pp. 254–256). Northvale, NJ: Jason Aronson.

Jones, E., & Wessely, S. (2003). "Forward psychiatry" in the military: Its origins and effectiveness. *Journal of Traumatic Stress, 16,* 411–419.

Jongedijk, R. A., Carlier, I. V. E., Schreuder, B. J. N., & Gersons, B. P. R. (1996). Complex posttraumatic stress disorder: An exploratory investigation of PTSD and DES DOS among Dutch war veterans. *Journal of Traumatic Stress, 9,* 577–586.

Kabat-Zinn, J. (1990). *Full catastrophe living.* New York: Delta.

Kaduson, H. G., & Schaefer, C. (1997). *101 favorite play therapy techniques.* Northvale, NJ: Jason Aronson.

Kaduson, H. G., & Schaefer, C. (2001). *101 more favorite play therapy techniques.* Northvale, NJ: Jason Aronson.

Kardiner, A. (1941). *The traumatic neuroses of war.* New York: Hoeber.

Karlamangla, A. S., Singer, B. H., McEwen, B. S., Rowe, J. W., & Seeman, T. E. (2002). Allostatic load as a predictor of functional decline: MacArthur studies of successful aging. *Journal of Clinical Epidemiology, 55,* 696–710.

Kataoka, S. H., Stein, B. D., Jaycox, L. H., Wong, M., Escudero, P., Tu, W., et al. (2003). A school-based mental health program for traumatized Latino immigrant children. *Journal of the American Academy of Child and Adolescent Psychiatry, 42,* 311–318.

Kaufman, G. (1989). *The psychology of shame.* New York: Springer.

Kaysen, D., Resick, P. A., & Wise, D. (2003). Living in danger: The impact of chronic traumatization and the traumatic context on posttraumatic stress disorder. *Trauma, Violence, and Abuse, 4,* 247–264.

Keane, T. M., Fairbank, J. A., Caddell, J. M., Zimmering, R. T., & Bender, M. E. (1985). A behavioral approach to assessing and treating posttraumatic stress disorder in Vietnam veterans. In C. R. Figley (Ed.), *Trauma and its wake* (pp. 257–294). New York: Brunner/Mazel.

Keane, T. M., Street, A. E., & Stafford, J. (2004). The assessment of military-related PTSD. In J. P. Wilson & T. M. Keane (Eds.), *Assessing psychological trauma and PTSD* (2nd ed., pp. 262–285). New York: Guilford Press.

Kendler, K. S., Walters, E. E., Neale, M. C., Kessler, R. C., Heath, A. C., & Eaves, L. J. (1995). The structure of the genetic and environmental risk factors for six major psychiatric disorders in women: Phobia, generalized anxiety disorder, panic disorder, bulimia, major depression and alcoholism. *Archives of General Psychiatry, 52,* 374–383.

Keren, M., & Tyano, S. (2000). A case-study of PTSD in infancy: Diagnostic, neurophysiological, developmental and therapeutic aspects. *Israel Journal of Psychiatric and Related Sciences, 37,* 236–246.

Kessler, R. C., Sonnega, A., Bromet, E., Hughes, M., & Nelson, C. B. (1995). Post-traumatic stress disorder in the National Comorbidity Survey. *Archives of General Psychiatry, 52,* 1048–1060.

Kessler, R. C., & Ustun, T. B. (2004). The World Mental Health (WMH) Survey Initiative version of the World Health Organization (WHO) Composite International Diagnostic Interview (CIDI). *International Journal of Methods in Psychiatric Research, 13,* 93–121.

Kilpatrick, D. G., & Acierno, R. (2003). Mental health needs of crime victims: Epidemiology and outcomes. *Journal of Traumatic Stress, 16,* 119–132.

Kilpatrick, D. G., Ruggiero, K. J., Acierno, R., Saunders, B. E., Resnick, H. S., & Best, C. L. (2003). Violence and risk of PTSD, major depression, substance abuse/dependence, and comorbidity: Results from the National Survey of Adolescents. *Journal of Consulting and Clinical Psychology, 71,* 692–700.

Kilpatrick, D. G., Saunders, B. E., Amick-McMullan, A., Best, C. L., Veronen, L. J., & Resnick, H. S. (1989). Victim and crime factors associated with the development of crime-related post-traumatic stress disorder. *Behavior Therapy, 20,* 199–214.

King, D. W., King, L. A., Erickson, D. J., Huang, M. T., Sharkansky, E. J., & Wolf, J. (2000a). Posttraumatic stress disorder and retrospectively reported stressor exposure: A longitudinal prediction model. *Journal of Abnormal Psychology, 109,* 624–633.

King, N. J., Tonge, B. J., Mullen, P., Myerson, N., Heyne, D., Rollings, S., et al. (2000b). Treating sexually abused children with posttraumatic stress symptoms: A randomized clinical trial. *Journal of the American Academy of Child and Adolescent Psychiatry, 39,* 1347–1355.

Klemm, W. R. (1977). Identity of sensory and motor systems that are critical to the immobility reflex (animal hypnosis). *Psychological Record, 1,* 145–159.

Koch, W. J., & Taylor, S. (1995). Assessment and treatment of motor vehicle accident victims. *Cognitive and Behavioral Practice, 2,* 327–342.

Koenen, K. C., Driver, K. L., Oscar-Berman, M., Wolfe, J., Folsom, S., Huang, M. T., et al. (2001). Measures of prefrontal system dysfunction in posttraumatic stress disorder. *Brain and Cognition, 45,* 64–78.

Koss, M. P., Tromp, S., & Tharan, M. (1995). Traumatic memories: Empirical foundations, forensic and clinical implications. *Clinical Psychology: Science and Practice, 2,* 111–132.

Krakow, B., Hollifield, M., Johnston, L., Koss, M., Schrader, R., Warner, T. D., et al. (2001a). Imagery rehearsal therapy for chronic nightmares in sexual assault survivors with posttraumatic stress disorder: A randomized controlled trial. *Journal of the American Medical Association, 286,* 537–545.

Krakow, B., Sandoval, D., Schrader, R., Keuhne, B., McBride, L., Yau, C. L., et al.

(2001b). Treatment of chronic nightmares in adjudicated adolescent girls in a residual facility. *Journal of Adolescent Health, 29*, 94–100.

Kubany, E. S. (1997). Application of cognitive therapy for trauma-related guilt (CT-TRG) with a Vietnam veteran troubled by multiple sources of guilt. *Cognitive and Behavioral Practice, 4*, 213–244.

Kubany, E. S. (1998). Cognitive therapy for trauma-related guilt. In V. M. Follette, J. I. Ruzek, & F. R. Abueg (Eds.), *Cognitive-behavioral therapies for trauma* (pp. 124–161). New York: Guilford Press.

Kubany, E. S., Haynes, S. N., Abueg, F. R., Manke, F. P., Brennan, J. M., & Stahura, C. (1996). Development and validation of the trauma-related guilt inventory (TRGI). *Psychological Assessment, 8*, 428–444.

Kubany, E. S., Hill, E. E., Owens, J. A., Iannce-Spencer, C., McCraig, M. A., Tremayne, K. J., et al. (2004). Cognitive trauma therapy for battered women with PTSD (CTT-BW). *Journal of Consulting and Clinical Psychology, 72*, 3–18.

Kubany, E. S., & Manke, F. P. (1995). Cognitive therapy for trauma-related guilt: Conceptual bases and treatment outlines. *Cognitive and Behavioral Practice, 2*, 27–61.

Kubany, E. S., & Watson, S. B. (2002). Cognitive trauma therapy for formerly battered women with PTSD: Conceptual bases and treatment outlines. *Cognitive and Behavioral Practice, 9*, 111–127.

Kulka, R. A., Schlenger, W. E., Fairbank, J. A., Hough, R. L., Jordan, B. K., Marmar, C. R., et al. (1990). *Trauma and the Vietnam war generation*. New York: Brunner/Mazel.

Lamberg, L. (2004). Psychiatrists strive to quell soldiers' nightmares of war. *Journal of the American Medical Association, 292*, 1539–1540.

Lamprecht, R., & LeDoux, J. (2004). Structural plasticity and memory. *Nature Reviews, Neuroscience, 5*, 45–54.

Lang, P. J., Bradley, M. M., & Cuthbert, B. N. (1998). Emotion, motivation, and anxiety: Brain mechanisms and psychophysiology. *Biological Psychiatry, 44*, 1248–1263.

Leahy, R. L. (2001). *Overcoming resistance in cognitive therapy*. New York: Guilford Press.

Leahy, R. L. (2003). *Cognitive therapy techniques: A practitioner's guide*. New York: Guilford Press.

LeDoux, J. E. (2000). Emotion circuits in the brain. *Annual Review of Neuroscience, 23*, 155–184.

Lee, D. A., Scragg, P., & Turner, S. (2001). The role of shame and guilt in traumatic events: A clinical model of shame-based and guilt-based PTSD. *British Journal of Medical Psychology, 74*, 451–466.

Lehman, D. R., Wortman, C. B., & Williams, A. F. (1987). Long-term effects of losing a spouse or child in a motor vehicle crash. *Journal of Personality and Social Psychology, 52*, 218–231.

Lerner, P. (2003). *Hysterical men: War, psychiatry, and the politics of trauma in Germany, 1890–1930*. New York: Cornell University Press.

Levitt, J. T., & Cloitre, M. (2005). A clinician's guide to STAIR/MPE: Treatment for PTSD related to childhood abuse. *Cognitive and Behavioral Practice, 12*, 40–52.

Linehan, M. M. (1993). *Cognitive-behavioral treatment of borderline personality disorder.* New York: Guilford Press.

Litz, B. T., Schlenger, W. E., Weathers, F. W., Caddell, J. M., Fairbank, J. A., & LaVange, L. M. (1997). Predictors of emotional numbing in posttraumatic stress disorder. *Journal of Traumatic Stress, 10,* 607–618.

Livanou, M., Başoğlu, M., Marks, I. M., de Silva, P., Noshirvani, H., Lovell, K., et al. (2002). Beliefs, sense of control and treatment outcome in post-traumatic stress disorder. *Psychological Medicine, 32,* 157–165.

Lonigan, C. J., Phillips, B. M., & Richey, J. A. (2003). Posttraumatic stress disorder in children: Diagnosis, assessment, and associated features. *Child and Adolescent Clinics of North America, 12,* 171–194.

Loo, C. M., Fairbank, J. A., Scurfield, R. M., Ruch, L. O., King, D. W., Adams, L. J., et al. (2001). Measuring exposure to racism: Development and validation of a race-related stressor scale (RRSS) for Asian American Vietnam veterans. *Psychological Assessment, 13,* 503–520.

Lovibond, P. F. (1998). Long-term stability of depression, anxiety, and stress syndromes. *Journal of Abnormal Psychology, 107,* 520–526.

Lucas, J. A., Telch, M. J., & Bigler, E. D. (1991). Memory functioning in panic disorder: A neuropsychological perspective. *Journal of Anxiety Disorders, 5,* 1–20.

Lyons, M. J., Goldberg, J., Eisen, S. A., True, W., Tsuang, M. T., Meyer, J. M., et al. (1993). Do genes influence exposure to trauma? A twin study of combat. *American Journal of Medical Genetics (Neuropsychiatric Genetics), 48,* 22–27.

Macklin, M. L., Metzger, L. J., Litz, B. T., McNally, R. J., Lasko, N. B., Orr, S. P., et al. (1998). Lower pre-combat intelligence is a risk factor for posttraumatic stress disorder. *Journal of Consulting and Clinical Psychology, 66,* 323–326.

Maercker, A. (2002). Life-review technique in the treatment of PTSD in elderly patients: Rationale and three single case studies. *Journal of Clinical Geropsychology, 8,* 239–249.

March, J. S., Amaya-Jackson, L., Murray, M., & Schulte, A. (1998). Cognitive-behavioral psychotherapy for children and adolescents with post-traumatic stress disorder following a single-incident stressor. *Journal of the American Academy of Child and Adolescent Psychiatry, 37,* 585–593.

Marks, I., Lovell, K., Noshirvani, H., Livanou, M., & Thrasher, S. (1998). Treatment of posttraumatic stress disorder by exposure and/or cognitive restructuring. *Archives of General Psychiatry, 55,* 317–325.

Marlatt, G. A., & Donovan, D. M. (Eds.). (2005). *Relapse prevention: Maintenance strategies in the treatment of addictive behaviors* (2nd ed.). New York: Guilford Press.

Marsella, A. J., Friedman, M. J., Gerrity, E. T., & Scurfield, R. M. (1996). Ethnocultural aspects of PTSD: Some closing thoughts. In A. J. Marsella, M. J. Friedman, E. T. Gerrity, & R. M. Scurfield (Eds.), *Ethnocultural aspects of posttraumatic stress disorder: Issues, research, and clinical applications* (pp. 529–538). Washington, DC: American Psychological Association.

Marshall, W. L., Laws, D. R., & Barbaree, H. E. (1990). *Handbook of sexual assault: Issues, theories, and treatment of the offender.* New York: Plenum Press.

Matsakis, A. (1996). *I can't get over it* (2nd ed.). Oakland, CA: New Harbinger.

Matsakis, A. (1998). *Trust after trauma*. Oakland, CA: New Harbinger.

Matsakis, A. (2003). *The rape recovery handbook*. Oakland, CA: New Harbinger.

McCall, G. J., & Resick, P. A. (2003). A pilot study of PTSD symptoms among Kalahari bushmen. *Journal of Traumatic Stress, 16*, 445–450.

McCann, I. L., & Pearlman, L. A. (1990). *Psychological trauma and the adult survivor*. New York: Brunner/Mazel.

McCarroll, J. E., Ursano, R. J., Fullerton, C. S., Liu, X., & Lundy, A. (2001). Effects of exposure to death in a war mortuary on posttraumatic stress disorder symptoms of intrusion and avoidance. *Journal of Nervous and Mental Disease, 189*, 44–48.

McCloskey, L. A., & Walker, M. (2000). Posttraumatic stress in children exposed to family violence and single-event trauma. *Journal of the American Academy of Child and Adolescent Psychiatry, 39*, 108–115.

McCrone, P., Knapp, M., & Cawkill, P. (2003). Posttraumatic stress disorder (PTSD) in the armed forces: Health economic considerations. *Journal of Traumatic Stress, 16*, 519–522.

McFarlane, A. C., Atchison, M., & Yehuda, R. (1997). The acute stress response following motor vehicle accidents and its relation to PTSD. *Annuals of the New York Academy of Sciences, 821*, 437–441.

McFarlane, A. C., Yehuda, R., & Clark, C. R. (2002). Biologic models of traumatic memories and post-traumatic stress disorder: The role of neural networks. *Psychiatric Clinics of North America, 25*, 253–270.

McLean, L. M., & Gallop, R. (2003). Implications of childhood sexual abuse for adult borderline personality disorder and complex posttraumatic stress disorder. *American Journal of Psychiatry, 160*, 369–371.

McMullin, R. E. (2000). *The new handbook of cognitive therapy techniques*. New York: Norton.

McNally, R. J. (1998a). Experimental approaches to cognitive abnormality in posttraumatic stress disorder. *Clinical Psychology Review, 18*, 971–982.

McNally, R. J. (1998b). Information-processing abnormalities in anxiety disorders: Implications for cognitive neuroscience. *Cognition and Emotion, 12*, 479–495.

McNally, R. J. (2003a). Psychological mechanisms in acute response to trauma. *Biological Psychiatry, 53*, 779–788.

McNally, R. J. (2003b). *Remembering trauma*. Cambridge, MA: Harvard University Press.

McNally, R. J., Amir, N., & Lipke, H. J. (1996). Subliminal processing of threat cues in posttraumatic stress disorder? *Journal of Anxiety Disorders, 10*, 115–128.

McNally, R. J., Lasko, N. B., Macklin, M. L., & Pitman, R. K. (1995). Autobiographical memory disturbance in combat-related posttraumatic stress disorder. *Behaviour Research and Therapy, 33*, 619–630.

McNally, R. J., Litz, B. T., Prassas, A., Shin, L. M., & Weathers, F. W. (1994). Emotional priming of autobiographical memory in post-traumatic stress disorder. *Cognition and Emotion, 8*, 351–367.

McNally, R. J., Metzger, L. J., Lasko, N. B., Clancy, S. A., & Pitman, R. K. (1998).

Directed forgetting of trauma cues in adult survivors of childhood sexual abuse with and without posttraumatic stress disorder. *Journal of Abnormal Psychology, 107,* 596–601.

Meadows, E. A., & Foa, E. B. (1998). Intrusion, arousal, and avoidance: Sexual trauma survivors. In V. M. Follette, J. I. Ruzek, & F. R. Abueg (Eds.), *Cognitive-behavioral therapies for trauma* (pp. 100–123). New York: Guilford Press.

Messman-Moore, T. L., & Long, P. J. (2003). The role of childhood sexual abuse sequelae in the sexual revictimization of women: An empirical review and theoretical reformulation. *Clinical Psychology Review, 23,* 537–571.

Metzger, L. J., Orr, S. P., Berry, N. J., Ahern, C. E., Lasko, N. B., & Pitman, R. K. (1999). Physiological reactivity to startling noises in women with PTSD. *Journal of Abnormal Psychology, 108,* 347–352.

Meyer, C., & Taylor, S. (1986). Adjustment to rape. *Journal of Personality and Social Psychology, 50,* 1226–1334.

Meyer, T. M. (2003). Psychological aspects of mutilating hand injuries. *Hand Clinics, 19,* 41–49.

Miller, W. R. (1995). *Motivational enhancement therapy with drug users.* Albuquerque, NM: University of New Mexico.

Miller, W. R., & Rollnick, S. (2002). *Motivational interviewing: Preparing people for change* (2nd ed.). New York: Guilford Press.

Mitchell, J. T., & Everly, G. S. (2000). Critical incident stress management and critical incident stress debriefings: Evolutions, effects and outcomes. In B. Raphael & J. P. Wilson (Eds.), *Psychological debriefing: Theory, practice and evidence* (pp. 71–90). New York: Cambridge University Press.

Mitchell, K. J., Finkelhor, D., & Wolak, J. (2001). Risk factors for and impact of online sexual solicitation of youth. *Journal of the American Medical Association, 285,* 3011–3014.

Mitchell, K. J., Finkelhor, D., & Wolak, J. (2003a). The exposure of youth to unwanted sexual material on the Internet: A national survey of risk, impact, and prevention. *Youth and Society, 34,* 330–358.

Mitchell, K. J., Finkelhor, D., & Wolak, J. (2003b). Victimization of youths on the Internet. *Journal of Aggression, Maltreatment, and Trauma, 8,* 1–39.

Mittal, D., Torres, R., Abashidze, A., & Jimerson, N. (2001). Worsening of posttraumatic stress disorder symptoms with cognitive decline: Case series. *Journal of Geriatric Psychiatry and Neurology, 14,* 17–20.

Mol, S. S. L., Arntz, A., Metsemakers, J. F. M., Dinant, G.-J., Vilters-van Monfort, P. A. P., & Knottnerus, J. A. (2005). Symptoms of post-traumatic stress disorder after non-traumatic events: Evidence from an open population study. *British Journal of Psychiatry, 186,* 494–499.

Mollica, R. F., Caspi-Yavin, Y., Bollini, P., Truong, T., Tor, S., & Lavelle, J. (1992). The Harvard Trauma Questionnaire. *Journal of Nervous and Mental Disease, 180,* 111–116.

Mollica, R. F., Sarajlic, N., Chernoff, M., Lavelle, J., Vukovic, I. S., & Massagli, M. P. (2001). Longitudinal study of psychiatric symptoms, disability, mortality, and emigration among Bosnian refugees. *Journal of the American Medical Association, 286,* 546–554.

Monnier, J., Elhai, J. D., Frueh, B. C., Sauvageot, J. A., & Magruder, K. M. (2002). Replication and expansion of findings related to racial differences in veterans with combat-related PTSD. *Depression and Anxiety, 16*, 64–70.

Moradi, A. R., Neshat-Doost, H. T., Taghavi, R., Yule, W., & Dalgleish, T. (1999). Performance of children of adults with PTSD on the Stroop color-naming task: A preliminary study. *Journal of Traumatic Stress, 12*, 663–671.

Morrow, B. A., Elsworth, J. D., Rasmusson, A. M., & Roth, R. H. (1999). The role of mesoprefrontal dopamine neurons in the acquisition and expression of conditioned fear in the rat. *Neuroscience, 92*, 553–564.

Moskowitz, A. K. (2004). "Scared stiff": Catatonia as an evolutionary-based fear response. *Psychological Review, 111*, 984–1002.

Mowrer, O. H. (1960). *Learning theory and behavior.* New York: Wiley.

Moyer, D. M., Burkhardt, B., & Gordon, R. M. (2002). Faking PTSD from a motor vehicle accident on the MMPI-2. *American Journal of Forensic Psychology, 20*, 81–89.

Moyers, T. B., & Rollnick, S. (2002). A motivational interviewing perspective on resistance in psychotherapy. *Journal of Clinical Psychology, 58*, 185–193.

Murdoch, M., Polusny, M. A., Hodges, J., & O'Brien, N. (2004). Prevalence of in-service and post-service sexual assault among combat and noncombat veterans applying for Department of Veterans Affairs posttraumatic stress disorder disability benefits. *Military Medicine, 169*, 392–395.

Murray, J., Ehlers, A., & Mayou, R. A. (2002). Dissociation and post-traumatic stress disorder: Two prospective studies of road traffic accident survivors. *British Journal of Psychiatry, 180*, 363–368.

Nader, K., Newman, E., Weathers, F., Kaloupek, D., Kriegler, J., Blake, D., et al. *Clinician-administered PTSD scale for children and adolescents.* Los Angeles, CA: Western Psychological Press.

Najavits, L. M. (2002). *Seeking safety: A treatment manual for PTSD and substance abuse.* New York: Guilford Press.

National Institute of Mental Health (2002). *Mental health and mass violence* (NIH Publication No. 02-5138). Washington, DC: U.S. Government Printing Office.

Nemeroff, C. B. (2004). Neurobiological consequences of childhood trauma. *Journal of Clinical Psychiatry, 65*(Suppl. 1), 18–28.

Neuner, F., Schauer, M., Klaschik, C., Karunakara, U., & Elbert, T. (2004). A comparison of narrative exposure therapy, supportive counseling and psychoeducation for treating posttraumatic stress disorder in an African refugee settlement. *Journal of Consulting and Clinical Psychology, 72*, 579–587.

Newman, E., Kaloupek, D. G., & Keane, T. M. (1996). Assessment of posttraumatic stress disorder in clinical and research settings. In B. A. van der Kolk, A. C. McFarlane, & L. Weisaeth (Eds.), *Traumatic stress: The effects of overwhelming experience on mind, body, and society* (pp. 242–275). New York: Guilford Press.

Nieves-Grafals, S. (2001). Brief treatment of civil war-related trauma: A case study. *Cultural Diversity and Ethnic Minority Psychology, 7*, 387–396.

Norris, F. H., & Hamblen, J. L. (2004). Standardized self-report measures of civilian trauma and PTSD. In J. P. Wilson & T. M. Keane (Eds.), *Assessing psychological trauma and PTSD* (2nd ed., pp. 63–102). New York: Guilford Press.

Norris, F. H., Kaniasty, K., Conrad, M. L., Inman, G. L., & Murphy, A. D. (2002). Placing age differences in cultural context: A comparison of the effects of age on PTSD after disasters in the United States, Mexico, and Poland. *Journal of Clinical Geropsychology, 8*, 153–173.

Novaco, R. W. (1975). *Anger control.* Lexington, MA: Lexington Books.

Nutt, D. J., & Malizia, A. (2004). Structural and functional brain changes in post-traumatic stress disorder. *Journal of Clinical Psychiatry, 65*(Suppl. 1), 11–17.

Olsen, C. K., Hogg, S., & Lapiz, M. D. S. (2002). Tonic immobility in guinea pigs: A behavioural response for detecting an anxiolytic effect? *Behavioural Pharmacology, 13*, 261–269.

Orr, S. P., Metzger, L. J., Lasko, N. B., Macklin, M. L., Peri, T., & Pitman, R. K. (2000). De novo conditioning in trauma-exposed individuals with and without posttraumatic stress disorder. *Journal of Abnormal Psychology, 109*, 290–298.

Orr, S. P., Metzger, L. J., Miller, M. W., & Kaloupek, D. G. (2004). Psychophysiological assessment of PTSD. In J. P. Wilson & T. M. Keane (Eds.), *Assessing psychological trauma and PTSD* (2nd ed., pp. 289–343). New York: Guilford Press.

Öst, L.-G. (1987). Applied relaxation: Description of a coping technique and review of controlled studies. *Behaviour Research and Therapy, 25*, 397–409.

Ozer, E. J., Best, S. R., Lipsey, T. L., & Weiss, D. S. (2003). Predictors of posttraumatic stress disorder and symptoms in adults: A meta-analysis. *Psychological Bulletin, 129*, 52–73.

Ozer, E. J., & Weiss, D. S. (2004). Who develops posttraumatic stress disorder? *Current Directions in Psychological Science, 13*, 169–172.

Palace, E. M., & Johnston, C. (1989). Treatment of recurrent nightmares by the dream reorganization approach. *Journal of Behavior Therapy and Experimental Psychiatry, 20*, 219–226.

Pare, D., Quirk, G. J., & LeDoux, J. E. (2004). New vistas on amygdala networks in conditioned fear. *Journal of Neurophysiology, 92*, 1–9.

Paterson, R. J. (2000). *The assertiveness workbook.* Oakland, CA: New Harbinger.

Paunovic, N., & Öst, L. G. (2001). Cognitive-behavior therapy vs exposure therapy in the treatment of PTSD in refugees. *Behaviour Research and Therapy, 39*, 1183–1197.

Paunovic, N., Lundh, L.-G., & Öst, L. G. (2002). Attentional and memory bias for emotional information in crime victims with acute posttraumatic stress disorder (PTSD). *Journal of Anxiety Disorders, 16*, 675–692.

Peri, T., Ben-Shakhar, G., Orr, S. P., & Shalev, A. Y. (2000). Psychophysiological assessment of aversive conditioning in posttraumatic stress disorder. *Biological Psychiatry, 47*, 512–519.

Persons, J. B. (1989). *Cognitive therapy in practice: A case formulation approach.* New York: Norton.

Persons, J. B., & Tompkins, M. A. (1997). Cognitive-behavioral case formulation. In T. D. Eells (Ed.), *Handbook of psychotherapy case formulation* (pp. 314–339). New York: Guilford Press.

Peters, J., & Kaye, L. W. (2003). Childhood sexual abuse: A review of its impact on older women entering institutional settings. *Clinical Gerontologist, 26*, 29–53.

Peterson, R. A., & Reiss, S. (1992). *Anxiety Sensitivity Index Revised Manual.* Worthington, OH: International Diagnostic Systems Publishing.

Pitman, R. K. (1989). Posttraumatic stress disorder, hormones and memory. *Biological Psychiatry, 26,* 645–652.

Pitman, R. K., Altman, B., Greenwald, E., Longpre, R. E., Macklin, M. L., Poire, R. E., et al. (1991). Psychiatric complications during flooding therapy for posttraumatic stress disorder. *Journal of Clinical Psychiatry, 52,* 17–20.

Pitman, R. K., van der Kolk, B. A., Orr, S. P., & Greenberg, M. S. (1990). Naloxone-reversible analgesic response to combat-related stimuli in posttraumatic stress disorder. *Archives of General Psychiatry, 47,* 541–544.

Pope, K. S., Butcher, J. N., & Seelen, J. (2000). *The MMPI, MMPI-2, and MMPI-A in court.* Washington, DC: American Psychological Association.

Prigerson, H. G., Maciejewski, P. K., & Rosenheck, R. A. (2002). Population attributable fractions of psychiatric disorders and behavioral outcomes associated with combat exposure among US men. *American Journal of Public Health, 92,* 59–63.

Pynoos, R. S., & Nader, K. (1993). Issues in the treatment of posttraumatic stress disorder in children and adolescents. In J. P. Wilson & B. Raphael (Eds.), *International handbook of traumatic stress syndromes* (pp. 535–549). New York: Plenum Press.

Rescorla, R. A. (1988). Pavlovian conditioning: It's not what you think it is. *American Psychologist, 43,* 151–160.

Resick, P. A., Nishith, P., & Griffin, M. G. (2003). How well does cognitive-behavioral therapy treat symptoms of complex PTSD? An examination of child sexual abuse survivors within a clinical trial. *CNS Spectrums, 8,* 351–355.

Resick, P. A., Nishith, P., Weaver, T. L., Astin, M. C., & Feurer, C. A. (2002). A comparison of cognitive-processing therapy with prolonged exposure and a waiting condition for the treatment of chronic posttraumatic stress disorder in female rape victims. *Journal of Consulting and Clinical Psychology, 70,* 867–879.

Resick, P. A., & Schnicke, M. K. (1993). *Cognitive processing therapy for rape victims.* Thousand Oaks, CA: Sage.

Ressler, K. J., Rothbaum, B. O., Tannenbaum, L., Anderson, P., Graap, K., Zimand, E., et al. (2004). Cognitive enhancers as adjuncts to psychotherapy: Use of D-cycloserine in phobic individuals to enhance extinction of fear. *Archives of General Psychiatry, 61,* 1136–1144.

Reviere, S. L., & Bakeman, R. (2001). The effects of early trauma on autobiographical memory and schematic self-representation. *Applied Cognitive Psychology, 15,* S89–S100.

Richards, D. A., & Lovell, K. (1999). Behavioural and cognitive behavioural interventions in the treatment of PTSD. In W. Yule (Ed.), *Post-traumatic stress disorders: Concepts and therapy* (pp. 239–266). New York: Wiley.

Riskind, J. H., & Williams, N. L. (2006). A unique vulnerability common to all anxiety disorders: The looming maladaptive style. In L. B. Alloy & J. H. Riskind (Eds.), *Cognitive vulnerability to emotional disorders* (pp. 175–206). Mahwah, NJ: Erlbaum.

Roemer, L., Litz, B. T., Orsillo, S. M., Ehlich, P. J., & Friedman, M. J. (1998). Increases in retrospective accounts of war-zone exposure over time: The role of PTSD symptom severity. *Journal of Traumatic Stress, 11,* 597–605.

Rosenberg, S. D., Mueser, K. T., Jankowski, M. K., Salyers, M. P., & Acker, K. (2004). Cognitive-behavioral treatment of PTSD in severe mental illness: Results of a pilot study. *American Journal of Psychiatric Rehabilitation, 7,* 171–186.

Rosenheck, R., & Fontana, A. (1996). Race and outcome of treatment for veterans suffering from PTSD. *Journal of Traumatic Stress, 9,* 343–351.

Rosenheck, R., Fontana, A., & Cottrol, C. (1995). Effect of clinician-veteran racial pairing in the treatment of posttraumatic stress disorder. *American Journal of Psychiatry, 152,* 555–563.

Rossman, B. B. R., & Ho, J. (2000). Posttraumatic response and children exposed to parental violence. *Journal of Aggression, Maltreatment, and Trauma, 3,* 85–106.

Roth, S., Newman, E., Pelcovitz, D., van der Kolk, B., & Mandel, F. S. (1997). Complex PTSD in victims exposed to sexual and physical abuse: Results from the DSM-IV field trial for posttraumatic stress disorder. *Journal of Traumatic Stress, 10,* 539–555.

Rothbaum, B. A., & Foa, E. B. (1991). Exposure treatment of PTSD concomitant with conversion mutism: A case study. *Behavior Therapy, 22,* 449–456.

Rothbaum, B. O., Foa, E. B., Riggs, D. S., Murdock, T., & Walsh, W. (1992). A prospective examination of post-traumatic stress disorder in rape victims. *Journal of Traumatic Stress, 5,* 455–475.

Rothbaum, B. O., Kozak, M. J., Foa, E. B., & Whitaker, D. J. (2001). Posttraumatic stress disorder in rape victims: Autonomic habituation to auditory stimuli. *Journal of Traumatic Stress, 14,* 283–293.

Rothbaum, B. O., & Mellman, T. A. (2001). Dreams and exposure therapy in PTSD. *Journal of Traumatic Stress, 14,* 481–490.

Rothbaum, B. O., Ruef, A. M., Litz, B. T., Han, H., & Hodges, L. (2004). Virtual reality exposure therapy of combat-related PTSD. In S. Taylor (Ed.), *Advances in the treatment of posttraumatic stress disorder* (pp. 93–112). New York: Springer.

Rothschild, B. (2000). *The body remembers.* New York: Norton.

Roy-Byrne, P., Berliner, L., Russo, J., Zatzick, D., & Pitman, R. K. (2003). Treatment preferences and determinants in victims of sexual and physical assault. *Journal of Nervous and Mental Disease, 191,* 161–165.

Ruggiero, K. J., Del Ben, K., Scotti, J. R., & Rabalais, A. E. (2003). Psychometric properties of the PTSD Checklist—Civilian Version. *Journal of Traumatic Stress, 16,* 495–502.

Ruscio, A. M., Ruscio, J., & Keane, T. M. (2002). The latent structure of posttraumatic stress disorder: A taxometric investigation of reactions to extreme stress. *Journal of Abnormal Psychology, 111,* 290–301.

Rusting, C. L., & Nolen-Hoeksema, S. (1998). Regulating responses to anger: Effects of rumination and distraction on angry mood. *Journal of Personality and Social Psychology, 74,* 790–803.

Ruzek, J. I., Riney, S. J., Leskin, G., Drescher, K. D., Foy, D. F., & Gusman, F. D.

(2001). Do posttraumatic stress disorder symptoms worsen during trauma focus group treatment? *Military Medicine, 166,* 898–902.

Şalcioğlu, E., Başoğlu, M., & Livanou, M. (2003). Long-term psychological outcome for non-treatment-seeking earthquake survivors in Turkey. *Journal of Nervous and Mental Disease, 191,* 154–160.

Salmon, K., & Bryant, R. A. (2002). Posttraumatic stress disorder in children: The influence of developmental factors. *Clinical Psychology Review, 22,* 163–188.

Salomons, T. V., Osterman, J. E., Gagliese, L., & Katz, J. (2004). Pain flashbacks in posttraumatic stress disorder. *Clinical Journal of Pain, 20,* 83–87.

Sapolsky, R. M. (2000). Glucocorticoids and hippocampal atrophy in neuropsychiatric disorders. *Archives of General Psychiatry, 57,* 925–935.

Schacter, D. L. (2002). *The seven sins of memory.* Boston, MA: Houghton Mifflin.

Schauer, M., Neuner, F., & Elbert, T. (2005). *Narrative exposure therapy: A short-term intervention for traumatic stress disorders after war, terror, or torture.* Gottingen, Germany: Hogrefe & Huber.

Scheeringa, M. S., Zeanah, C. H., Drell, M. J., & Larrieu, J. A. (1995). Two approaches to the diagnosis of posttraumatic stress disorder in infancy and early childhood. *Journal of the American Academy of Child and Adolescent Psychiatry, 34,* 191–200.

Scheeringa, M. S., Zeanah, C. H., Myers, L., & Putnam, F. W. (2003). New findings on alternative criteria for PTSD in preschool children. *Journal of the American Academy of Child and Adolescent Psychiatry, 42,* 561–570.

Schiraldi, G. R. (2000). *The post-traumatic stress disorder sourcebook.* Los Angeles: Lowell.

Schnurr, P. P., Friedman, M. J., Foy, D. W., Shea, T., Hsieh, F. Y., Lavori, P. W., et al. (2003). Randomized trial of trauma-focused group therapy for posttraumatic stress disorder. *Archives of General Psychiatry, 60,* 481–489.

Schnurr, P. P., Rosenberg, S. D., & Friedman, M. J. (1993). Change in MMPI scores from college to adulthood as a function of military service. *Journal of Abnormal Psychology, 102,* 288–296.

Seligman, M. E. P., & Johnston, J. C. (1973). A cognitive theory of avoidance learning. In F. J. McGuigan & D. B. Lumsden (Eds.), *Contemporary approaches to learning and conditioning* (pp. 69–145). Washington, DC: Winston.

Sharp, T. J., & Harvey, A. G. (2001). Chronic pain and posttraumatic stress disorder: Mutual maintenance? *Clinical Psychology Review, 21,* 857–877.

Shipherd, J. C., & Beck, J. G. (1999). The effects of suppressing trauma-related thoughts on women with rape-related posttraumatic stress disorder. *Behaviour Research and Therapy, 37,* 99–112.

Shrestna, N. M., Sharma, B., van Ommeren, M., Regmi, S., Makaju, R., & Komproe, I. (1988). Impact of torture on refugees displaced within the developing world. *Journal of the American Medical Association, 280,* 443–448.

Silove, D., Steel, Z., McGorry, P., Miles, V., & Drobny, J. (2002). The impact of torture on post-traumatic stress symptoms in war-affected Tamil refugees and immigrants. *Comprehensive Psychiatry, 43,* 49–55.

Silva, R. C. B., Gargaro, A. C., & Brandao, M. L. (2004). Differential regulation of the expression of contextual freezing and fear-potentiated startle by 5–HT mechanisms of the median raphe nucleus. *Behavioural Brain Research, 151,* 93–101.

Silverman, W. K., & Albano, A. M. (1996). *Anxiety disorders interview schedule for DSM-IV, child version.* New York: Graywind.

Simon, R. I. (2003). *Posttraumatic stress disorder in litigation: Guidelines for forensic assessment* (2nd ed.). Washington, DC: American Psychiatric Publishing.

Simpson, C., & Papageorgiou, C. (2003). Metacognitive beliefs about rumination in anger. *Cognitive and Behavioral Practice, 10,* 91–94.

Söchting, I., Fairbrother, N., & Koch, W. J. (2004). Sexual assault of women: Prevention efforts and risk factors. *Violence against Women, 10,* 73–93.

Solomon, Z., & Benbenishty, R. (1986). The role of proximity, immediacy, and expectancy in frontline treatment of combat stress reaction among Israelis in the Lebanon War. *American Journal of Psychiatry, 143,* 613–617.

Soravia, L. M., Heinrichs, M., Aerni, A., Maroni, C., Schelling, G., Ehlert, U., et al. (2006). Glucocorticoids reduce phobic fear in humans. *Proceedings of the National Academy of Science, 103,* 5585–5590.

Sotres-Bayon, F., Bush, D. E. A., & LeDoux, J. E. (2004). Emotional perseveration: An update on prefrontal-amygdala interactions in fear extinction. *Learning and Memory, 11,* 525–535.

Southwick, S. M., Krystal, J. H., Bremner, J. D., Morgan, C. A., Nicolaou, A. L., Nagy, L. M., et al. (1997a). Noradrenergic and serotonergic function in posttraumatic stress disorder. *Archives of General Psychiatry, 54,* 749–758.

Southwick, S. M., Morgan, C. A., Nicolaou, A. L., & Charney, D. S. (1997b). Consistency of memory for combat-related traumatic events in veterans of Operation Desert Storm. *American Journal of Psychiatry, 154,* 173–177.

Spiegel, D. (1996). Dissociative disorders. In R. E. Hales & S. C. Yudofsky (Eds.), *Synopsis of psychiatry* (pp. 583–604). Washington, DC: American Psychiatric Press.

Spielberger, C. D. (1988). *State-trait anger expression inventory.* Odessa, FL: Psychological Assessment Resources.

Stapleton, J. A., Taylor, S., & Asmundson, G. J. G. (2006). Effects of three PTSD treatments on anger and guilt: Exposure therapy, eye movement desensitization and reprocessing, and relaxation training. *Journal of Traumatic Stress, 19,* 19–28.

Steil, R., & Ehlers, A. (2000). Dysfunctional meaning of posttraumatic intrusions in chronic PTSD. *Behaviour Research and Therapy, 38,* 537–558.

Stein, M. B., Jang, K. L., Taylor, S., Vernon, P. A., & Livesley, W. J. (2002). Genetic and environmental influences on trauma exposure and posttraumatic stress disorder symptoms: A general population twin study. *American Journal of Psychiatry, 159,* 1675–1681.

Stowe, R., & Taylor, S. (2002). Posttraumatic stress disorder. In *Encyclopedia of life sciences.* Oxford, UK: Elsevier. (Available online at www.els.net.)

Streeck-Fischer, A., & van der Kolk, B. A. (2000). Down will come baby, cradle and all: Diagnostic and therapeutic implications of chronic trauma on child development. *Australian and New Zealand Journal of Psychiatry, 34,* 903–918.

Sutker, P. B., Davis, J. M., Uddo, M., & Ditta, S. R. (1995). War zone stress, personal resources, and PTSD in Persian Gulf War returnees. *Journal of Abnormal Psychology, 104,* 444–452.

Switzer, G. E., Dew, M. A., Thompson, K., Goycoolea, J. M., Derricott, T., & Mullins, S. D. (1999). Posttraumatic stress disorder and service utilization among urban mental health center clients. *Journal of Traumatic Stress, 12,* 25–39.

Tangey, J. P. (1990). Assessing individual differences in proneness to shame and guilt: Development of the self-conscious affect and attribution inventory. *Journal of Personality and Social Psychology, 59,* 102–111.

Tangey, J. P. (1991). Moral affect: The good, the bad and the ugly. *Journal of Personality and Social Psychology, 61,* 598–607.

Tarrier, N. (2001). What can be learned from clinical trials? Reply to Devilly and Foa (2001). *Journal of Consulting and Clinical Psychology, 69,* 117–118.

Tarrier, N., & Humphreys, A.-L. (2004). PTSD and the social support of the interpersonal environment: The development of social cognitive behaviour therapy. In S. Taylor (Ed.), *Advances in the treatment of posttraumatic stress disorder: Cognitive-behavioral perspectives* (pp. 113–127). New York: Springer.

Tarrier, N., Pilgrim, H., Sommerfield, C., Faragher, B., Reynolds, M., Graham, E., et al. (1999a). A randomized trial of cognitive therapy and imaginal exposure in the treatment of chronic posttraumatic stress disorder. *Journal of Consulting and Clinical Psychology, 67,* 13–18.

Tarrier, N., Sommerfield, C., & Pilgrim, H. (1999b). Relatives' expressed emotion (EE) and PTSD treatment outcome. *Psychological Medicine, 29,* 801–811.

Taylor, S. (1999). *Anxiety sensitivity.* Mahwah, NJ: Erlbaum.

Taylor, S. (2000). *Understanding and treating panic disorder: Cognitive-behavioural approaches.* New York: Wiley.

Taylor, S. (2004). *Advances in the treatment of posttraumatic stress disorder: Cognitive-behavioral perspectives.* New York: Springer.

Taylor, S., & Asmundson, G. J. G. (2004). *Treating health anxiety: A cognitive-behavioral approach.* New York: Guilford Press.

Taylor, S., Carleton, R. N., & Asmundson, G. J. G. (2006). Simple versus complex PTSD: A cluster analytic investigation. *Journal of Anxiety Disorders, 20,* 459–472.

Taylor, S., Fedoroff, I. C., Koch, W. J., Thordarson, D. S., Fecteau, G., & Nicki, R. (2001). Posttraumatic stress disorder arising after road traffic collisions: Patterns of response to cognitive-behavior therapy. *Journal of Consulting and Clinical Psychology, 69,* 541–551.

Taylor, S., Frueh, B. C., & Asmundson, G. J. G. (in press). Detection and management of malingering in people presenting for treatment of posttraumatic stress disorder: Methods, obstacles, and recommendations. *Journal of Anxiety Disorders.*

Taylor, S., & Rachman, S. (1994). Stimulus estimation and the overprediction of fear. *British Journal of Clinical Psychology, 33,* 173–181.

Taylor, S., & Thordarson, D. (2002). Behavioural treatment of posttraumatic stress disorder associated with recovered memories. *Cognitive Behaviour Therapy, 31,* 8–17.

Taylor, S., Thordarson, D. S., Maxfield, L, Fedoroff, I. C., Lovell, K., & Ogrodniczuk, J. (2003). Comparative efficacy, speed, and adverse effects of three treatments for PTSD: Exposure therapy, EMDR, and relaxation training. *Journal of Consulting and Clinical Psychology, 71,* 330–338.

Tedstone, J. E., & Tarrier, N. (2003). Posttraumatic stress disorder following medical illness and treatment. *Clinical Psychology Review, 23,* 409–448.

Terr, L. (1991). Childhood traumas: An outline and overview. *American Journal of Psychiatry, 148,* 10–20.

Thompson, A. J. (1995). Phenylketonuria: An unfolding story. In M. M. Robertson (Ed.), *Movement and allied disorders in childhood* (pp. 83–103). New York: Wiley.

Thorn, B. E. (2004). *Cognitive therapy for chronic pain: A step-by-step guide.* New York: Guilford Press.

Tremblay, C., Hebert, M., & Piche, C. (1999). Coping strategies and social support as mediators of consequences in child sexual abuse victims. *Child Abuse and Neglect, 23,* 929–945.

Trent, C. R., Rushlau, M. G., Munley, P. H., Bloem, W., & Driesenga, S. (2000). An ethnocultural study of posttraumatic stress disorder in African-American and White American Vietnam war veterans. *Psychological Reports, 87,* 585–592.

Tromp, S., Koss, M. P., Figueredo, A. J., & Tharan, M. (1995). Are rape memories different?: A comparison of rape, other unpleasant and pleasant memories among employed women. *Journal of Traumatic Stress, 8,* 607–627.

True, W. R., Rice, J., Eisen, S. A., Heath, A. C., Goldberg, J., Lyons, M. J., et al. (1993). A twin study of genetic and environmental contributions to liability for posttraumatic stress symptoms. *Archives of General Psychiatry, 50,* 257–264.

Tull, M. T., & Roemer, L. (2003). Alternative explanations of emotional numbing of posttraumatic stress disorder: An examination of hyperarousal and experiential avoidance. *Journal of Psychopathology and Behavioral Assessment, 25,* 147–154.

Turner, S. M., Beidel, D. C., & Frueh, B. C. (2005). Multicomponent behavioral treatment for chronic combat-related posttraumatic stress disorder. *Behavior Modification, 29,* 39–69.

Ursano, R. J., & McCarroll, J. E. (1990). The nature of a traumatic stressor: Handling dead bodies. *Journal of Nervous and Mental Disease, 178,* 396–398.

van Achterberg, M. E., Rohrbaugh, R. M., Southwick, S. M. (2001). Emergence of PTSD in trauma survivors with dementia. *Journal of Clinical Psychiatry, 62,* 206–207.

van der Kolk, B. A. (1994). The body keeps the score: Memory and the evolving psychobiology of posttraumatic stress. *Harvard Review of Psychiatry, 1,* 253–265.

van der Kolk, B. A., Greenberg, M. S., Boyd, H., & Krystal, J. (1985). Inescapable shock, neurotransmitters, and addiction to trauma: Toward a psychobiology of posttraumatic stress. *Biological Psychiatry, 20,* 314–325.

van der Kolk, B. A., Greenberg, M. S., Orr, S. P., & Pitman, R. K. (1989). Endogenous opioids, stress induced analgesia, and posttraumatic stress disorder. *Psychopharmacology Bulletin, 25,* 417–421.

van der Kolk, B. A., McFarlane, A. C., & Weisaeth, L. (Eds.). (1996). *Traumatic stress: The effects of overwhelming experience on mind, body, and society.* New York: Guilford Press.

van Emmerik, A. A. P., Kamphuis, J. H., Hulsbosch, A. M., & Emmelkamp, P. M. G. (2002). Single session debriefing after psychological trauma: A meta-analysis. *The Lancet, 360,* 766–771.

van Etten, M., & Taylor, S. (1998). Comparative efficacy of treatments for post-traumatic stress disorder: A meta-analysis. *Clinical Psychology and Psychotherapy, 5,* 126–145.

van Minnen, A., Arntz, A., & Keijsers, G. P. J. (2002). Prolonged exposure in patients with chronic PTSD: Predictors of treatment outcome and dropout. *Behaviour Research and Therapy, 40,* 439–457.

van Minnen, A., & Hagenaars, M. (2002). Fear activation and habituation patterns as early process predictors of response to prolonged exposure treatment in PTSD. *Journal of Traumatic Stress, 15,* 359–367.

Vasterling, J. J., Brailey, K., Constans, J. I., & Sutker, P. B. (1998). Attention and memory dysfunction in posttraumatic stress disorder. *Neuropsychology, 12,* 125–133.

Vermetten, E., & Bremner, J. D. (2002a). Circuits and systems in stress: I. Preclinical studies. *Depression and Anxiety, 15,* 126–147.

Vermetten, E., & Bremner, J. D. (2002b). Circuits and systems in stress: II. Applications to neurobiology and treatment in posttraumatic stress disorder. *Depression and Anxiety, 16,* 14–38.

Vermetten, E., & Bremner, J. D. (2003). Olfaction as a traumatic reminder in post-traumatic stress disorder: Case reports and review. *Journal of Clinical Psychiatry, 64,* 202–207.

Vermetten, E., Vythilingam, M., Southwick, S. M., Charney, D. S., & Bremner, J. D. (2003). Long-term treatment with paroxetine increases verbal declarative memory and hippocampal volume in posttraumatic stress disorder. *Biological Psychiatry, 54,* 693–702.

Vernberg, E. M., & Johnston, C. (2001). Developmental considerations in the use of cognitive therapy for posttraumatic stress disorder. *Journal of Cognitive Psychotherapy, 15,* 223–227.

Vernberg, E. M., La Greca, A. M., Silverman, W. K., & Prinstein, M. J. (1996). Prediction of posttraumatic stress symptoms in children after hurricane Andrew. *Journal of Abnormal Psychology, 105,* 237–248.

Vrana, S. R., Roodman, A., & Beckham, J. C. (1995). Selective processing of trauma-relevant words in posttraumatic stress disorder. *Journal of Anxiety Disorders, 9,* 515–530.

Wald, J., & Taylor, S. (2005a). Interoceptive exposure therapy combined with trauma-related exposure therapy for posttraumatic stress disorder: A case report. *Cognitive Behaviour Therapy, 34,* 34–40.

Wald, J., & Taylor, S. (2005b). *Interoceptive exposure in the treatment of posttraumatic stress disorder: An open trial.* Manuscript submitted for publication.

Wald, J., Taylor, S., & Fedoroff, I. C. (2004a). The challenge of treating PTSD in the context of chronic pain. In S. Taylor (Ed.), *Advances in the treatment of posttraumatic stress disorder: Cognitive-behavioral perspectives* (pp. 197–222). New York: Springer.

Wald, J., Taylor, S., & Scamvougeras, A. (2004b). Cognitive-behavioural and neuropsychiatric treatment of posttraumatic conversion disorder: A case study. *Cognitive Behaviour Therapy, 33*, 12–20.

Walker, D. L., & Davis, M. (2002). The role of glutamate receptors within the amygdala in fear learning, fear-potentiated startle, and extinction. *Pharmacology, Biochemistry, and Behavior, 71*, 379–392.

Walker, D. L., Ressler, K. J., Lu, K.-T., & Davis, M. (2002). Facilitation of conditioned fear extinction by systemic administration or intra-amygdala infusions of D-cycloserine as assessed with fear-potentiated startle in rats. *Journal of Neuroscience, 22*, 2343–2351.

Walker, E. A., Katon, W., Russo, J., Ciechanowski, P., Newman, E., & Wagner, A. W. (2003). Health care costs associated with posttraumatic stress disorder symptoms in women. *Archives of General Psychiatry, 60*, 369–374.

Waller, N., Putnam, F. W., & Carlson, E. B. (1996). Types of dissociation and dissociative types: A taxometric analysis of dissociative experiences. *Psychological Methods, 1*, 300–321.

Watson, D. (2003). Investigating the construct validity of the dissociative taxon: Stability analyses of normal and pathological dissociation. *Journal of Abnormal Psychology, 112*, 298–305.

Weathers, F. W., Litz, B. T., Huska, J. A., & Keane, T. M. (1994). *PTSD Checklist—Civilian Version.* Boston: National Center for PTSD.

Weaver, A. (2001). Can post-traumatic stress disorder be diagnosed in adolescence without a catastrophic stressor? A case report. *Clinical Child Psychology and Psychiatry, 5*, 77–83.

Wegner, D. M. (1994). Ironic processes of mental control. *Psychological Review, 101*, 34–52.

Weintraub, D., & Ruskin, P. E. (1999). Posttraumatic stress disorder in the elderly: A review. *Harvard Review of Psychiatry, 7*, 144–152.

Wells, A. (1997). *Cognitive therapy of anxiety disorders.* New York: Wiley.

Williams, J. B. W., Gibbon, M., First, M. B., Spitzer, R. L., Davis, M., Borus, J., et al. (1992). The Structured Clinical Interview for DSM-III-R (SCID): II. Multisite test-retest reliability. *Archives of General Psychiatry, 49*, 630–636.

Williams, J. M. G., & Scott, J. (1988). Autobiographical memory in depression. *Psychological Medicine, 18*, 689–695.

Williams, J. M. G., Watts, F. N., MacLeod, C., & Mathews, A. (1997). *Cognitive psychology and emotional disorders* (2nd ed.). New York: Wiley.

Williams, M. B., & Poijula, S. (2002). *The PTSD workbook.* Oakland, CA: New Harbinger.

Wilson, J. P. (2001) An overview of clinical considerations and principles in the treatment of PTSD. In J. P. Wilson, M. J. Friedman, & J. D. Lindy (Eds.), *Treating psychological trauma and PTSD* (pp. 59–93). New York: Guilford Press.

Wittchen, H.-U. (1996). Critical issues in the evaluation of comorbidity of psychiatric disorders. *British Journal of Psychiatry, 168*(Suppl.), 9–16.

Wolfe, J., Keane, T. M., Kaloupek, D. G., Mora, C. A., & Wine, P. (1993). Patterns of positive stress adjustment in Vietnam combat veterans. *Journal of Traumatic Stress, 6*, 179–193.

Yehuda, R. (2002a). Clinical relevance of biologic findings in PTSD. *Psychiatric Quarterly, 73,* 123–133.

Yehuda, R. (2002b). Current status of cortisol findings in post-traumatic stress disorder. *Psychiatric Clinics of North America, 25,* 341–368.

Yehuda, R. (2004). Risk and resilience in posttraumatic stress disorder. *Journal of Clinical Psychiatry, 65*(Suppl. 1), 29–36.

Yehuda, R., McFarlane, A. C., & Shalev, A. Y. (1998). Predicting the development of posttraumatic stress disorder from the acute response to a traumatic event. *Biological Psychiatry, 44,* 1305–1313.

Yehuda, R., & Wong, C. M. (2001). Etiology and biology of post-traumatic stress disorder: Implications for treatment. *Psychiatric Clinics of North America, 8,* 109–134.

Young, E. A., & Breslau, N. (2004). Cortisol and catecholamines in posttraumatic stress disorder: An epidemiologic community study. *Archives of General Psychiatry, 61,* 394–401.

Yule, W. (2001). Posttraumatic stress disorder in the general population and in children. *Journal of Clinical Psychiatry, 62*(Suppl. 17), 23–28.

Zoellner, L. A., Alvarez-Conrad, J., & Foa, E. B. (2002). Peritraumatic dissociative experiences, trauma narratives, and trauma pathology. *Journal of Traumatic Stress, 15,* 49–57.

Zoellner, L. A., Feeny, N. C., Fitzgibbons, L. A., & Foa, E. B. (1999). Response of African American and Caucasian women to cognitive behavioral therapy for PTSD. *Behavior Therapy, 30,* 581–595.

Index

Triggers, 140
    patient education about, 171
    trauma-related, postexposure processing
        of, 254

u

Uncertainty, intolerance of, 186–187, 194,
    201, 242

v

Veterans. *See* Combat veterans
Veterans Center group therapy, for African
    Americans, 129

Violence, patient, 132
Virtual reality exposure, 250
Virtually Better, website for, 250

w

Witnessed events, 9–10
Workbooks, 127, 129
Working memory, in PTSD, 25
World Assumptions Scale, 109
Worry Can, 189
Worry diary, 184
Worry management, 188–190
    stimulus control for, 199
Wrongdoing analysis, 214–215